DATA COMPRESSION IN DIGITAL SYSTEMS

Roy Hoffman

Join Us on the Internet

WWW: http://www.thomson.com
EMAIL: findit@kiosk.thomson.com

thomson.com is the on-line portal for the products, services and
resources available from International Thomson Publishing (ITP).
This Internet kiosk gives users immediate access to more than 34 ITP
publishers and over 20,000 products. Through *thomson.com* Internet
users can search catalogs, examine subject-specific resource centers
and subscribe to electronic discussion lists. You can purchase ITP
products from your local bookseller, or directly through *thomson.com*.

Visit Chapman & Hall's Internet Resource Center for information on our new publications,
links to useful sites on the World Wide Web and an opportunity to join our e-mail
mailing list. Point your browser to: **http://www.chaphall.com** or
http://www.thomson.com/chaphall/electeng.html for Electrical Engineering

---

A service of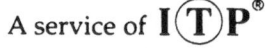

Digital Multimedia Standards Series

City of Westminster College
Paddington Learning Centre
25 Paddington Green
London W2 1NB

DATA COMPRESSION IN DIGITAL SYSTEMS

Roy Hoffman

Former IBM Senior Technical Staff Member
and a member of the
IBM Academy of Technology

 SPRINGER-SCIENCE+BUSINESS MEDIA, B.V.

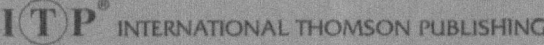 INTERNATIONAL THOMSON PUBLISHING

Cover design: Curtis Tow Graphics

Copyright © 1997 Springer Science+Business Media Dordrecht
Originally published by Chapman & Hall in 1997
Softcover reprint of the hardcover 1st edition 1997

1 2 3 4 5 6 7 8 9 10 XXX 01 00 99 98 97

Library of Congress Cataloging-in-Publication Data

Hoffman, Roy (Roy L.)
     Data compression in digital systems / by Roy Hoffman.
        p.   cm.
     Includes bibliographical references and index.
        ISBN 978-1-4615-6795-0   ISBN 978-1-4615-6793-6 (eBook)
        DOI 10.1007/978-1-4615-6793-6
     1. Data compression (Computer science).   2. Digital electronics.
I. Title.
QA76.9.D33H64   1996
005.74'6--dc20   96-9522
                                                     CIP

British Library Cataloguing in Publication Data available

Warning and Disclaimer

Some of the clip art contained herein was obtained from CorelDraw™.

Preface

This book is about compressing data to make digital systems work more efficiently. According to the dictionary, when something is compressed, it is condensed, squeezed, constricted, or pressed together to fit into less space. Air is compressed for a variety of useful purposes. Businesses are downsized to make them more efficient. We pack our daily schedules tighter and tighter to accomplish more. Who has not crushed an empty soda can for recycling? Many different things can be compressed, including the data in computers, communications links, consumer-electronics gear, and all sizes and shapes of digital systems. Are you curious about how data compression squeezes the "air" out of digital bits? Would you like to know where it is used and, increasingly, why the marketplace demands it be used? Would you like to learn the right way to build data compression into your products? Then, this book is for you.

This exciting technology and its importance for current and future digital systems are explained in easy to understand terms. No previous knowledge of data compression is required because the necessary technical background is carefully developed. Neither is an extensive understanding of mathematics because there are few equations and important ideas are graphically illustrated. If you read any of the popular or professional monthly magazines that cover the latest advances in digital systems, your background is adequate. If you understand this preface, you are ready to tackle this book.

This book explains why and how data compression went from being an obscure technology, known by few, to one used every day by millions of people. Not long ago, only people with specialized skills in information theory, computer science, or communications knew of data compression, much less understood its workings or its importance. Today, almost everyone interested in the latest advances in digital information technology knows something about data compression. Magazine and newspaper articles dealing with progress in consumer electronics and communications mention it frequently. Data compression is fast becoming, not just a household word, but a household servant. Everyone who views a direct broadcast satellite television program, uses a facsimile machine, or waits patiently while their personal computer downloads image-laden pages from the World Wide Web experiences the magic of data compression. It is all around us in computer-based products and services from many industries. Like computers and communications, the consumer-electronics, publishing, entertainment, and healthcare industries, to name a few, find data compression is now indispensable, not just to be competitive, but, often, to deliver practical products and services.

Anyone interested in the *digital revolution* now bringing sweeping changes in electronic information handling should buy and read this book. That includes purchasers, administrators, system managers, product and market analysts, consultants, manufacturers, sales personnel, planners, designers, engineers, programmers, and all who are involved in creating an ever-expanding universe of products and services that depend on data compression. Also included are technologists who know data compression well, students just learning about it, technically-oriented consumers experiencing its power, or anyone who simply wants to know more. All will discover how data compression is used in real-world applications and gain insight for its future application and development.

The material is organized in four parts: Marketplace, Algorithms, Applications, and Digital Systems. *Marketplace* explores the user requirements for data compression and the marketplace constraints and rules that effect its application. *Algorithms* provides the background needed to understand how the most important data compression algorithms operate. *Applications* contains a comprehensive industry-by-industry guide to modern data compression applications. *Digital Systems* describes important decisions and techniques for incorporating data compression in current and future digital information-handling systems.

The inspiration for this book came from a study sponsored by the IBM Academy of Technology. The Academy, whose members are key technical professionals drawn from all locations in the worldwide IBM family of companies, each year commissions studies on technical matters of importance to IBM. The reports that result from these studies are directed to two audiences, to the IBM technical community and to IBM management. Therefore, while focused on technology, Academy studies give equal treatment to the marketplace, application, system, and implementation issues influencing successful deployment of technology. It was my good fortune to be selected to lead an Academy study of data compression for digital computer systems and computer-based products. Going into that assignment, my qualifications were those of as an engineer who had applied data compression to midrange IBM business computers. I knew about data compression for business computers, but not of other applications, much less what data compression technology might be appropriate for those applications, and certainly not of many factors relating to its deployment. Consequently, I needed to learn everything there is to know about data compression—fast!

In a frenzied effort to become a worthy study leader, I set out to gather information from within and outside the IBM Corporation. It was easy to find a wealth of sources that explain how data compression works. For those who are technically adept, there are books filled with the theory and equations for data compression algorithms and professional society journals that convey recent work. Within organizations devoted to digital system research and development, such as IBM, there are knowledgeable technologists who can explain the latest happenings. All are very helpful if you too are a technologist, at or near the forefront of research, or hope to become one. Similarly, there is a growing abundance of information for practitioners interested in using data compression products such as disk compression software for personal computers and video compression software for CD-ROM application development. Popular how-to-do-it books and magazines, along with conversations with fellow practitioners, are very helpful if your intent is to apply existing products. For technically-oriented consumers, or anyone interested in the societal impacts of data compression, the people and publications devoted to consumer electronics have a lot to offer. Unfortunately, it is but one area for data compression application and, while the discussions and publications are numerous, too often little is explained about data compression technology beyond the buzzwords. Perhaps the people who must invest the most time learning about it are those who design the products and services that use data compression. It was difficult to locate the kind of information needed to make design, development, and deployment decisions and even more difficult to unearth the marketplace factors that (as you will learn) have important influences on data compression.

After making a considerable investment of time, and with much help from many study participants, I did get the overview of data compression that I desperately needed. Out of this experience came my observation that there ought to be an easier way to get the whole picture. There should be a reference one could turn to for learning the vocabulary and the concepts of data compression. It should explain where modern-day data compression came from, what is happening today, and, equally important, what to expect in the future. This source should also provide a perspective on marketplace dynamics and how data compression influences what is taking place in computers, communications, or any of the other industries it touches. Conversely, it should explain how data compression technology is influenced by the marketplace. Finally, it should also speak to the issues system designers face when incorporating data compression in their products and services.

The search for a comprehensive introduction to data compression continued without much success while the Academy study was in progress. When the study was completed, it was time to write the final report, which we realized must include an introduction that would reach out to the report's diverse readers, many of whom would be learning about data compression for the first time. Having no other choice, we wrote an introduction to data compression from scratch. Shortly after the Academy report was published, one warm summer day in 1994 I was mowing the lawn. Suddenly, it occurred to me: "Ah-ha, parts of the Academy report have the makings of an introductory book about data compression!" To be sure that it was more than an aberration of thought induced by heat stress, I consulted with Dr. Joan Mitchell, an IBM Researcher and coauthor of a recent book on data compression [Penn93], who agreed with my observation. To shorten a long story, as Academy reports are not distributed outside IBM, I asked for and received the Academy's permission to use material from its data compression report. As the saying goes, the rest is history, and you are now about to read the book that resulted.

And now a few words about what you will find in this book: Data compression is a very dynamic field. Many applications described in this book are still evolving, as is the data compression technology needed to support them. This is particularly true for compressing speech, audio, image, and video data where the development of new applications and new data compression technology goes hand-in-hand. Standards for applying data compression are still being created. New data compression methods are still being discovered that someday may be included in new standards. Consequently, what this book contains is a snapshot of important developments and events as they happened up to the time of writing (1996). By the time you read this, the picture for some applications, particularly in the fast-paced world of consumer electronics, surely will have changed. Thus, you should use this book as the beginning of your education on data compression. To keep up, you (and I) must continue to read and learn about this dynamic technology.

Acknowledgments

This book would not have been possible without the support and encouragement of many people at IBM. For rekindling my interest in data compression, I would especially like to thank Al Cutaia who for many years was my manager at IBM. At his urging, I accepted the assignment to lead the IBM Academy of Technology study of this subject. To the members of the Academy and many other IBM people who were involved in that effort, whose knowledge greatly expanded my understanding of data compression, my sincere thanks. I am also grateful to the Academy and IBM management for allowing portions of the data compression report to be used in writing this book. I am particularly indebted to Dr. Joan Mitchell of IBM Research for first encouraging me to write this book and then, while serving as technical editor, guiding me throughout the publication process. I also want to thank Polly Frierson and all the staff at the IBM Rochester Site Library for making research materials available and for their unwavering support, both during my IBM days and afterward; I could not have done it without you!

I am also grateful to many other people for their help in writing this book. These include Dr. Hartwig Blume of Philips Medical Systems for information on the DIACOM-3 medical imaging standard; Dr. Nicholas Hangiandreou of the Mayo Clinic for information on Mayo PACS and discussion of compression in medical applications; Joseph Hull and Mark Davis of Dolby Laboratories Inc. for information on Dolby AC-3 coding; Don Manuell of Storage Technology Corporation for information on the ICEBERG 9200 Storage Subsystem; Herb Squire of WQXR Radio in New York City, Tom Jones of KNXR Radio in Rochester, Minnesota, and Bill Davis of KROC Radio in Rochester, Minnesota for information on the use of lossy codecs in radio broadcasting. I am also indebted to the reviewers, Dave Liddell and Mike Fleischman, for their many comments and suggestions, and especially to Tom Paska for reviewing the communications chapters. To all the people at Chapman & Hall involved with producing this book, especially MaryAnn Cottone and Barbara Tompkins whose help in preparing the manuscript was invaluable, a special thanks. And to the many others whose names I have overlooked, my apologies.

Trademarks

Advanced Hardware Architectures— AHA

Aladdin Systems, Inc.—Suffit

AlphaStar Television Network Inc.— AlphaStar

America Online, Inc.—America Online

Apple Computer Inc.—Apple, Macintosh, QuickTime

Atari Corp.—Atari, Pong

AT&T Corp.—Picasso Still-Image Phone, Picturephone, VideoPhone 2500

Audio Processing Technology Inc.— APT-X

Compression Laboratories Inc.—CLI

CompuServe Inc.—CompuServe, GIF, Graphics Interchange Format

Digital Equipment Corp.—ALPHA AXP, DEC, DECnet, VAX

Digital Theater Systems, Inc.—Coherent Acoustics, DTS

DirecTV Inc. (a unit of GM Hughes Electronics Corp.)**—**DSS

Discovision Associates, Inc.—LaserDisc

Dolby Laboratories Inc.—AC-2, AC-3, Dolby, Dolby Pro Logic, Dolby Surround, DSD

DSP Group, Inc.—Truespeech

Duck Corp. / Horizon Technologies— TrueMotion-S

Eastman Kodak Co.—FlashPix, Image Pac, Kodak, PhotoYCC, Photo CD

EchoStar Communications Corp.— EchoStar

EWB & Associates Inc.—capaCD

Fox News Inc.—Fox Movietone News

Global Network Navigator, Inc.—Web-Crawler

Hewlett-Packard Corporation—H-P, Image Adapt

IBM Corporation—ADLC, AIX, APPN, Aptiva, AS/400, BDLC, DB2, ES-CON, ES/9000, ES/9000 Sysplex, IBM, Mwave, OS/2, OS/400, PC-XT, PowerPC, PS/2, RISC System/6000, Scalable POWERparallel Systems, SNA, SP1, SP2, System/38

Intel Corp.—DVI, INDEO, Intel, i486, Native Signal Processing, PCI, Pentium, PentiumPro

Intersecting Concepts Inc.—DiskMizer

Iterated Systems Inc.—Fractal Video Pro

Media Vision Inc.—Captain Crunch, Video 1

Microsoft Corp.—AVI, Microsoft, MS-

DOS, Video for Windows, Windows, Windows 95

Motorola Inc.—Motorola

MPC Marketing Council (Software Publishers Association)—MPC

NEC Corp.—Silicon Audio

Nintendo Co.—Nintendo

Philips Consumer Electronics Co.—CD-I, PASC, Philips

Philips Consumer Electronics Co. and **Matsushita Corp.**—Compact Cassette

PictureTel Corporation—PictureTel, SG3

PKWare—PKZIP

Primestar Partners, L.P.—PrimeStar

Scientific Atlanta Inc.—SEDAT

Sega Enterprises, Ltd.—Sega

Softkey International Inc.—PC Paintbrush

Sony Inc.—ATRAC, Betamax, DCC, Digital Betacam, Digital Compact Cassette, MiniDisc, SDDS, Sony

Stac Electronics—Stac, Stacker

Storage Technology Corp.—Iceberg

Sun Microsystems Inc.—Cell

SuperMac Technologies—Cinepak

System Enhancement Associates—ARC

UNIX System Laboratories, Inc.—UNIX

Victor Company of Japan—D-VHS

3M Corp.—3M

Contents

1

Overview

Information, the computers to process it, and the communications infrastructure to transmit it are essential in today's global economy. Distance, time, even differences in spoken language are no longer barriers thanks to advances in computers and communications technology. Routinely, we accept as everyday events in our lives the acquisition and use of information from distant sources. Online credit card validation, international banking transactions, news reports from around the world, E-mail, or videoconferencing all have become commonplace. Some of us cannot remember a world without these services.

These advances in information handling are tangible results achieved by integrating computers and communications. In the 1970s and 1980s, computers learned to communicate, and communications networks learned to speak the language of digital computers. It was a time when the computer and communications industries converged on standard data representations, digital data representations. Today, combinations of data processing equipment (computers) and data communication (transmission and switching) equipment form integrated information systems that seamlessly handle data encoded in digital formats. Convergence continues in the 1990s as other industries discover the advantages of computer technology and digital data. Music on compact discs (CDs), books on CD-ROM, digitally enhanced motion pictures, products and services offered from video kiosks, and, soon, interactive television—these are but a few applications joining what might be called the digital revolution.

1.1   Representation of Information

Information comes to us in many forms from many sources: text in books, numbers in reports, a person speaking, music, photographs, images, motion pictures, television, and computer-generated video are but a few examples. To *electronically* process, store, or communicate information, the facts, concepts, or instructions each information source conveys must be represented as data.

There are many ways to represent data. One choice is to use a representation that mimics the information itself. Some information is discrete: text and integer numbers take on discrete values (A, B, C, . . ., 0, 1, 2, . . .). For discrete information, a *digital* representation is the natural choice. Some information is continuous: speech, audio, video, and most information collected by data sensors come to us as continuously varying values. Speech and audio are ever-changing patterns of sound-pressure level amplitudes and frequencies. Video is a continuous sequence of image "snapshots" (frames) depicting lighting and color. For continuous information, where data take on a continuous range of values, an *analog* representation is the natural choice. Indeed, most early information-handling systems including telephone, radio, and television used analog.

Now, with the availability of low-cost VLSI (very large-scale integration) digital (computer) technology, it is becoming practical to represent both discrete and continuous information in digital form. Processing, storing, and transmitting data in digital format offers many advantages. Digital data is easily manipulated and digital allows the use of many signal processing and enhancement techniques not available in the analog world. Most all information processing operations—including data compression—are easier to do and more effective in digital. As for storage and transmission, unlike analog data, digital data can be stored and transmitted with essentially no degradation. Copies of digital audio or video can be identical to the original. A received signal can be identical to the original signal when digital transmission links are used. Not only are digital signals less susceptible to noise than analog signals, but errors that occur during storage or transmission are easily corrected.

Five common types of information—text, speech, audio, image, and video—are shown in Figure 1.1. Each is digitally represented by doing the following: For each character of text, a bit pattern code is selected from a set of characters. Common character sets for computer systems include the 8-bit ASCII and EBCDIC character sets or, less common, the 16-bit DBCS (double byte character set) character set.[1] For speech and audio, digitized samples are extracted from the analog signal at regular intervals of time. Each sample typically contains from 4 to 20 bits; using more bits provides higher-quality reproduction. For example, telephone-quality speech uses 8-bit samples, whereas music-oriented

---

[1] A *bit* (binary digit) that takes on values of 0 or 1 is the basic unit of information in digital systems. A *byte* is an 8-bit group used to represent a character or other information.

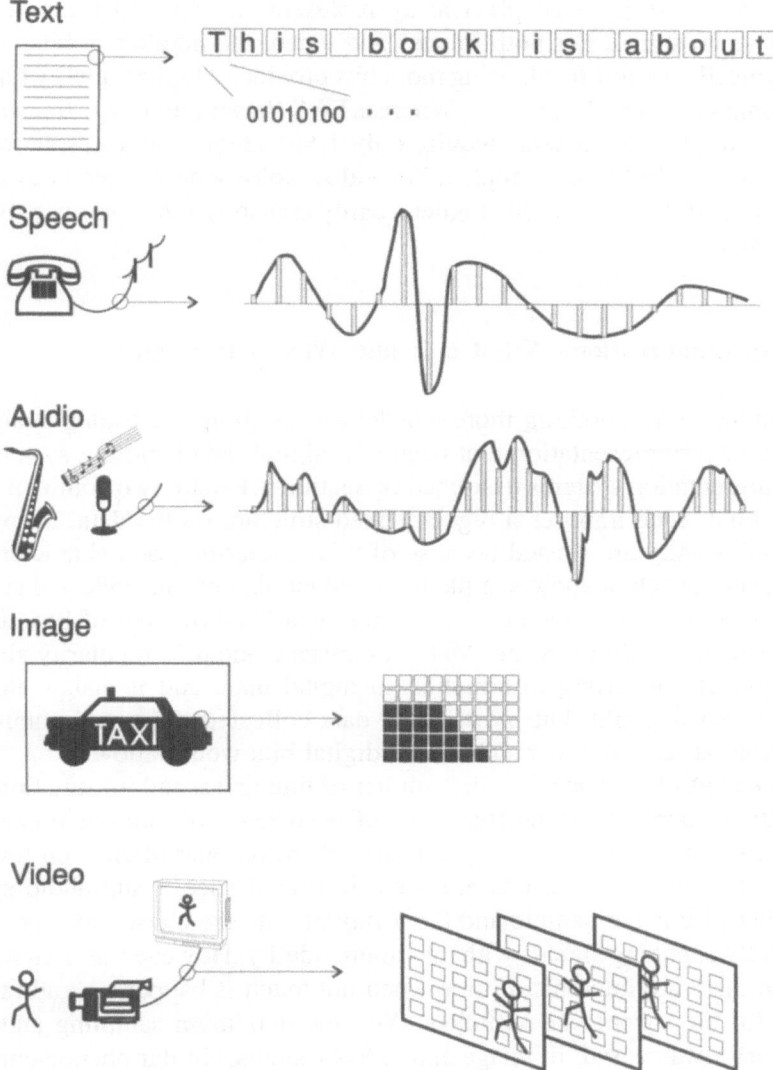

Figure 1.1   Digital representation.

compact discs use 16-bit samples. For images (and video too), the image is scanned in a predefined pattern, say left-to-right, top-to-bottom, and samples are collected at regular intervals. These samples are called *pixels* (picture elements) for obvious reasons.[2] They are organized as a two-dimensional array of points. Whereas a single pixel array is needed to represent a still image, for video a time-ordered sequence of pixel arrays must be used to capture motion within a

---

[2] Some authors use the term *pels*.

televised scene. Here, each pixel array represents a digitized image captured from the video signal. For both images and video, the number of bits per pixel varies, typically, from 1 to 24; using more bits provides a higher-quality reproduction of complex images and scenes. Whereas FAX (facsimile) image transmissions of black-and-white documents require only 1-bit samples, high-resolution color images may require 24-bit samples. For video, color videoconferences are captured with 12-bit samples, but higher-quality transmissions may use 16-bit or 24-bit samples.

1.2   Data Compression—What Is It and Why Is It Needed

Data compression is nothing more—or less—than efficient coding designed to correct the overrepresentation that occurs in digital data-handling systems.[3] All of the representation systems described in Section 1.1 share two common characteristics. First, each imposes a regular, fixed structure on the data. Second, bits can be and usually are wasted because of this regularity. Each character is 8 or 16 bits. Each speech or audio sample is a fixed number of bits collected at regular intervals of time. Each video or image pixel is a fixed number of bits collected at regular points within a scene. Make no mistake about it, regularity simplifies the process of converting information to digital data, and it makes electronic systems easier to build; but most of the data collected does not contain much information, at least not as much as the digital bits would allow.

To make this clear, consider what studies of linguistics and information theory tell us: By accounting for the frequency of occurrence of individual characters, text usually can be represented by not more than four and often even fewer bits per character. Yet, 8 or 16 bits are used. In digital speech and audio systems, the number of bits per sample and the sampling rate are chosen to represent the most rapidly changing signals with maximum fidelity. However, as seen in Figure 1.1, often there are intervals of time when not much is happening and far fewer samples (or bits) would be sufficient. Yet, the maximum sampling and digital bit rates are always used. In image and video systems, similar phenomena occur. The image and video digitization process is designed to capture changes in the scene with some prespecified fidelity. However, some parts of the image may have the same light intensity or color and, consequently, all the pixels within a spatial region will have similar digital values. In video, a sequence of frames will not change much if there is little movement in the scene and pixels within a region will not change much from frame to frame. Yet, the maximum prespecified space and time pixel sampling rates are always used.

What data compression strives to do is find innovative ways to represent

---

[3] Other names for data compression are source coding (an information theory term), data compaction, and data reduction (when there is information loss).

information using as few bits as possible for storage and transmission. The two main techniques data compression uses are redundancy reduction and, sometimes, intelligent removal of unusable information. When too many bits are used to represent data, those that are excessive can be discarded. When information is collected that cannot or will not be used, it can be discarded. Although these may seem simple tasks, they are not. In reality, data compression is complex; complex enough that people write books about the subject!

In digital systems, there are three reasons to use data compression:

- Storage efficiency
- Transmission bandwidth conservation
- Transmission time reduction

Both the storage capacity and the transmission bandwidth available for digitized data have grown and continue to grow at remarkable rates. But the amount of data to be stored and transmitted is growing even faster. Existing business applications require ever-larger, often geographically distributed databases. New applications—particularly those for home and office that use digitized speech, audio, image, and video—require exponentially increasing amounts of storage and bandwidth. Meeting the needs of end users, who are always looking to do more things in less time, is rarely easy. Digital system designers know there is never enough storage, bandwidth, or time, and none of them are cheap enough to waste. Data compression allows each of these precious commodities to be used more efficiently, creating more opportunity for innovative new products and services. This is accomplished by adding software and, sometimes, hardware for data compression processing. The result, from a system cost perspective, is a more balanced system. As Figure 1.2 indicates, modest increases in processing cost usually are offset by greatly reduced costs for storage and bandwidth.

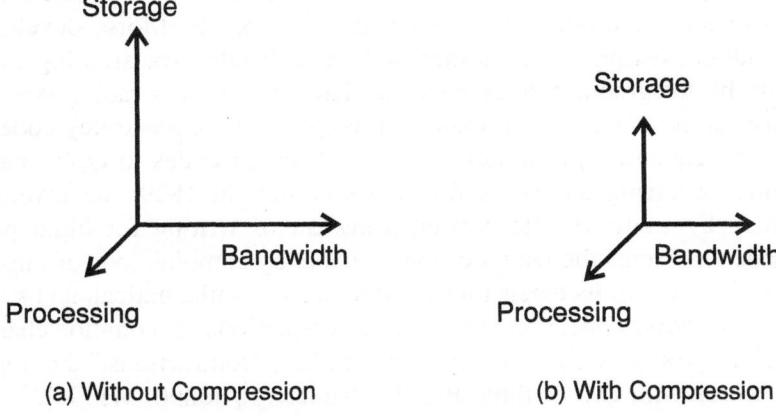

Figure 1.2   System costs.

1.3   Historical Origins of Data Compression

The need to efficiently represent information, particularly text, has been with us since man learned to write. Stenography, the art of writing in shorthand can be traced back to the first century B.C. when a form of shorthand was used to record the speeches of the Roman orator Cicero. Shorthand is a system that uses simple strokes, abbreviations, or symbols to represent letters of the alphabet or even words and phrases. It is a form of data compression for writing. Over the centuries, various shorthand systems have been introduced. With the invention of electronic recording equipment, the need to write as fast as someone speaks has all but disappeared, except for court reporters.

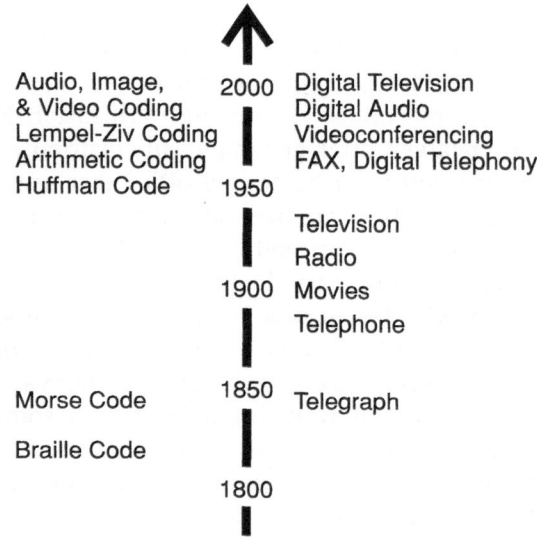

Figure 1.3   Data compression timeline.

More recent data compression developments are shown in Figure 1.3. Two important events occurred in the 1800s. In 1843, S.F.B. Morse developed an efficient code consisting of dots, dashes, and spaces to allow transmitting messages electrically by telegraph, first by wire and later by wireless radio. Morse code uses a basic form of data compression. It assigns short easy-to-key codes to E, I, and other frequently transmitted letters, and longer codes to Q, Z, and other infrequently occurring letters. A few years earlier, in 1829, the invention of Braille code by Louis Braille created a system of writing for blind persons. Braille code represents the letters of the alphabet by combinations of raised dots that are read by touch. Its extensions include music, mathematical, and scientific notation. Like Morse code, it uses shorter representations for common characters. It also includes a second form of data compression, "contractions," that represent common words with two or three Braille characters [Bell90, Witt94].

The ideas of Morse and Braille are the basis for many modern-day text compression schemes. Beginning in the 1950s, information theory and probability concepts formed the backdrop for creating a class of statistical data compression algorithms. As with Morse code, these algorithms use variable-length bit patterns to encode individual symbols based on their frequency of occurrence. Two statistical codes, Huffman coding [Huff52] and arithmetic coding [Riss79], are now in widespread usage. In the 1970s, a second class of data compression algorithms, dictionary algorithms, was formalized by the work of Lempel and Ziv [Ziv77, Ziv78]. Dictionary algorithms encode, as does Braille code, sequences of symbols into shorter codes that are found in a "dictionary."

Data compression for other forms of information has a much shorter history. Before the 1950s, systems for transmitting and storing speech, audio, image, and video information primarily used analog technology. Analog signal (data) compression techniques were employed in some of these systems, particularly for speech transmission over telephone lines. However, analog signals and analog technology greatly limit what can be accomplished with compression.[4] It was not until the 1950s that technology advances allowed exploring digital systems for speech, audio, image, and video. Only then did the need for and power of data compression—digital data compression—became clear. In the 1970s, telephone networks began to go digital. It was at this time when, for transmission efficiency, the telecommunications industry began developing digital coding and compression techniques to allow packing more voice channels into digital telephone links.

Another early application was FAX transmission of images, an idea stretching back to the mid-1800s. In the early 1980s, FAX became a reality with the development of digital technology and standards for compressing and transmitting black-and-white, bi-level images over ordinary analog telephone lines. Data compression is essential for transmitting an FAX image in a reasonable amount of time. But image compression applications did not end with FAX; by the mid-1980s, business and consumer applications for high-quality, digitized photographs and all types of continuous-tone images began to appear. These applications were supported by the development of a new standard for compressing continuous-tone, still images, and an improved standard for compressing bi-level images.

Audio and video applications are the most recent to be invaded by data compression technology. In the 1980s, the digital revolution washed over the consumer audio marketplace and digital audio compression techniques began to appear. In this era, data compression also enabled the production of reasonably

---

[4] Analog signal compression, which is not what this book is about, takes several forms. One is to improve transmissions over noisy channels where, for instance, an analog electrical signal representing light or sound is compressed by applying gain control to increase small values and limit large values; this is somewhat akin to the way that humans handle wide variations in the light levels reaching their eyes or the sound levels impinging on their ears. Analog compression is also used to conserve bandwidth, particularly for speech, where the original analog signal is analyzed and processed into a few essential frequency components.

priced digital videoconferencing gear for businesses. Now, in the 1990s, broadcast television and all forms of video are going digital and here, more than for any other type of information, data compression is essential because video generates immense amounts of data. Standards for compressing audio and video are, depending on the application, in various states of development.

1.4   Marketplace Trends Relating to Data Compression

Three important trends are enabling affordable data compression that will change substantially how digital systems handle text, speech, audio, image, and video data, and that will nurture the creation of many new products and services. These trends are as follows:

- The development of effective techniques for compressing all types of data
- The commercial availability of fast, low-cost, single-chip, microprocessors, DSPs (digital signal processors), and VLSI hardware data compressors
- The convergence of the computer, communications, consumer electronics, publishing, entertainment, and other industries on standards for digital data representation

These trends have long-term impacts that are not limited to just products and services and what they do or how they operate. The industries themselves are affected, for converging on digital data changes the ground rules for doing business. The common underpinning of digitized text, speech, audio, image, and video data opens new opportunities for each industry. It allows sharing of technology, tools, processes, and ideas across the industries. This, in some cases, blurs the boundaries between computer, communications, consumer electronics, publishing, entertainment, and other applications, but it allows each application and industry to leverage the strengths of the others. For the computer industry, as an example, this means a wider application of computing technology, access to better multimedia computing application technology, and access to low-cost, low-power VLSI technology (such as data compression chips) developed for mass-consumption, consumer-electronics products. For the communications industry, this means access to computing technology (RISC microprocessors for set-top boxes, disk[5] storage devices for servers, and more), new opportunities to transport data such as for the entertainment industry, and opportunities to enable new applications such as interactive video. A similar list exists for each of the other industries caught up in digital convergence.

All of the converging industries are moving rapidly to define the technology, applications, and products that will capture the promised riches of digital data.

---

[5] In this book, we will follow industry convention and use *disk* for magnetic disk storage and *disc* for any disc that is read using a light beam.

Although most of the focus is on video, the opportunities for innovative applications, products, and services based on text, speech, audio, or images are not to be overlooked.

1.5 Data Compression Algorithms

As students of this subject soon learn, the variety of data compression algorithms is almost endless, ranging from ad hoc to highly formalized, employing a diversity of theories and mathematical techniques from various branches of science. To promote understanding, most authors choose to group data compression algorithms into a few classes based on the techniques used to do compression[6] [Lync85, Netr95]. Unfortunately, there is no one standard classification scheme. Adding to the confusion, many algorithms combine techniques and do not fit neatly into any one class. This book takes a different approach: Data compression algorithms are organized according to the data they compress, and all the algorithms that apply to each type of data are examined as a group.

As to classifying the data itself, there are various views of the universe of data encountered in digital systems. The communications industry classifies data in the following ways: Services are provided for voice, data, image, and video (where "data" means the symbols found on a terminal keyboard). Communications deals with information sources that either produce digital data (which takes on discrete values) or that produce analog data (which takes on continuous values in some interval) [Stal94A, Stal94B]. Sometimes the terms discrete media (such as text and digital images) and continuous media (such as audio and video) are used when describing the timing requirements for the (data transport) services provided [Gemm95, Lieb95]. Within the computer industry, all data is considered to be digital (because that is how it is processed), and data is referred to by its type, such as text, speech, audio, image, video, and so on. The consumer-electronics, publishing, and entertainment industries also follow this convention, at least when dealing with digital data.

For this book, we have chosen the unifying view of data described in [Arps79]. As shown in Table 1.1, there is *symbolic data*, where a letter, a figure, or other character or mark, or a combination of letters or the like, represents something that a human would recognize. The alphanumeric and special characters in the EBCDIC, ASCII, and DBCS codes for computer systems are familiar examples of symbolic data. There is also *diffuse data*, where the meaning and structural properties have not yet been extracted (i.e., remain widely spread, scattered, or dispersed—diffused) and not yet converted to something a human would recog-

---

[6] The term *algorithm* refers to a collection of techniques used for any particular data compression application. In contrast, a data compression *technique* is a particular method of compression, usable by itself, but likely to be used in combination with other techniques [Luth91].

Table 1.1   Data types.

Symbolic	Diffuse
Character text	Speech
Numeric	Audio
Computer program code	Image
Graphics and Icons	• Binary (bi-level)
	• Gray scale
	• Color
	Video
	• Black-and-white
	• Color

nize. Speech, audio, image, and video information, when represented as digital samples from the original analog data, are examples of diffuse data.

Data compression algorithms for symbolic and diffuse data operate differently. To compress symbolic data, only *lossless* data compression applies, because an exact, bit-identical reproduction of the original data usually is required. For business, computer programming, database, electronic mail, and scientific applications, which deal with exact representations of information, the loss of even a single bit in character text, numeric data, or computer programs is unacceptable.

Compressing diffuse data may involve *lossy* data compression that throws away bits which are not needed for reproducing speech, audio, image, and video. True, some information may be lost, but humans usually are the recipients, and their auditory and visual limits make lossy data compression acceptable for many applications. Also, often in succeeding phases, special forms of lossless data compression are applied for more efficient storage or transmission of compressed diffuse data.

How much a data collection will compress is a property of the data. It also depends on the data compression algorithm employed and, moreover, on how much and what kind of information loss is acceptable. For symbolic data, where no information loss is acceptable, *compression ratios* of 2:1 or 3:1 are typical.[7] In contrast, diffuse data can compress up to 100:1 or more depending on the type of data, the effectiveness of the compression algorithms, and the information loss acceptable.

Data compression does not come free; there is a cost. It trades processing

---

[7] Compression ratio is a measure of the amount of compression achieved. It is computed by dividing the original number of bits or bytes by the number of bits or bytes remaining after data compression is applied.

power and processing time for storage capacity, transmission bandwidth, or transmission time. How quickly data can be compressed is determined by the data, the data compression algorithms, and the processor speed. Data compression algorithms are compute-intensive, and performance (or more properly the lack of it) has sometimes restricted the opportunities for data compression. With the availability of high-performance microprocessors, data compression for many applications can be done in software. Sometimes more performance is required, and for those applications single-chip, high-performance DSPs and VLSI hardware data compressors are available. This range of implementations provides powerful data compression algorithms at a reasonable cost that execute fast enough to process the main dataflows of almost all applications in almost all digital systems.

1.6 Applications for Data Compression

Some applications for data compression from five key industries are show in Table 1.2.[8] Many text-based applications in the computer and communications industries are well established. In contrast, applications dealing with speech, audio, image, and video data are just emerging or are still being defined. This diversity reflects the state of the art for data compression technology. Compression for digitized text, as noted earlier, has decades of development history, and most computer-based applications that handle text data are fully committed to data compression. Compression for digitized speech is widely deployed, too, but mostly in the telecommunications industry and not in others. Compression for digitized audio, image, and video data is, by comparison, relatively new for everyone. In many instances, the compression technology is still being defined along with the applications that will use it.

1.7 Integrating Data Compression in Digital Systems

The advantages of using data compression for storage efficiency, transmission bandwidth conservation, and transmission time reduction are obvious. What sometimes is not so obvious is how to integrate data compression into new or existing digital systems. First, we need to define what a *digital system* is and does. A digital system is a collection of elements for processing digital information. In this book, we are considering digital systems that include data compression facilities. Figure 1.4 shows a simplified representation of a digital system that

---

[8] These industries and applications are examined in detail later in this text. In addition, some brief examples will be provided to show how data compression is applied in other industries.

Table 1.2   Data compression applications.

Computers	Communications	Consumer Electronics	Publishing	Entertainment
Tape	Voice • Telephones • Cellular telephony	Digital audio • CD • Tape • Home theater	CD-ROM multimedia publications	Media • Production • Distribution • Storage and archiving
Magnetic disc				
Optical disc	Data communications networks		Online multimedia publications	
Solid-state storage	• WAN • LAN	Digital video • HDTVs • Set-top boxes • Digital VCRs • Digital video discs		
Software distribution	FAX			

Software execution
• System
  software
• Database
• User data and
  programs
	Teleconferencing
	• Audiographics
	• Videophones
	• Videoconferencing
		Digital photography
		• Digital cameras
		• Photo CD		

Chip and system interconnections	Broadcasting • Terrestrial SDTV, HDTV • Satellite DBS • Cable TV • Telco video • Digital radio	Interactive multimedia set-top boxes • Education • Arcade games • Karaoke players		
Servers • Text • Speech • Audio • Image • Video	Telemetry	Multimedia PCs Multifunction office machines Digital speech products		

captures, encodes, and compresses data which it stores and/or transmits; it also decompresses, decodes, and displays or presents data to end users. A digital system can be as small as a hand-held audio/video product or as large as a worldwide computer network. Each digital system that uses compression performs the information processing steps shown in Figure 1.4. Digital systems obviously do more than manipulate compressed data; those information processing steps have not been shown.

It is important to know that the compression process, the compressed data it produces, and the decompression process interacts with the physical system and with all other logical functions performed by the system software. These interactions may not affect system operation, or how users perceive the system, but all too often they do, as examples throughout this book will show. Consequently, when data compression is driven into the main dataflows of digital systems, many technical, operational, and marketplace issues arise and must be

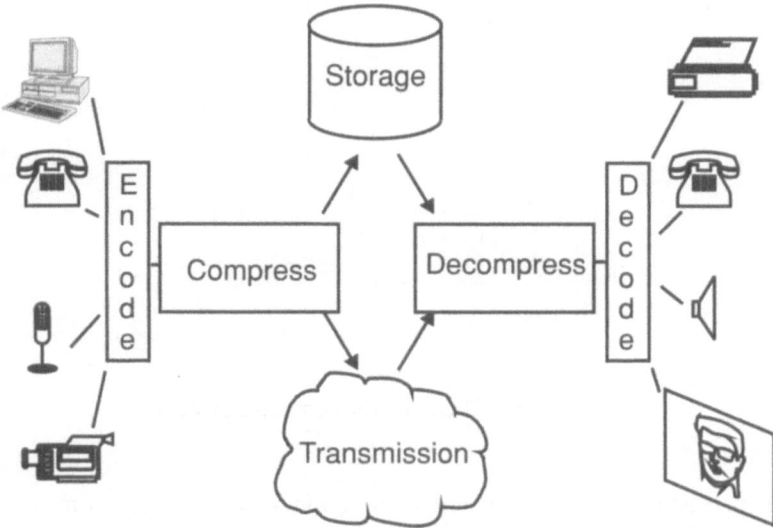

Figure 1.4   Integrating data compression in digital systems.

addressed. Often these issues override what many involved with data compression consider as the most important issue, selecting the data compression algorithm. Although assuredly an important step, algorithm selection is often the easiest decision facing digital system designers because the marketplace has made the choice for them. This is particularly true in a world of increasingly "open systems" (a computer industry term meaning that components and products of various origins can interoperate), where the choice of compression algorithm often is mandated by agreed-to standards.

A more difficult technical decision in digital system design is where to place the compression and decompression functions. As later chapters of this book will clarify, there are solutions that are either technically correct or market-driven but usually not both. Prudent design tells us to place data compression close to the producer or source of data, then compress the data and do not decompress it until it is delivered to the end user. This, the optimum system design for compression, provides the maximum storage and transmission efficiency. But the marketplace sometimes dictates other choices, especially in complex systems consisting of many components, from different manufacturers, perhaps even from different industries.

For example, consider the client-server computer system shown in Figure 1.5.[9]

_____

[9] Client-server computing was developed for LAN-based computer systems in the 1980s. Application programs on client computers communicate with server computers that provide services including access to information stored in databases. The processing workload in the clients is reduced at the expense of increased network traffic and increased work load on the servers [Laro94].

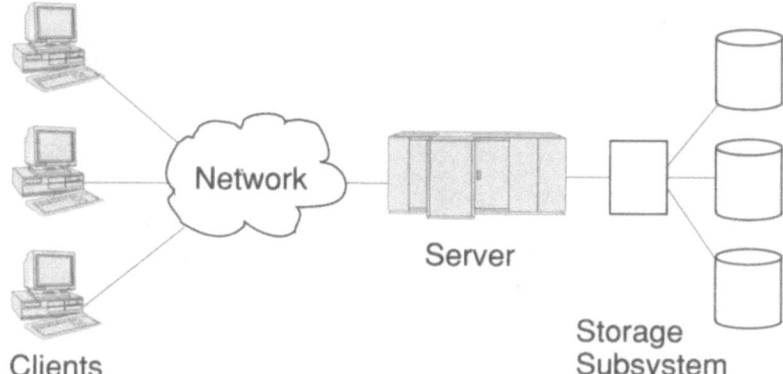

Figure 1.5   Client-server computer system.

End-user personal computer systems are connected to a telecommunications network that delivers data from a server—really another computer system—where the data is stored in a disk storage subsystem. Not only are each of these four components digital systems in their own right, but each has its own technical and marketing objectives, which, not surprisingly, may include compression optimized for the product or service. So, in complex digital systems, such as this example, it is not unusual that compression and decompression can take place several times between data capture and delivery to the end user.

Continuing to explore this example, we can appreciate that each component of the system needs to process the data in some way. Consider a simple data retrieval operation. The disk storage subsystem must package data for efficient storage and retrieval. The server needs to manage the data in a database. The telecommunications network needs to encode and possibly encrypt the data for transmission. Finally, the clients must prepare the data for presentation to end users. Complex systems, including this one, lead to a set of design decisions about handling compressed information. In removing redundancy from data (and sometimes information too), the compression process also destroys the fixed, regular storage structures that other digital data processing operations have come to expect. Fixed-length computer text records are no longer of fixed length. Depending on their content, images are a variable number of bits or bytes with no fixed storage structure corresponding to rows and columns of pixels. Fixed-rate video bit streams become variable rate, with each frame allocated a variable number of bits depending on the video content. How to process compressed data—short of decompressing, processing, and recompressing it in each component of a complex digital system—is a subject explored in later chapters of this book.

1.8 Summary

In this chapter we learned the following:

- The computer, telecommunications, consumer-electronics, publishing, entertainment, and other industries are converging on digital data.
- Digital data-handling systems overrepresent data, using more bits than required.
- Data compression employs innovative ways to represent data, using as few bits as possible for storage and transmission.
- The history of data compression traces back to the 1800s and much earlier times.
- Advances in data compression algorithms, VLSI technology, and standards for digital data representation are enablers for new products and services that take advantage of data compression.
- Digital data can be classified as symbolic (text, etc.) or diffuse (speech, audio, image, video, etc.).
- Lossless compression is applicable to symbolic data; lossless and lossy compression are applicable to diffuse data.
- Lossless data compression removes redundancy; lossy compression removes unneeded information.
- Symbolic data may compress by 2:1 or 3:1 whereas some types of diffuse data may compress by 100:1 or more.
- Many applications already use data compression and many more will in the future.
- Important digital system design decisions include where to compress and how to handle compressed data.

Part I—Marketplace

This first part of the book explores what users of digital systems want and need from data compression. Also, it explores the marketplace constraints and rules that affect data compression.

Chapter 2 provides an overview of the requirements that users of digital systems have for data compression technology. The chapter begins with trends for digital systems and their applications. Next, the role of data compression for delivering multimedia information is described. Then user expectations for data compression are examined. The chapter concludes with a short history of successful applications of data compression.

Chapter 3 continues to expand the discussion of marketplace factors that are important influences on data compression technology. First, industry convergence on digital data representation and its effect on data compression technology is examined. Then standards for data compression and their increasing importance in a world of open systems are analyzed. This is followed by a discussion of data compression for closed processes, situations where data compression standards are not all-important. The chapter concludes with a look at the restrictions on using proprietary, patented, and shared data compression technology.

2

Data Compression in the Marketplace

Table 1.2 in Chapter 1 presents an extensive list of applications that use data compression to store or transmit data more efficiently or to transmit it in less time. This chapter examines what the end users of those applications require, expect, and will get from data compression. It explores why data compression is *the* enabler for new, innovative products and services.

2.1 Digital Systems and Applications Trends

Processors, storage (electronic, magnetic, and optical), communications channels, and I/O devices—along with software—are the essential technologies for building computers and all systems that handle digital information. For several decades, each of these technologies have grown in capacity and performance while shrinking in size and/or cost. The good news is these trends are predicted to continue throughout the 1990s [Cuta90, Lewi94]. The bad news is technology advances alone are not sufficient to enable many new applications, particularly those that use video data. "Smart" processing techniques, including data compression, are needed too. This section looks at some important trends in digital systems and their applications, trends that accelerate the need for data compression.

Shrinking computers and expanding markets

The single-chip microprocessor has forever changed the computing industry. Computing tasks once confined to large, expensive computers now are done on the desktop. Computing costs have dropped by orders of magnitude, and computers are now mass-marketed products. In 1994, some 16 million personal computers, about the same as the number of automobiles, were sold in the United States, and nearly 50 million were sold worldwide [Juli95]. In the United States, almost half were sold as home computers [Arms94]. At the other end of the scale, microprocessors are increasingly the building blocks for large-scale computing systems where they are organized into teams and operate in parallel [Kher95]. The microprocessor has revolutionized other industries too. Automobiles, industrial equipment, communications gear, microwave ovens, stereos, VCRs, and a variety of home electronics products—all are controlled by microprocessors.

Microprocessors are becoming more powerful too. A frequently cited statistic is that the speed of Intel™ microprocessors has improved by nearly 50% each year for the past two decades. As shown in Figure 2.1, the PentiumPro™ chip

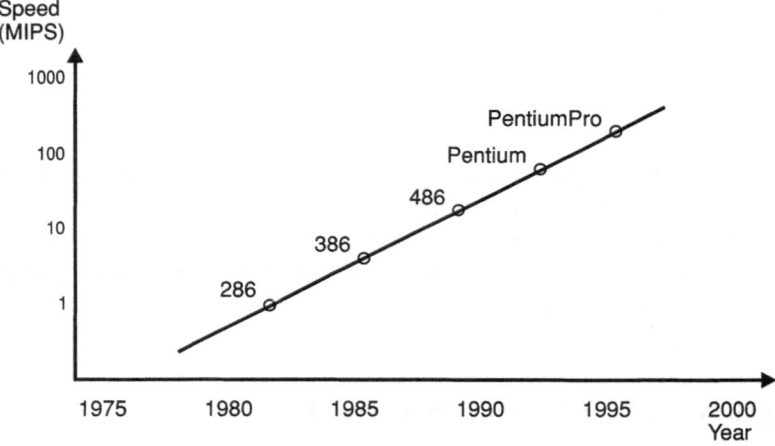

Figure 2.1   Intel microprocessors.

introduced in 1995 is some 250 times faster than its counterpart from the early 1980s [Hof95].[1] Every 18 months or so, the performance of silicon doubles at no increase in cost, thanks to improvements in chip-making technology. Smaller line widths make the circuitry more compact, which, in turn, makes the chips run faster (fewer nanoseconds per cycle) and allows denser chips (more logic circuits per chip). With each new chip generation, designers have given microprocessors more powerful dataflows by using wider data paths, more registers, parallel instruction execution, and other techniques to make them run faster. As a result, the instructions for manipulating text and numbers—the work of traditional processors—require less time, but there is some evidence that future improvements must take a different direction.

---

[1] MIPS (millions of instructions per second) is a measure of processor speed.

New applications for microprocessors such as in set-top cable boxes, HDTV (high-definition television) receivers, a variety of digital audio/video consumer-electronics products, and especially multimedia computers have growing needs for processing diffuse data. All spend less time doing text and numbers and more time with graphics, images, and handling real-time speech, audio, and video data. Consequently, these products need a microprocessor that can quickly process both symbolic and diffuse data. However, even the fastest microprocessors are not yet fast enough to do all graphics operations or image and video processing—particularly video compression—in software.

One solution is to continue to use separate chips for programmable DSPs, specialized data compressors, graphics accelerators, and video processors (which do data compression too). For products that do not need microprocessor programmability, this is an effective solution. But for personal computers, it is an expensive solution, especially when, as in present-day personal computers, those chips are mounted on separate boards. A more cost-effective solution for personal computers, one that some believe will lead to the microprocessor of the future, is to build a specialized multimedia microprocessor. This new type of microprocessor, as shown in Figure 2.2, uses the increasing number of logic circuits on future-

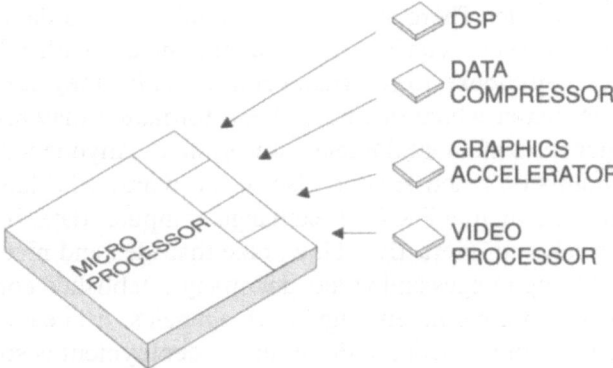

Figure 2.2   Multimedia microprocessor.

generation VLSI chips to integrate the function of DSPs, data compressors, graphics accelerators, and video processors. Not everyone agrees that a single microprocessor chip can or should do all these functions. However, following various tradepress reports of pending product announcements [Webb93, Wils94A, Wils95A, Wils95B, Slat95], a new generation of microprocessors with integrated multimedia functions has arrived. (Further discussion of this and many other multimedia processing options appears in Section 9.11.)

Communications for everyone

Communications are an integral part of modern society. The end-user demand for communications, which is fueled by widely available, low-cost personal computers, telephones, and television sets, has spurred all branches of the communications industry. Thanks to intensive competition and technology advances like fiber optics and high-power satellites, the number of telecommunications networks, computer data networks, cable television systems, terrestrial broadcast channels, and satellite transponders continues to grow. All are providing increased bandwidth and more choice to end users. However, just as computing has become more personal, so too will communications become more personal. Much as everyone expects a private line for telephone conversations, users are looking forward to private communications channels that can deliver all types of data—including images and video—customized to meet their needs. All signs point to a future where communications bandwidth will remain a scarce (or expensive) commodity. In brief, the number of users continues to grow, the demand for private communications is increasing, and more data must be transmitted, which translates to more excess bits and more need for data compression.

As important as these communications activities and trends are, some would say they are just the warm-up acts for the headline event of the 1990s. The Information Superhighway, Infobahn, National Information Infrastructure (NII), and Global Information Infrastructure (GII): in the 1990s no one can avoid hearing these terms and everyone involved with communications is trying to define them. The idea is simple: There should be available an affordable information infrastructure that everyone can access, to communicate with whomever they choose, whenever they choose, to get whatever information they need, in whatever form it may be, no matter where that person or information may reside [Wein94, Nesd95]. Consider for a moment the telephone system: Anyone with a telephone can dial a few numbers, reach anyone else in the world who has a telephone, speak with them, send them a FAX, or exchange computer data. It is affordable, accessible, universal, and interactive. Now, take that idea and mix in a few new types of data, including images and video, and many established communications providers, politics, and government regulatory agencies. It is easy to appreciate why moving the NII from concept to definition to deployment is so complicated.

Figure 2.3 shows some of many users and activities proposed for the NII. It is not clear whether there will be a single infrastructure for the NII—a universal "information pipe" that homes and businesses can plug into—or whether there will be, as now, many different delivery channels [Wirb94]. Nor is it clear what services will be available. What is clear is that there are two loosely clustered groups of providers, each intent on defining a new information infrastructure [Pres93]. Each plans to use client-server computing technology to provide all types of information—text, voice, audio, images, video, and whatever else can be digitized and transported.

The first group believes the personal computer is the "information appliance" for today and the future [Arms94]. For this group, the Internet is the model for the NII. They may be correct. The Internet experienced tremendous growth in the early 1990s. Homes, businesses, universities, and government agencies; all rushed to be connected. Clients now number in the millions, and many host

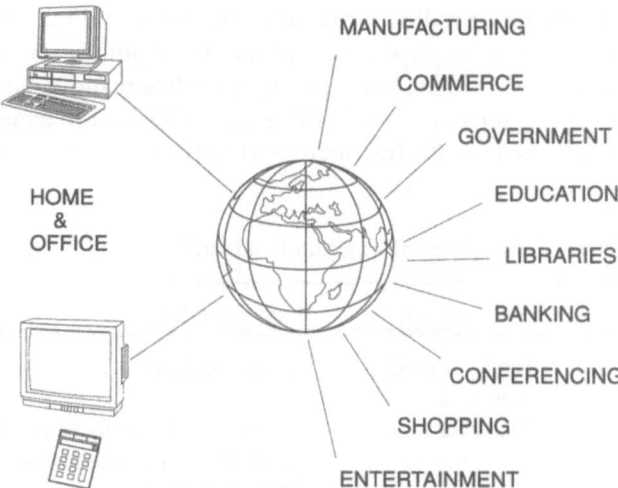

Figure 2.3   National Information Infrastructure (NII).

servers are online. What started as a computer network for research organizations in the United States has taken on a commercial flavor and has become global. Text-based communications have been augmented with graphics, voice, audio, images, and video. However, Internet bandwidth, although adequate for text and, perhaps, audio, severely limits transmissions of images and video—even compressed images and video.

The second group believes an *interactive* television receiver is the information appliance of the future. This device combines a standard-resolution television receiver or (in the future) an HDTV receiver and a set-top box. Actually a low-cost, microprocessor-driven computer, the set-top box is envisioned to be a product that provides functions ranging from channel selection and video decompression to controlling a camera for picking up and transmitting compressed video images back into the network. The knottiest question about interactive television is—what is the network? None of the existing communications systems—telephone networks, cable systems, nor broadcasting systems—meets all the requirements for fully-interactive television.

Increasing information bandwidth
for the end user

Digital systems continue, as in the past, to undergo continuous change. Thanks to advances in image and video displays, graphics devices, audio gear, and all I/O devices, and the software that drives them, digital systems are providing more information bandwidth to end users. This trend in digital systems reflects the rising expectations end users have about electronic media. One constant in all that has gone before, and what is to come, is the growing demand for information. Once, end users were happy to speak via telephone and to be entertained or informed by listening to radio or records; television and computers changed their expectations. End users expect to communicate and be entertained or informed by text, graphics, images, high-quality speech and audio, and video. Their demands have not gone unanswered. Table 2.1 provides some examples to show how the information bandwidth has increased between digital systems and the end users.

Table 2.1   More information bandwidth for end users.

Industry	Old Function	New Function
Computers	Black-and-white monitors	Color monitors
	Character text	Graphic user interfaces (GUIs) using text plus icons, graphs, and tables
		Speech and audio
		Images and video
Communications	Text-only	Computer networks carrying text data, audio, images, and video
	Voice-only	Telecommunications channels carrying voice, FAX, images, and video
Consumer electronics	Stereo audio	Surround sound 5.1 channel audio
	Television	HDTV
Publishing	Paper	Multimedia publications with text plus sound, images, and video
Entertainment	Movies on film	Digital special-effects movies
	Video games	Virtual reality

How does this relate to data compression? With each advance that increases the information bandwidth which a digital system can deliver to its end users, there are more bits to be stored and transmitted. Whatever form that information may take, whether video or something totally different, some of those bits will be excess bits that can be eliminated by data compression.

Interactive Multimedia

End users are intrigued by what interactive multimedia has to offer. It is more than just the bright colors and sound. End users can deal with information more efficiently when all their senses are involved, and they can use information more effectively by being interactive controllers of what they see and hear, not just passive observers and listeners. So goes the argument for why all digital systems of the future will be interactive multimedia systems. Let us explore some reasons why interactive multimedia is attractive.

It began innocently enough—a few icons, a splash of color, a snippet of sound, a bouncing ball.[2] At first only computer wizards and, soon, kids were attracted. Then, gradually, ever so slowly, the rest of us learned what they already knew—computers are fun to use and educational too! Interactivity and multimedia (plus good programming!) makes them that way. Gone are the drab black-white or gray-green screens with only a few lines of text and a blinking cursor to tell us what is happening inside the box. In their place are colors, meaningful icons, and windows to help us organize and display information. In those windows, not only is there text, but graphics, animation, images, and video too. Computers talk and listen to us. Stereo speakers provide audio playback and a microphone allows entering commands or capturing whatever sounds we choose.

Multimedia computing mixes text, graphics, animation, voice, audio, images, and video in whatever way works best to capture and deliver information. Interactivity involves the end users in a two-way dialog with the computer. Although, in the future, multimedia information will be delivered by high-speed networks, such as those foreseen for the NII, now most multimedia information is stored locally on CD-ROMs. Multimedia CD-ROM software for reference, education, and entertainment became a billion-dollar industry in 1994 [Cort95, Juli95]. Judging from sales figures, 1994 can be marked as the year of the multimedia computer. In that year, at least in the home computer market, machines without multimedia capability piled up in warehouses while those with CD-ROM players, sound cards, and speakers moved briskly off dealers' shelves.

Interactive multimedia is slowly finding its way into business applications too. Visions of workers playing video games or multimedia-retrofitting accounting and other traditional applications do not stir much interest, but new applications do. Desktop videoconferencing, video E-mail, and information kiosks are some examples. Multimedia has already established itself as an effective, highly productive tool for selling complex products, whereas a multimedia-equipped laptop computer (see Figure 2.4) can produce a dazzling customer presentation [Howa95, Moha95].

In the home market, personal computers are not the only vehicles for delivering multimedia information. The consumer-electronics industry continues to pump out hand-held video games and an expanding collection of products based on CD-ROMs. However, some believe even bigger opportunities exist for television-based products. In the United States, some 98% of homes have television, whereas in 1994, only about one-third of those homes had computers. Home computers are more complex and costly that television, and, therefore, they are not projected to ever achieve the same level of penetration [Arms94]. The problem with television—plain old television—is that it is a broadcast medium without infrastructure

---

[2] Remember Pong,™ from Atari™, circa 1972?

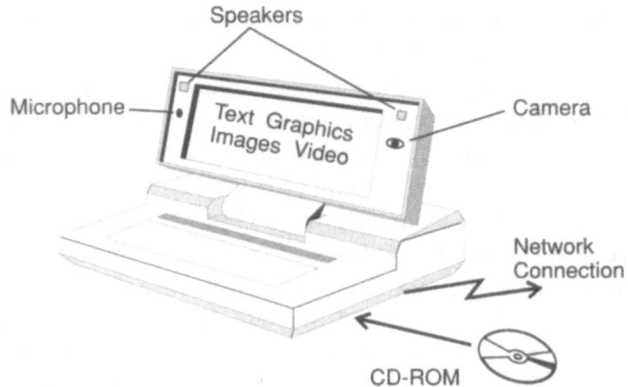

Figure 2.4   Multimedia laptop computer.

for two-way, interactive communications. Consequently, television cannot offer end users the full multimedia experience that computers provide. Chapters 8 and 9 describe the plans for making television interactive, but the real question is, once it is interactive, what multimedia-based services should it deliver? Suffice it to say that what consumers will want to do with interactive television probably are not the same things they already are doing with multimedia computers.

2.2   The Role of Data Compression

Let us now examine the role of data compression in delivering multimedia information. Even the most effective compression that it is practical to deploy today cannot overcome all the storage and bandwidth demands of text, graphics, speech, audio, image, and video data. This can be illustrated by a simple multimedia application. Our "application" presents the ideas on one page of this book using different presentation media ranging from text on paper to HDTV with 5.1-channel CD-quality audio. Figure 2.5 shows the storage required (assuming a single FAX page, image, or slide, and 5-minute audio or video presentations). Figure 2.6 shows the bandwidth required (for compressed data). For detailed information about channel bandwidth, and the storage and bandwidth required by various media used in this application, see Appendices 2A and 2B at the end of this chapter.

One may choose to change the presentation media, the presentation quality, or the length of presentation to best convey the ideas on one page of this book. But whatever your choice, the storage for uncompressed audio, images, and video exceeds by one or more orders of magnitude that needed for text. Also the transmission bandwidth required for transmitting uncompressed audio, images, and video would overload all available networks and broadcast channels.

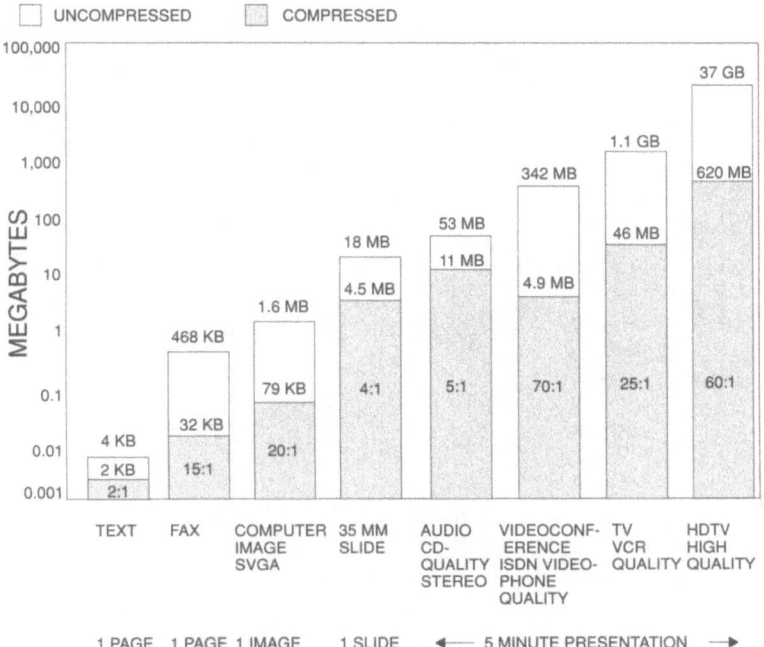

Figure 2.5 Storage required to present the ideas on a typical page of this book.

With data compression, the situation is more manageable—except for video. Multimedia applications that use video, even compressed video, stress the storage capacity of personal computers (the clients) and larger computers (the servers) and stress the bandwidth of all but the fastest available networks and broadcast channels. Consequently, the multimedia applications that have appeared do not deliver all that interactive multimedia can offer. If video storage is required, CD-ROM is the only economical storage media currently available for personal computers. Because it is read-only, authoring applications like the one above, which require writable storage, are problematical. If networking is required, high-bandwidth, two-way networks to connect clients and servers are still expensive and often unavailable. This has slowed the introduction of networked, interactive multimedia applications. To live within storage and bandwidth limitations, most multimedia applications for personal computers compromise video quality. Small video windows, low frame rates, and limited color depth are common. All are obvious and annoying limitations.

What does the future hold? Both home and business multimedia applications will benefit from advances in storage and networking technology. Storage density and capacity will continue to increase for both read-only and read-write storage with advances in optical and magnetic technology. High-density optical storage will likely continue to be the media of choice for video storage. Network band-

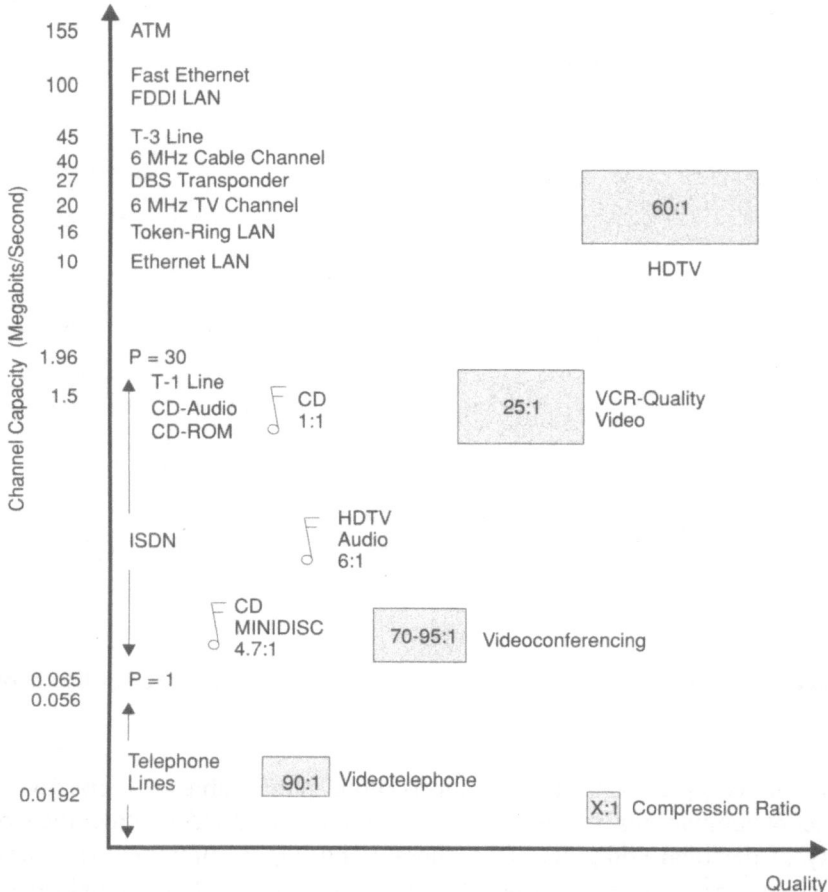

Figure 2.6   Quality and channel-capacity relationships for various media.

width, cost, and availability will continue to improve with increasing deployment of optical fiber. But even with these improvements, it will not be economical to store or transmit uncompressed data.

The consumer-electronics industry will exert an even stronger influence on the future of multimedia. Consumers, the end users, are accustomed to 30 frames-per-second video and ever-better speech, audio, and image quality. They expect multiple simultaneous image viewing options, special control and processing capabilities, and all the other capabilities provided by TVs and VCRs. It follows that consumers are likely to demand those same capabilities for the multimedia products in their homes and businesses too. If true, computer manufacturers, communications providers, and all other providers of multimedia products and services must meet the norms of the consumer-electronics industry for performance, function, and data quality.

It would be comforting to think data compression is the magic bullet that erases all the storage capacity and transmission bandwidth problems that multimedia information creates—that with a little more invention, time, and dollars these will be past issues. But this is not true. Throughout the 1990s, data compression technology will improve for all types of data. Data compression algorithms that are considered leading edge today will give way to newer algorithms that provide more compression, more quality, and faster operation, causing old standards to be revised or give way to new standards. However, although it is always hazardous to predict the future, experts and observers do not foresee breakthroughs that will increase compression ratios by orders of magnitude. For symbolic data, such as text, decidedly modest improvements are forecast. For diffuse data, image and video in particular, expect perhaps an order of magnitude in general-purpose and somewhat more in special-purpose applications, but not orders of magnitude [Habi92]. Economical delivery of full-function solutions for multimedia applications can only be assured when data compression is teamed with advances in VLSI technology, storage capacity, and communications bandwidth—plus lower costs for all.

2.3 End-User Expectations for Data Compression

End-user expectations for data compression are simple but demanding. Consider the following analogy: Automobiles operate more efficiently with fuel injection, stop more reliably with antilock brakes, and are more crash worthy with air bags. Each of these technologies contributes, in the eyes of the consumer, to making a better automobile. However, none of these technologies could address the mass market for automobiles until it was proven effective, demonstrated to be reliable, unobtrusively integrated, and, when integrated, still yield an automobile that consumers could afford.

So it is also for data compression, a technology for making better digital systems. End users expect data compression to be nothing short of totally invisible and invincible. They do not want to understand how it works, manage it, or experience anything except its positive effects; specifically:

- Data compression must be completely integrated, not an add-on or afterthought visible to end users.
- Data compression must not change how end users perceive digital system operation; there can be no slowdowns, no performance glitches, no changes in function.
- Data compression must predictably compress data with no surprises, no exceptions.
- Data compression must not compromise data in any way observable to end users.
- Data compression must be reliable; data should not be lost, but if it is, end users should not be involved in its recovery.

End users also expect that data compression will make products and services more affordable. This does not mean that the extra processing power or added hardware logic for data compression always must be provided at no additional cost. Rather, end users must recognize how the savings they realize from reduced storage or transmission costs (or time) reduces the total cost of the product or service.

Finally, end users expect that, like any new technology, data compression will enable new products and services that provide added value, other than just pure economics. This can mean products that are smaller, lighter, or faster. Also it can mean products and services that contain new functions. Sometimes, as the marketplace has demonstrated, end users view these as advances, and they are willing to pay for them.

2.4   Applications: From Dreams to Mass Markets

Every market has its (to use the vernacular of the computer software industry) "killer" applications; those applications, so attractive, so essential, customers will stand in line to buy. The trouble with killer applications, once you know what they are, is making them happen. This section presents some killer applications from the recent past that were impossible (or at least impractical) without data compression.

In the 1960s and 1970s, both the computer and communications industries were growing rapidly. The amount of digital data to be stored and transmitted (mostly text and voice) had grown to the point where computer disk storage and telecommunications network bandwidth were seen as technology constraints looming on the horizon. It was a time to experiment, using the then-fledgling data compression technology to relieve those constraints. Computer manufacturers, telecommunications providers, and large customers for computers and telecommunications were involved. The literature records many proposals and some products for compressing databases, computer files, and voice for storage or transmission [Snyd70, Regh81, Coop82, Hark82, Rait87, Held91]. But none of these efforts elevated data compression to the status of being an essential technology, in part, because solutions could still be found by throwing more money at the problem—buy more storage, contract for more bandwidth—and customers were willing and able to do so. By the 1980s, changes were afoot. Money became scarcer. Computer and telecommunications customers became more sophisticated. The applications that captured their attention grew increasingly more functional, more complex. Digital technology took on more importance for delivering the right products, but only if the price was right. In the 1990s, these trends continued.

That brings us to the applications shown in Table 2.2. The common thread is that data compression not only made (or is making) these applications possible, but it also revolutionized the marketplace. When these new products using data compression were introduced, they had readily discernible, easily measurable competitive advantages over older products, and demand quickly followed availability. Part III of this book (Applications) explores how data compression is used in each of these applications.

Table 2.2   Killer applications for data compression.

Application	Date	Constraint
FAX	1980	Telephone line bandwidth
Videoconferencing	1982-1985	Telecommunications bandwidth
Cartridge tapes for small computers	1989	Tape cartridge capacity and tape-drive data rate
Disk storage for personal computers	1990	Disk storage capacity
Direct broadcast satellite (DBS) TV	1994	Satellite transponder bandwidth
HDTV	2000	Broadcast channel bandwidth

2.5   Summary

This chapter explored trends in digital systems and their applications along with what end users expect and will get from data compression and how it is the enabler for many of those applications. We learned the following:

- Technology growth for processors, storage, and communications channels will continue but will be outpaced by application demand.
- Microprocessors are key to economical data compression implementation.
- A National Information Infrastructure (NII) is being defined that will provide wider access to all types of information—text, voice, audio, image, video, and whatever can be digitized and transported.
- Personal computers and interactive television receivers are contending to be the future information appliances for tapping into the NII.
- Users not only expect information to be more accessible but are using more bandwidth to access it.
- Interactive multimedia is becoming pervasive.
- Data compression alone cannot solve all storage and bandwidth limitations but must be used in combination with technology advances.
- End users expect data compression to be transparent, to make products and services more affordable, and to enable innovative new products and services.
- Data compression is essential to FAX, videoconferencing, computer tapes and disks, DBS television, and HDTV.
- Data compression will continue to become more pervasive.

Appendix 2A—Channel Bandwidth

Table 2A.1 summarizes the bandwidth of some important information storage and transmission channels encountered throughout this book.

Table 2A.1   Channel bandwidth.

Information Channel	Bandwidth	Comments
Standard telephone line	64 Kbps	
ISDN telephone line	P * 64 Kbps	P = 1 - 30
CD-ROM	1.248 Mbps	2 - 8X enhanced products
CD audio	1.4112 Mbps	
T-1 communications line	1.566 Mbps	
Digital video disc (DVD)	3.5 - 11 Mbps	Average - maximum rates
Ethernet LAN	10 Mbps	
Token-ring LAN	16 Mbps	
6-MHz terrestrial TV channel	20 Mbps	
DBS satellite transponder	27 Mbps	Transmits 4 - 8 channels
6-MHz cable TV channel	40 Mbps	
T-3 communications line	45 Mbps	
FDDI LAN	100 Mbps	
Fast ethernet LAN	100 Mbps	
ATM	155 Mbps	

Appendix 2B—Media Characteristics

Tables 2B.1, 2B.2, and 2B.3 summarize the characteristics of various media encountered throughout this book.

Table 2B.1   Speech and audio.

Media	Resolution	Data Rate	Channel Bandwidth[1]	Compression Ratio[2]	Compression Algorithm
Telephone speech	8 KHz x 8 bits/sample	0.065 Mbps	< 0.065 Mbps	2 - 16:1	See Table 5.2(a)
Wideband speech	16 KHz x 8 bits/sample	0.131 Mbps	< 0.065 Mbps	2 - 4:1	See Table 5.2(b)
CD audio	2 x 44.1 KHz x 16 bits/sample	1.4112 Mbps	1.4112 Mbps	-	Uncompressed
CD MiniDisc™	2 x 44.1 KHz x 16 bits/sample	1.4112 Mbps	0.292 Mbps	5:1	ATRAC™, See Table 5.3
DCC™ audio tape	2 x 44.1 KHz x 16 bits/sample	1.4112 Mbps	0.384 Mbps[3]	4:1	PASC™, See Table 5.3
HDTV audio	5.1 (6) x 48 KHz x 16 bits/sample	4.608 Mbps	0.384 Mbps	12:1	MPEG-Audio, See Table 5.3

Notes:
[1]   Bandwidth of existing channels and networks.
[2]   Compression ratio objective to meet the limitations of existing channels and networks.
[3]   Audio + ECC data = 0.768 Mbps.

Table 2B.2   Still image.

Media	Resolution[1]	Original Image	Typical Compressed Image	Typical Compression Ratio	Compression Algorithm
FAX	8.5 in. x 11 in. @ 200 x 200; 1 bit/pixel	3.74 Mb	0.250 Mb	15:1	ITU-T T.4/6
Computer VGA (black-and-white)	640 x 480; 8 bits/pixel	2.46 Mb	0.123 Mb	20:1	JPEG and others
Computer SVGA (color)	1024 x 768; 16 bits/pixel	12.58 Mb	0.629 Mb	20:1	JPEG and others
Kodak Photo CD™ 35-mm slide	3072 x 2048; 24 bits/pixel	151 Mb	48 Mb[2]	4:1	Proprietary; See Section 9.9

Notes:
[1]   Pixels/line x lines/image.
[2]   The original image and four smaller images are stored at various resolutions and compression ratios. Each 650-MB CD-ROM contains 100 - 110 images.

Table 2B.3   Video.

Media	Resolution[1]	Data Rate	Channel Bandwidth[2]	Compression Ratio[3]	Compression Algorithm
Videophone (AT&T VideoPhone 2500™)	128 x 112; 12 bits/pixel @ 2-10 fps	0.344 - 1.72 Mbps	0.0192 Mbps (Analog telephone line)	18:1 - 90:1	Proprietary
Video-conferencing (ISDN videophone)	QCIF 176 x 144; 12 bits/pixel @ 10-30 fps	3.04 - 9.12 Mbps	128 Kbps (ISDN; P = 2)	23:1 - 70:1	H.261
Video-conferencing (high quality)	CIF 352 x 288; 12 bits/pixel @ 10-30 fps	12.2 - 36.5 Mbps	384 Kbps (ISDN; P = 6)	32:1 - 95:1	H.261
VCR-Quality (VHS equivalent MPEG-1 video)	SIF 352 x 240; 12 bits/pixel @ 30 fps	30.4 Mbps	1.248 Mbps (CD)[4]	25:1	MPEG-1
SDTV	MAIN profile 720 x 480 16 bits/pixel @ 30 fps	166 Mbps	4 Mbps (DBS channel)	42:1	MPEG-2
HDTV	HIGH profile 1920 x 1080 16 bits/pixel @ 30 fps	995 Mbps	15-20 Mbps (6-MHz TV channel)	50:1 - 66:1	MPEG-2

Notes:
[1] Pixels/line x lines/frame.
[2] Bandwidth of existing channels and networks.
[3] Compression ratio objective to meet the limitations of existing channels and networks.
[4] 1.248 Mbps of 1.4112 Mbps bandwidth is available for video.

3

Marketplace Factors

In Chapter 2, we learned that data compression is the enabling technology for many highly visible applications and services. We also learned of the increasing importance of digital systems that offer high information bandwidth, provide interactive multimedia capability, and are widely connected. This chapter looks at a marketplace in which several industries and the products and services they offer are caught up in the transition to digital data. The factors affecting this activity and exerting important influences on data compression technology are shown in Figure 3.1.

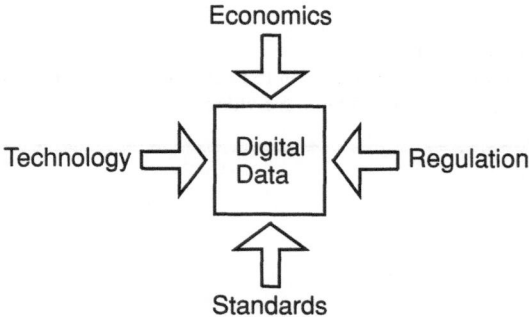

Figure 3.1 Marketplace factors.

3.1 Industry Convergence on Digital Data Representation

Mergers, acquisitions, the formation of alliances and consortiums, announcements of revolutionary new products and services: in the 1990s these events shape and define the industries affected by the transition to digital data. Although visionaries see a future with abundant new products and opportunities for all these industries, that future will not be reached without problems and delays. The adoption of digital data representation and digital processing technology creates many complex problems. Basic incompatibilities between the various industries, including different cost sensitivities, user bases, government regulations (the list goes on and on), will make convergence slow and perhaps difficult. To date, the convergence process has not been without a touch of chaos, and sometimes it has been anything but peaceful. And it certainly is taking longer than many expected. Let us briefly explore how the marketplace is affected.

Convergence on digital data representation within the communications industry teaches a valuable lesson: In the digital bit business, revolutions do not happen overnight! Telephone communications networks began going digital in the 1970s; yet, in the mid-1990s, it is rare to find any home connected to a digital telephone line. There are several reasons why it has taken so long. First, the investment in old (analog) telephone network technology is immense. One estimate says that to replace copper lines and switching equipment and bring a high-bandwidth fiber-optic cable into every home in the United States would cost more than $100 billion [Beac94]. Second, the customer demand for digital telecommunications has developed slowly because users have been satisfied with plain old analog telephone service. Their needs for more bandwidth and the kinds of services digital telephony can offer are just now emerging. Third, there is the cost to customers. Consider the deployment of IDSN (Integrated Services Digital Network), a service that delivers modest to moderate amounts of digital bandwidth over existing copper lines. Until the mid-1990s, any customer needing a digital ISDN line for their home or business found that, if available, it was (as new technology often is) expensive.

There are other examples where the convergence process (maybe it should be called the conversion process) most likely will take a long time: the transformation of cable television to become an interactive service, the transformation of terrestrial television broadcasting to HDTV, the transformation of business computing to interactive multimedia. In all these examples, old must give way to new, consumer demand must be generated for the new, and costs for the new product or service must be reasonable.

Another effect of convergence is that the boundaries between applications and between industries becomes fuzzy. For example, consider videoconferencing. Within the communications industry, PictureTel Corporation, CLI (Compression Laboratories Inc.), and other pioneers have grown to become large, independent companies offering videoconferencing products and services. The question is whether videoconferencing products and services can continue to be independent offerings once video capabilities are commonplace in computers, or whether videoconferencing will become just another desktop or portable computer application. A second example comes from the cable television industry where it appears that the next major advance depends on digital video and computer technology.

What is not clear is who will build and introduce what, and how it will be done. Who will provide the digital video servers that will replace traditional analog storage devices? Who will build the (television) set-top boxes and, beyond decoding, decompressing, and descrambling video, what computing functions will they have?

Not incidentally, the blurring of boundaries between traditional applications and industries may have a delaying effect. The introduction of new technology may be delayed as established product and service providers seek to maintain their market positions.

Another observation is that convergence increases contention in the market-place. The convergence of the computer and communications industries has been a more-or-less harmonious affair where, together, their individual products and services complement each other. But consider what is happening in the communications and consumer-electronics industries with the delivery of full-motion video.

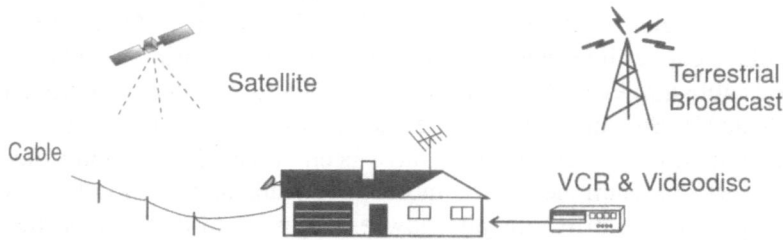

Figure 3.2   Analog television home delivery.

As shown in Figure 3.2, at present no fewer than four approaches compete to deliver analog television pictures to our homes. Each provider—over-the-air terrestrial broadcasting, cable, satellite, and in-home boxes (VCRs and video disc players)—has established a market niche. However, the prospects of using full-motion *digital* video are stimulating these providers to explore new products and are encouraging others to enter the competition.

A few of many future possibilities for digital video delivery include multimedia computers offering live television; also included are telephone companies distributing television signals and cable television companies providing 500 channels of video (plus games, home shopping, other computer-based video services, and some telephone services). In-home boxes, not to be left out, will exploit digital video too. In reality, each player from the computer, communications, consumer-electronics, publishing, and entertainment industries sees digital video as enabling enormous opportunities to get into new businesses or, perhaps, to gain a share of each other's old business. Now, and for some time to come, it is a turbulent situation fueled by the glitz and glamor of being able to handle compressed full-motion digital video.

In the United States, thanks to deregulation, a striking change is taking place in the telecommunications industry [Leop96]. Not only is the business environment for existing and new electronic media companies vastly different in the

1990s, but changing the rules also means regulators must cope with the unknown. Who should regulate the cable television or telephone company that offers television, telephone, and computer-based services? Should the FCC (Federal Communications Commission) continue to be the sole regulator of over-the-air television broadcasters who now realize that, if they choose, they can be in the bit-radiation business and can deliver any form of digitized information, whether text, speech, audio, image, or video? No longer are the dividing lines between communications domains so clearly defined as they once were when the regulatory agencies were put in place. Decisions by a regulatory agency in one area may affect many other areas, thus contributing to the destabilization and blurring of the marketplace. A key example is the 1992 FCC decision which allowed telephone companies to offer video dial-tone service [UPI92].

Underlying these complex and heady issues is one issue this book must deal with, standards. In the simplest terms, convergence means that products and services from various industries must work together. Consider the digital system

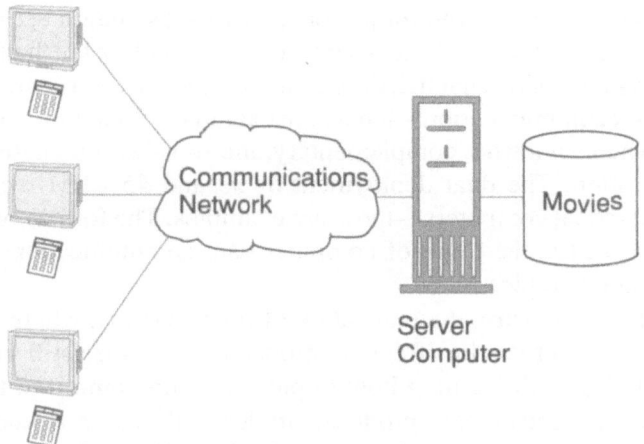

Figure 3.3 On-demand movies.

shown in Figure 3.3 for on-demand delivery of digital movies. The movies, produced in digital format, are stored on digital storage devices. A server computer and its database software manage user requests for viewing the films, do billing, and control delivery. A communications network transports the bits to home television receivers and transports user commands back to the server. In some sense, this might be considered the prototype for many future NII applications, for no one industry or organization controls all elements of this application. Products and services from the computer, communications, consumer-electronics, and entertainment industries are involved. They all must and can work together, cooperatively, thanks to defined interfaces and rules for creating, storing, processing, transmitting, and displaying digital data. In a word, they must conform to standards—including standards for audio and video data compression.

3.2   Standards for Open Systems

Without question, the 1990s have ushered in a new business paradigm for companies and industries dependent on hi-tech electronics. For many players, the costs to go it alone and develop new proprietary products are becoming prohibitive; sharing development expense with partners or competitors may be the only answer. Increasingly, too, companies are finding their survival depends on making products that are part of multivendor systems. The hardware and software they produce must work with that from other manufacturers in their own and other industries. Competition takes on new meaning in, this, a new era of cooperation, compromise, and compatibility.

In this atmosphere, standards are needed to assure that mass markets will develop. The lesson is old but often unlearned, causing mistakes to be repeated; standards are important! The communications industry knows it well. So, too, do the publishing and entertainment industries. The consumer-electronics industry has relearned it several times in the 20th century. The computer industry is still learning it. Often, there is a need for just one, universal standard because anything else is unworkable. Choosing to drive on the right-hand or left-hand side of the road, the 6-MHz television channel, the common physical, electrical, and signaling standards for telecommunications—these are examples. Sometimes, mass markets can develop when somewhat complementary, more-or-less compatible standards exist, but not often. The dual deployment of 33 and 45 RPM records, IBM™ and Apple™ personal computers—these are examples. The format "war" between VHS and Beta VCRs, the maze of computer data communications protocols—these are counterexamples.

In the computer industry, the realization of *open systems*, where products and services from different vendors freely interoperate, is an idea still in the making. As an industry, it is still learning how to put forth and commit to the degree of standardization required of mass-produced products. This is particularly important to our subject, data compression, because all information-oriented industries are looking to the computer industry for much of the technology—including data compression—to make digital data universal. True to form, the computer industry (with some outside help) has created a plethora of data compression algorithms for each type of data encountered in later chapters of this book. For example, there are many algorithms competing to compress video on multimedia computers. There will need to be a shakeout—which, incidentally, has already begun.

The need for successful standards

Standards can make markets bigger and help markets develop faster. They define products, solving chicken/egg problems, and provide name recognition for products that conform to the standards. Standards encourage competition and a wider range of solutions. They contribute to lower costs by stimulating mass production and permitting, in some cases, adoption of low-cost but expensive-to-develop VLSI technology. They also contribute to lower cost by assuring that interchangeable components will conform to uniform interfaces and operating procedures. Standards are required for open systems and they encourage interoperability through, to use a computer industry term, cross-platform compatibility. They simplify the complex relationships that exist between various parties involved in multi-industry (or multinational) ventures such as the NII described in Chapter 2. They ensure interchange of data, allowing information to be exchanged freely between standards-conforming products. For programmable products, when standards exist, suppliers are encouraged to create a wealth of high-quality program material. Finally, standards are mandatory to bid government contracts and some large-industry accounts.

The characteristics of successful standards can be summarized as follows: They are important in satisfying market requirements by providing clear, concise documentation for widely applicable, readily implementable technology. Successful open standards are required for interoperability. Successful standards are embraced by producers, users, and marketers because they are timely and they do not render existing products or services into instant obsolescence, or they offer prospects for supporting future enhancements, and, most of all, they are easy to implement and have reasonable licensing fees. They make economic sense.

Why standards fail

Not every standard is successful. There are many reasons why a standard can fail to take hold. Creating standards for emerging technologies, video data compression for example, can be especially difficult. By their very nature, standards attempt to freeze technology, which is difficult to do while the technology is still evolving. For this reason, and the very nature of the standards-making process itself, standards can take a long time to make. Waiting for a standard to emerge can mean being late to market, and when products that do conform to the standard are introduced, they may find themselves competing with entrenched technology.

A standard may be used as a tool of economic warfare to carve up the market. The very act of creating a widely useful standard sometimes involves compromises in performance, function, and complexity. Manufacturers may choose to stay with their proprietary technology and convince their customers that this is the wisest choice because it offers better performance, richer function, or lower cost. This was the situation in the videoconferencing marketplace for many years during the evolution leading to the ITU-T H.261 video coding standard.

Standards may overspecify, leaving little room for innovation. Worse yet, a standard may specify little-used features and require they be implemented. This kind of standard results, it is argued, when the standards-making process drags on and on. One operable theory is that good standards are made expeditiously; bad standards are not—and the examples are numerous [Coy95]. That theory may or may not be true. After two false starts, more than 5 years were spent making ITU-T H.261 the video coding standard for videoconferencing. Not incidentally, ITU-T H.261 is quite free of overspecification; it addresses only picture decoding which allows considerable room for innovation in how pictures are encoded—even allowing two videoconferencing participants to negotiate and use a proprietary compression algorithm of their choosing [Port94, Trow94]!

There are additional reasons why standards are not always successful. Cooperative standards may produce complex licensing arrangements due to excessive patents. When many parties contribute their proprietary technology to a standard, the intellectual property issues become complex. Then, too, standards sometimes are too expensive to implement, at least more expensive than nonstandard technology. Backers of early videoconferencing standards faced this situation as did early supporters for using the ISO MPEG (Motion Picture Experts Group) video standard to provide full-motion video on multimedia computers.

Standards sometimes are not all that long lasting, not all that widely applicable. Fast-moving technologies can rapidly make a standard obsolete. This was the situation in the 1980s, when rapid improvement in video compression technology caused the two standards for videoconferencing that preceded ITU-T H.261 to be quickly abandoned. In the 1990s, the ISO MPEG–1 compression standard, created for compact-disc-based distribution of audio and video, experienced a similar fate, at least for its intended application. Almost everyone concluded that, although the video quality (at the 1.5 Mbps rate it specified) might be marginally acceptable, the 74-minute playing time of compact discs was not sufficient for feature-length motion pictures. Quickly, the DVD (digital video disc), a new high-capacity optical disc was developed. This disc format provides both the longer playing times needed for movies and the higher data rates needed for the superior quality of ISO MPEG–2 compression. Interest in ISO MPEG–1 soon faded away as ISO MPEG–2 became the algorithm of choice.[1] Without question, a standard created for a niche product or market will not be very important when the marketplace moves on. In a worst-case scenario, a standard may be obsolete before it is completed and not address an (or any) application of interest.

The standards-making process

It has been said that the wonderful thing about standards is that there are so many from which to choose. The decision to standardize or not to standardize depends on many factors. It is binding on all involved to be sure that a standard is really needed before embarking on the lengthy and often difficult process to create one. For technology, such as a data compression algorithm, that will be used in an open systems environment, there really is no choice but for the parties involved to agree to a standard. Reaching a consensus among many interested

---

[1] ISO MPEG–1 has gone on to become the standard for other applications, as will be learned in Chapter 5.

parties can be a lengthy process, and moving a standard through a standards organization can take several years. The process usually begins with the formation of an "ad hoc group" or "experts group." This group may be chartered by an international or national formal standards-making organization (e.g., ANSI, IEC, ISO, and ITU-T) or by an industry organization, association, or consortium (e.g., QIC and many others) [Mcco92, Sher92, Stal94A]. See Table 3.1 for a description of the organizations mentioned in this paragraph. It is the job of the participants to evaluate proposals from one or several members of the group, to make compromises when there are conflicts, and to prepare a technical specification for the standard. The draft proposal they present to the voting members of the standards organization will go through one and usually more cycles of balloting and technical comments. During this process of refinement, the objective is to get all parties affected by the standard to buy-in, to gain a consensus, so that when the final standard is approved it will have the widest possible support and usage.

Table 3.1   Examples of standards organizations.

Organization	Description
ANSI	The American National Standards Institute is a nonprofit, nongovernment U.S. standards group that acts as a clearinghouse for standards developed by its members who include professional societies, trade associations, governmental and regulatory bodies, industrial organizations, and consumer groups.
IEC	The International Electrotechnical Commission is a nongovernmental standards organization devoted to standards for data processing and office equipment. It is concerned with functions such as interconnection, component measures, and safety.
ISO	The International Organization for Standardization, a nontreaty agency of the United Nations, is an international, nongovernmental body. It develops standards for industry and trade relating to a wide range of subjects. Most of its members are designated standards-making groups from the participating nations. Membership is voluntary.
ITU-T	The International Telecommunications Union - Telecommunications standardization sector, a United Nations treaty organization formerly known as the CCITT, develops standards relating to the end-to-end compatibility of international telecommunications connections. Membership is open to standards-making groups and also other government agencies, industry representatives, and those who will use the standards.
QIC	The Quarter-Inch Cartridge Drive Standards, Inc. is an industry trade association devoted to standards for computer tape drives.

It is important for all interested parties to participate in the standards-making process. Not only does this assure that the final standard has the widest possible support, but it also affords each of them the opportunity to be fully aware of the decisions leading up to the final standard and to know what the standard will contain long before it final. Participants have the opportunity to inject their views, making sure their interests and sensitivities are considered by the standard, and to shorten the time-to-market window for their standards-conforming products; nonparticipants do not have these advantages.

3.3   Data Compression Standards and Standards Compliance

In this book, the only standards considered are those for data compression algorithms and their implementations in digital systems.[2] From a standards perspective, there are three classes of data compression algorithms:

- The *official standards* for data compression embody algorithms arrived at by an official, national or international consensus process.
- The *de facto* standards for data compression employ algorithms that were originally created as single-vendor proprietary technology but have been adopted by manufacturers or customers and are in widespread usage within a marketplace segment for a particular application.
- The *proprietary* nonstandard algorithms for data compression are many and varied. They may not have been put before any standards group or adopted by more than one vendor, but some of these algorithms are the dominant (or the only player) in niche applications.

Those data compression algorithms that are official or de facto standards can be further classified by how they are used [Stal94B]. There may be the following:

- Voluntary compliance with standards created by international, national, or industry standards groups. A manufacturer or user of products or services to which the standard applies may choose to comply with all, part, or none of the standard. Compliance depends on business and technical advantages, not legal requirements.
- Mandatory compliance with standards created by international, national, or industry standards groups. A business organization or government agency may use these standards to define or limit acceptable products or services. For example, ITU-T H.261-compliant video compression may be specified for all videoconferencing product purchases.
- Mandatory compliance with regulatory standards developed by government regulatory agencies or authorities such as the FCC. Products and services that operate

---

[2] For in-depth discussions of data compression algorithms and their standards, see Chapters 4 and 5.

within the context in which the standard applies must conform, and there are penalties for noncompliance.

The standards picture in a world of emerging markets and technology is hardly clear or simple. In some applications—those where regulatory agencies direct what industries can or cannot do—official standards reign supreme and compliance is mandatory. HDTV is an example: If a manufacturer wants to participate in HDTV, its products and services must conform to the ISO MPEG–2 data compression standard. In other applications, regulatory mandates are not needed to motivate participants to voluntarily adopt official standards; economics is the only motivation needed. In the computer industry, voluntary compliance with the QIC standards for a compressed ¼-inch cartridge tape is an example.

Multimedia computers are a different story. Multimedia computing is in its infancy, at least when it comes to having an official standard for video data compression. There is a plethora of de facto standards and proprietary nonstandard algorithms for video data compression, each challenging the official standards. Each caters to the special needs of multimedia computing, and each claims to require fewer computing resources than the official standard algorithms, thereby allowing existing personal computers to execute a limited form of motion video in software. The function they offer may not be equal to that of the official standard algorithms such as ITU-T H.261 or ISO MPEG, but, their backers argue, it is appropriate for multimedia computing.

In other industries and applications, the use of proprietary nonstandard data compression algorithms preceded the introduction of official standards by several years. Videoconferencing is a prime example, for it might be argued that proprietary data compression was the cornerstone technology that launched the industry. Even today, proprietary algorithms for videoconferencing still have an edge (higher picture quality for a given data transmission rate, more tolerant of transmission errors, and so on) over the official standard ITU-T H.261 algorithm [Trow94]. For videoconferencing equipment manufacturers who have achieved some degree of market dominance, thanks in part to their proprietary algorithms, it is an interesting balancing act. Currently most offer both the official standard ITU-T H.261 algorithm to participate in "openness" and proprietary algorithms to differentiate themselves. For videoconferencing and other industries with established products, the rush to exclusively embrace official standards may, indeed, be leisurely.

3.4   Data Compression for Closed Processes

Not all applications for data compression are of the open systems variety described in Sections 3.2 and 3.3. This book describes many data compression applications where one manufacturer, one product, or one software program controls all the steps—from the time when data is first compressed until it is finally decompressed.

In fact, in the computer industry, where modern digital data compression originated, the most important applications operate in this way. Let us define these
as *closed processes* or, if you prefer, closed applications.

A variety of data compression technology is employed in the closed processes
that will be explored. Because these processes are closed, many reasons for
standardizing the data compression algorithm (or anything else) disappear, or at
least become less important. However, what we will learn is that, when given
the option, some product developers choose to go with official standards for their
compression technology, whereas others choose de facto standards or highly
proprietary, nonstandard compression algorithms. We will examine the reasons
for their choices in each application involving a closed process.

3.5 Proprietary, Patented, and Shared Data Compression Technology

Questions of intellectual property ownership take on increasing importance as
data compression moves from being merely an interesting technology to being
an essential element of commercial, for-profit products and services. Data compression algorithms come from many sources, including individuals working
on their own, academia, and industry. Details of some algorithms and their
implementations have been maintained as closely guarded trade secrets, the
property of their creators for use in proprietary products and services. Other
algorithms have been widely published by their creators, complete with prototypes
for executable code. Books, magazine articles, libraries on the Internet; all are
rich sources. One might assume that because an algorithm is well known, it can
be freely used, but that is not always true. Many algorithms or their implementations (and deciding where the algorithm definition leaves off and implementation
begins is not always easy) are covered by patents. Although it may be permissible
to create or obtain (either free or for a one-time shareware fee) a copy of a
patented algorithm for noncommercial, nonprofit use, a licensing agreement must
be negotiated with the patent owners before any patented algorithm can be used
in commercial, for-profit products or services.

Manufacturers or anyone contemplating the use of data compression in a
commercial, for-profit product or service would be wise to investigate the origins
of the data compression technology and to seek competent legal counsel. As the
following examples show, the consequences for not paying heed to intellectual
property rights can be serious.

LZW compression algorithm

Dictionary algorithms have proven to be effective for compressing general
text and some types of graphics data. Lempel and Ziv [Ziv77, Ziv78] formalized
the algorithms but left the implementation to others, and there have been lots of

them, each with subtle—and sometimes patented—variations. The LZW algorithm is one such variation on the work of Lempel and Ziv; it was first published by Terry Welch in 1984 [Welc84]. It was awarded a patent, since assigned to the Unisys Corporation who has agreed to license the algorithm. Modem manufacturers were among the first licensees, as LZW is part of the ITU-T V.42bis standard for data compressing modems [Thom92]. Because the LZW algorithm is effective, many software developers also chose LZW for their products. They believed (falsely) that it was in the public domain, for details of LZW were widely published, and so they were free to use it. They were wrong.

One of the software products that elected to use LZW is GIF™ (Graphics Interchange Format™) from CompuServe™, a standard format for storing bit-mapped graphical images.[3] CompuServe introduced GIF in 1987. Since then, many developers have licensed GIF for use in their products, and it has become a worldwide de facto standard in its own right. In 1993, Unisys advised CompuServe that it would have to license LZW technology and pay royalties on all code which created GIF-format files. In 1994, CompuServe became a licensee with authority to grant sub-licenses to GIF developers [Wueb95]. CompuServe advised application developers using GIF that their for-profit products and services would be affected by licensing and royalty fees. They were encouraged to register with CompuServe to obtain a sublicense. This was not good economic news for many graphics software developers, leading to speculation that they would drop GIF in favor of other graphics file formats that have no licensing requirements [Hine95]. Reportedly, Unisys chose not seek payment for noncommercial, nonprofit software that uses GIF; only for-profit products marketed after 1995 will require licensing [Crot95, Gaff95, Wolf95A].

LZS compression technology

A high-profile intellectual property rights case involving Stac Electronics Inc. and Microsoft Corporation received nationwide publicity during 1993–1994. According to tradepress articles of that era [ElTi93, Mall93, NSci93, Rohr93, Doyl94, FTL94, John94, Mall94A, Mall94B, Mall94C, Scan94, Wald94], a sequence of events began in January 1993 when, after licensing negotiations between the two companies had reportedly broken down, Stac™ filed a patent infringement suit against Microsoft™. The suit alleged that the disk data compression algorithm planned for the then-upcoming 6.0 release of MS-DOS™ violated Stac's patent on its LZS (Lempel-Ziv-Stacker) technology. In February 1993, Microsoft filed a countersuit containing several charges, one of which stated that Stac had misappropriated and used a Microsoft trade-secret MS-DOS preloading feature in its Stacker™ disk data compression products for PCs (personal computers).

---

[3] A few of the many other software products that use the LZW algorithm include the UNIX™ Compress code, ARC™ from System Enhancement Associates, Stuffit™ from Aladdin Systems, Inc., and PKZIP™ from PKWare [Apik91, Nels92].

The case came to trial, and in February 1994 a jury awarded Stac $120 million in compensatory damages for patent infringement and awarded Microsoft $13.6 million on its trade-secret counterclaim.

The story did not end there. Following the trial, Microsoft stopped shipments of its current MS-DOS 6.0 and 6.2 products and, in April 1994, began shipping MS-DOS 6.21, which contained no data compression. Microsoft also announced it was working on new data compression technology that subsequently was released as part of MS-DOS 6.22 in June 1994. In early June 1994, responding to injunction requests from both parties, the United States District Court in Los Angeles denied Microsoft's request to have Stacker 4.0 withdrawn from distribution. The court also ordered a recall of all MS-DOS 6.0 and 6.2 products shipped into distribution and retail channels after the date of the jury award. Microsoft promptly filed an appeal. In late June 1994, after months of legal maneuvering, with new rounds of appeals looming on the horizon and no apparent end in sight, the case came to a surprising and sudden conclusion. The two companies announced they would drop their court-awarded judgments and cross-license each other's technologies, with Microsoft agreeing to purchase 15% of Stac for $39.9 million, to pay Stac an additional $1 million in royalties per month for 43 months, and to use Stac data compression algorithms in its software.

In related matters, after winning a similar suit in 1993, Stac signed a licensing agreement with IIT (Integrated Information Technology), a manufacturer of data compression coprocessor cards and chips [Mall94B]. In 1994, after the court ruling in the Microsoft case, Stac signed licensing agreements with PC hardware vendors including Compac Computer Corporation, the IBM PC Company, and Packard Bell [Wald94].

Arithmetic coding

Arithmetic coding provides yet another example showing that widely published data compression algorithms sometimes have constraints on their usage. Although dictionary algorithms have grown to be the most popular choice for lossless compression of symbolic text data, arithmetic coding, in combination with dictionary and many other algorithms, can improve coding efficiency for a wide range of data types. Arithmetic coding is an option specified by the ISO JPEG (Joint Photographic Experts Group) standard for still-image compression and is specified by the ITU-T JBIG (Joint Bi-level Image Group) standard for bi-level image compression. Arithmetic coding is also patented (by IBM, Mitsubishi, and AT&T™). Therefore, for commercial ventures, a license must be negotiated to use arithmetic coding in connection with the JPEG and JBIG standards.

MPEG compression

In the cases cited above it, was quite clear who owned the patent and intellectual property rights. What if the product in question (or in the case to be described, a standard) was created by a committee and contained bits and pieces of patented technology from many sources? What if ownership belonged to multiple individuals or companies, perhaps spanning multiple industries, perhaps from different countries where patent rules and regulations differ? Such was the situation the Motion Picture Experts Group faced when creating the ISO MPEG–2 video compression standard. Sometimes experts groups chartered by standards organizations have a relatively easy task when the official standard they are creating is evolved from a preexisting de facto standard put forth by one or a few of the group members. In that circumstance, negotiating for reasonably priced licensing rights is straightforward. But this was not the situation the MPEG committee faced [Yosh94A, Yosh94B].

Standards organizations are not charged with licensing. To resolve the intellectual-property rights issues surrounding MPEG–2, an independent group known as the MPEG Intellectual Property Rights Group composed of users and manufacturers of MPEG compression products was set up to study the situation. The plan they devised was to create a separate licensing entity and, by placing all patents in a pool, provide a one-stop-shopping center for licensing MPEG technology [EET95B, EET96]. The alternatives, for potential users to negotiate with individual patent holders, or to work around those patents too difficult or too expensive to obtain, could delay widespread deployment of products based on MPEG–2. The group's charter was to focus on the MPEG–2 standard as a whole when defining reasonable royalties, so that licensing fees for the sum of its parts would not be exorbitant. To accomplish this, their first task was to sort out who owned what pieces of the technology that went into making MPEG–2, in itself a complex job, as many patents were involved. The next task was to convince each of the patent owners to make their technology available for reasonable licensing fees. In some instances, this meant convincing them to sacrifice potential patent revenue in hopes of creating a larger market for MPEG–2. As of this writing, complete agreement had not been reached, and arrangements for one-stop licensing were still in progress.

3.6 Summary

This chapter examined important influences that the marketplace exerts on the adoption of digital technology, data compression included. We learned the following:

- The digital revolution is impeded by investments in old analog technology, the need to stimulate customer demand for new digital technology, and the cost of digital technology.
- Industry convergence on digital data representation and processing may be a slow and perhaps difficult process because of basic incompatibilities between various industries, including different cost sensitivities, user bases, government regulations, and many other factors.

- Convergence blurs the boundaries between traditional applications and between traditional industries; the marketplace will require time to adjust to the new technology.
- Convergence has a destabilizing effect on the marketplace, causing contention among established players and generating new requirement for regulation.
- Standards are essential in a marketplace where economics and complex new applications dictate that products and services must interoperate in open systems environments.
- Successful standards are required for mass-marketed products and services.
- Successful standards get adopted because they are timely, do not make existing products or services obsolete, offer prospects for future enhancement, are easy to implement, and have reasonable licensing fees.
- Standards can fail for all the same reasons that go into making them successful.
- The standards-making process is lengthy, requiring a great deal of discipline and participation from all who are involved.
- From a standards perspective, there are three classes of data compression algorithms: official standards, de facto standards, and proprietary nonstandard algorithms.
- Standards compliance can be voluntary, mandatory, or regulatory agencies can use voluntary standards to define or limit acceptable products or services.
- Some applications involve closed processes that do not require the use of standard data compression algorithms.
- Data compression algorithms may be proprietary, patented, or (rarely) free of intellectual property constraints. Intellectual property rights must be respected. To not do so can be expensive!

Part II—Algorithms

This second part of the book introduces the algorithms that the marketplace has chosen for compressing symbolic and diffuse data.

Chapter 4 begins with an overview of data compression algorithms—what types there are, what they do, and how they are structured. The chapter continues with descriptions of the algorithms most frequently used for symbolic data—text, numbers, computer programs, and the like.

In Chapter 5, the discussion continues with descriptions of the data compression algorithms for diffuse data—speech, audio, image, and video.

Part II—Algorithms

4

Compression Algorithms
for Symbolic Data

In Chapters 4 and 5, we will learn how some important data compression algorithms work. The marketplace has selected these algorithms for its de facto and official standards because they are effective and implementable, allowing many other compression techniques to languish or remain subjects for further investigation. This chapter begins by looking at how data compression algorithms are constructed. Then it examines algorithms for compressing symbolic data, including character text, numbers, computer programs, and so on. In Chapter 5, the discussion continues with algorithms for compressing diffuse data, including speech, audio, image, and video. The simplest, most general algorithms for each data type are described first, followed by more powerful or more specialized algorithms.

An algorithm is a set of rules or procedures for solving a problem in a finite number of steps. The job of a digital data compression algorithm is to transform a stream of data symbols into a stream of codewords. If the transformation is effective, the codewords occupy fewer bits than the original data symbols. Decompression reverses the transformation. If the data compression is *lossless*, only redundancy is removed, and the decompressed data exactly matches the original data before compression. This is the kind of compression needed for symbolic data. If the data compression is *lossy*, noncritical information is removed, and the decompressed data may not exactly match the original data. However, the result must be an acceptable approximation, where human observers often are called upon to judge what "acceptable" means. This, along with lossless compression, is the kind of compression needed for diffuse data.

4.1 Modeling and Coding

To appreciate how data compression algorithms work, we need to understand how they are structured. Figure 4.1 shows that data compressors and decompress-

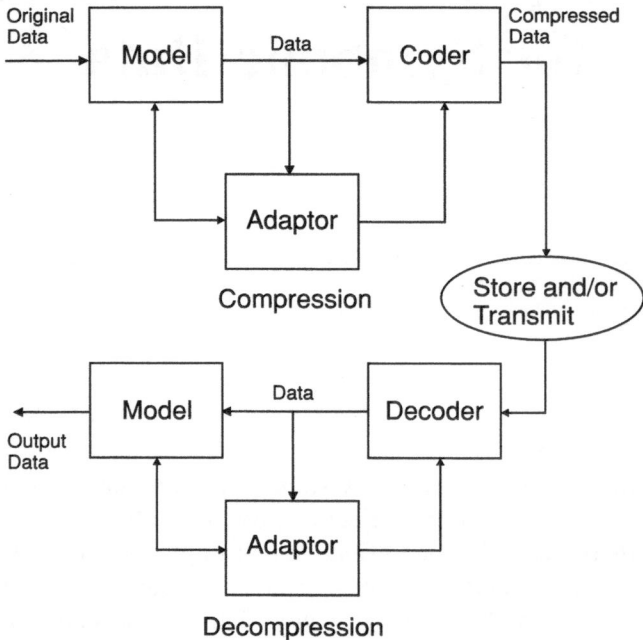

Figure 4.1 Adaptive data compression.

ors each contain three major building blocks. During compression, the following operations occur.

The *model* analyzes the input symbols and tells the coder which codeword(s) to output. The model is a collection of rules and data generated from knowledge about the structure of the input data and the probabilities of the individual symbols.[1] It allows redundancy and—if the compression is lossy—noncritical information to be removed from the input data stream during compression. For symbolic data, often, the data structure is no more complex than a stream of characters (or bits). Therein, the statistical frequency of characters and the occurrence of runs of identical characters, strings, or sequences of symbols such as common words in a language are used to remove redundancy. For diffuse data, each data type has its own complex structure and each requires an especially designed model to deal with removing redundancy and, usually, noncritical information. Specifically, speech is modeled as a time-ordered sequence of voice

---

[1] The probability of a symbol is a number between 0 and 1.0 that measures how frequently it occurs relative to all possible symbols.

parameters or, like audio, as a time-ordered sequence of waveform samples. Images are modeled as two-dimensional arrays of pixels, video is modeled as a time-ordered sequence of two-dimensional images, and so on.

The *coder* produces a compressed bit stream using information supplied by the model to generate codewords for input symbols. The coder matches the length of the codewords it produces with the statistics of the source symbols, generally trying to use the fewest bits to represent the input data. If the compression is effective, the coded output will be smaller than the original input data.

The *adaptor*, if the compression is adaptive, uses the data itself or information from the model to continuously adjust the model and/or the coder to reflect changes in the input data. If the compression is not adaptive, the adaptor function is missing, and the model and/or the coder statistics (having been determined by some a priori process) remain fixed throughout the compression process. Another possibility is semiadaptive compression where the adaptor operates at intervals, for example, when a new data file is encountered.

Once compressed, the data may be stored or transmitted. Later, during decompression, the compression process is undone by three building blocks that complement those in the compressor. The data and rules needed for decompression are identical to those used by the compressor. If the compression algorithm is nonadaptive, information about the input data and its structure is built into the decompressor's model and coder. If the compression is semiadaptive, this information is communicated to the decompressor along with the compressed input data. For adaptive compression algorithms, the decompressor creates this information on the fly from the decoded input data.

Not all data compression algorithms are adaptive, nor do their descriptions show well-separated modeling and coding functions. As noted in Chapter 1, modern-day digital data compression began in the 1950s with information theory and statistical probability concepts that led to "coders" for losslessly compressing symbolic data. Some of today's important lossless compression techniques—Huffman coding and others—are from that era when the whole compression process was called coding. It was not until the 1980s that the ideas of (1) viewing modeling as a separate step preceding coding and (2) making the compression process adaptive began to take root [Bell90]. These proved to be significant advances in both data compression theory and practice. Not coincidentally, it was during this same period that effective algorithms powerful enough to take on audio, image, and video were developed.

4.2 Symbolic Data Compression

Lossless compression of symbolic data is accomplished by creating codewords that are shorter than the corresponding symbols they encode, if those symbols are common. This is done at the expense of making the codewords longer for those symbols that are uncommon. (Nature does not let you get something for

Table 4.1 Symbolic data encoding.

Encoding Method	Input	Output
Fixed to variable	A symbol	Variable number of bits
Variable to fixed	Symbol string	Fixed number of bits (bytes)
Variable to variable	Symbol string	Variable number of bits

nothing!) As shown in Table 4.1, data compression algorithms implement these length changes as fixed-to-variable, variable-to-fixed, or, by combining both, variable-to-variable-length encoding. Historically, fixed-to-variable-length changes were first exploited for compression and were described by the term coder or entropy coder. From that perspective, any compression processing ahead of such a coder was viewed as a front-end model. This includes the aforementioned variable-to-fixed-length processing, which was formalized later as another technique for designing compression algorithms.

Run-length coding and the front-end models of Lempel-Ziv dictionary algorithms are examples of variable-to-fixed-length encoding. Huffman and arithmetic coding are examples of fixed-to-variable-length encoding. Variable-to-variable-length algorithms, such as a Lempel-Ziv front-end model followed by Huffman encoding, are appropriate if the first stage is not completely optimized to maximize compression (for example, if it is primarily optimized to maximize speed).

In the sections that follow we will examine how these algorithms work.

4.3 Run-Length Coding

A run-length coder replaces sequences of consecutive identical symbols with three elements: a single symbol, a run-length count, and an indicator that signifies how the symbol and count are to be interpreted. Run-length coding applies equally well to sequences of bytes, such as characters in text, and to sequences of bits, such as black-and-white pixels in an image.

To illustrate run-length coding, consider the HDC (Hardware Data Compression) algorithm used by the IBM 3430 and many other tape drives connected to the IBM AS/400™ computer system [IBM1]. This algorithm is a form of the character-oriented IBM SNA™ (IBM System Network Architecture) run-length compression algorithm for data communications. The HDC algorithm operates as follows:

- Strings of consecutive blanks (between 2 and 63 bytes long) are compressed to a single control byte containing a code signifying "blanks" and a count.

- Strings of consecutive characters other than blanks (between 3 and 63 bytes long) are compressed to 2 bytes: a control byte containing a code signifying "consecutive characters" and a count, and a byte containing a copy of the repeated character.
- Strings of nonrepeating characters (between 1 and 63 bytes long) are expanded by having a control byte added at the beginning of the nonrepeated character string. The control byte contains a code signifying "nonrepeating characters" and a count.

In the example shown in Figure 4.2, the HDC algorithm has been used to encode a character sequence where the first six blanks are compressed to a single control byte. Next in the compressed string is a control byte appearing before ABCDEF, designating a string not compressed. Another control byte for the string of two blanks follows. Then a control byte appears before 33GHJKbMN, designating another string not compressed. (The two consecutive 3's and the single blank cannot be compressed.) Finally, the nine consecutive 3's are compressed to a control byte and a single 3.

bbbbbbABCDEFbb33GHJKbMN333333333

(a) Uncompressed

ABCDEF33GHJKbMN*3

(b) Compressed

b - Blank
* - Control byte

Figure 4.2   Run-length coding.

Run-length coding is highly effective when the data has many runs of consecutive symbols. For example, computer data files may contain repeated sequences of blanks or 0's. Run-length coders are also effective during the final stages of image and video data compression where, after suitable transformations, many long runs of 1's and 0's occur. Run-length coding is not adaptive. Therefore, parameters of these algorithms must be carefully selected to match the data. For example, the algorithm shown in Figure 4.2 assigns the shortest possible codeword to runs of blanks. For this algorithm, the maximum compression only occurs when blanks are the most frequent character found in repeated sequences.

4.4 Huffman Coding

Huffman coding is the best known, most widely used *statistical* (entropy) coding technique to result from studies of information theory and probability. The general idea of statistical coding is that by observing how often particular symbols occur, compression can be obtained by assigning shorter codewords to frequently occurring, more-probable symbols, and assigning longer codewords to infrequently occurring, less-probable symbols. This technique, which was used in the Morse code, was formalized by the work of Shannon, Fano, Huffman, and many others beginning in the late 1940s [Bell90, Held91, Nels92, Witt94]. Huffman coding assigns variable-length codewords to symbols according to their individual probability of occurrence. If those probabilities happen to be negative powers of 2 (½, ¼, and so on), the Huffman coder is optimal in the sense that it uses the minimum amount of bits to represent the information in a message.[2]

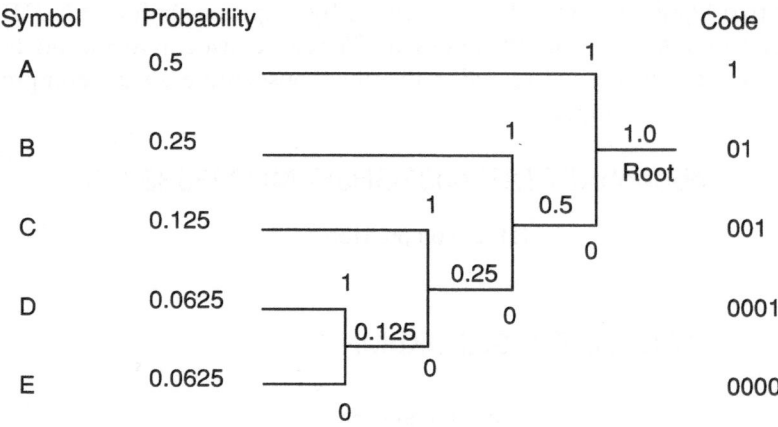

(a) Code tree construction

Symbols	AECBD
Huffman code	10000001010001
Parsed	1 | 0000 | 001 | 01 | 0001

(b) Encoding and decoding

Figure 4.3   Huffman coding example.

A simple example of Huffman coding is shown in Figure 4.3. The Huffman code is constructed by building a binary tree where the leaves of the tree are the probabilities of the symbols to be coded. The tree is built starting at the leaves and working toward the root of the tree. To begin the process, the symbols are ranked in order of their frequency of occurrence. Next, the two symbols with

---

[2] The information content of a message is measured by *entropy*, giving rise to the term entropy coding. If the probabilities of individual symbols are p_i, the entropy calculation tells us the minimum number of bits for coding the message is $-\sum \log_2 p_i$ bits.

the smallest probabilities are replaced by an intermediate node representing a subgroup whose probability is the sum of both symbols. Then the next least-frequent pair of symbols or subgroups is located and replaced by an intermediate node. The process continues until all the symbols have been combined into a single structure called a Huffman code tree. The final step is to assign codewords to the symbols. This is accomplished by tracing the tree beginning at the root node and continuing to the leaf node for each symbol.

A sequence of symbols is encoded left to right, symbol by symbol. An encoded sequence is decoded left to right, bit by bit. Huffman codes have the desirable prefix property which assures no codeword is the prefix of the codeword for another symbol. This property is illustrated when decoding the bit stream shown in Figure 4.3(b), where the first encoded bit encountered is a 1. In Figure 4.3(a), the symbol "A" is assigned the only codeword that begins with a 1. Therefore, "A" can be uniquely decoded as the first symbol in Figure 4.3(b). The next sequence of 0's decodes unambiguously to "E" and so on.

Huffman codes are easy to generate and, instantaneously, symbol by symbol, they are easy to decode, but there are some limitations. As stated earlier, Huffman code is only optimal when all symbol probabilities are negative powers of 2, a situation not guaranteed to occur in practice. Clearly, Huffman codes can be generated no matter what the symbol probabilities are, but they may not be very efficient. The worst case is if one symbol occurs very frequently (i.e., its probability approaches 1.0). Information theory tells us that, according to the entropy calculation, only a fraction of a bit is needed to code the symbol, but the best Huffman coding can do is assign a one-bit codeword. In this situation, other coding techniques are better, and we will look at one shortly, arithmetic coding.

The Huffman coding technique described above uses a static data model to build the Huffman code tree. This means that all the symbol probabilities must be known in advance. In practice, with a new data collection, one pass through the data is required to collect statistics, and, then, after the codewords are generated, a second pass is required to do the encoding. One of many extensions to Huffman code is to make it adaptive, whereby the Huffman code tree is updated whenever symbol probabilities change. Several adaptive Huffman coders have been developed [Held91, Mukh91]. However, by comparison, adaptive Huffman coding is more complex and not always as effective as adaptive arithmetic coding or adaptive Lempel-Ziv coding [Witt94]. Consequently, these adaptive techniques are far more popular.

Another limitation of Huffman coding is that when the number of symbols to be encoded grows very large, the Huffman coding tree and storage for it grow large too. Such a situation occurs in facsimile transmission (described in Chapter 7), where each scan line of the image is represented by 1728 pixels. A particular scan line could contain 1728 white pixels (represented as 0's), 1728 black pixels (represented as 1's), or runs of white and black pixels arranged in any order. Normally, within the scan line, a white pixel is followed by a long run of white pixels before a black pixel is encountered, whereas runs of black pixels tend to be much shorter. When directly applied to facsimile compression, Huffman coding requires 1728 codewords for runs of white pixels plus 1728 additional codewords for runs of black pixels to cover all possible combinations within the scan line. The storage requirements for facsimile coding can be dramatically reduced by combining run-length and Huffman coding to create a modified Huffman code. It operates by breaking up each black or white run into a long run containing a multiple of 64 pixels and a residual that contains 63 or fewer pixels. Encoding is a two-step process: Long runs are Huffman coded using one table; short runs are Huffman coded using a second table. In this way, only 92 codewords are needed for black runs plus 92 more for white runs. Separate pairs of tables are used for black and white pixels because the probability of finding them in runs is different. Detailed descriptions of modified Huffman coding for facsimile are found in [Held91] and [Mcco92]. We will return to this subject when the standards and coding techniques for image compression are examined in Chapter 5 and the facsimile application is examined in Chapter 7.

4.5 Arithmetic Coding

Arithmetic coding, a more recent statistical entropy coding technique, overcomes key limitations of Huffman coding. First, consider encoding a frequently occurring symbol, say one whose probability is 0.95. The shortest codeword that Huffman coding can assign is 1 bit when, according to information theory and the entropy calculation, only slightly more than 0.074 bits are needed. Arithmetic coding achieves near-optimal results for this and all other symbol probabilities. The trick it uses is to merge entire sequences of symbols and encode them as a single number. Another advantage of arithmetic coding is it makes adaptive compression much simpler, as will be discussed later in this section. Also, it applies to a variety of data, not just characters or a particular kind of image but to any information that can be represented as binary digits.

An example of nonadaptive arithmetic coding is shown in Figure 4.4, where "COMPRESSOR" is the message to be coded. To begin the encoding process, we first create a model for the message by assigning probabilities to symbols in the message such that the total probability for all symbols is 1.0. In this example, the symbol probabilities are determined from the message; in practice, average values from a larger body of text would be used. The next step is to arrange the symbols and assign each a unique, nonoverlapping symbol range in the interval 0 to 1. The width of each symbol range is determined by the probability of the symbol. What has been accomplished, effectively, is to map all symbols in the message onto the fractional number line from 0 to 1 in preparation for encoding. The ordering of the symbol ranges is unimportant; however, the encoder and decoder must use the same ordering and the same symbol ranges. Now, message encoding can begin.

Encoding the message proceeds symbol by symbol. The result of encoding

Message ————————➤ Modeling

| COMPRESSOR |

Symbol	Observed Probability	Symbol Range
C	0.1	0.0 - 0.1
E	0.1	0.1 - 0.2
M	0.1	0.2 - 0.3
O	0.2	0.3 - 0.5
P	0.1	0.5 - 0.6
R	0.2	0.6 - 0.8
S	0.2	0.8 - 1.0

Coding ◄————————

New Symbol	Symbol Range	Interval Width	Message Interval after encoding symbol
			0.0 - 1.0
C	0.0 - 0.1	1.0	0.0 - 0.1
O	0.3 - 0.5	0.1	0.03 - 0.05
M	0.2 - 0.3	0.02	0.034 - 0.036
P	0.5 - 0.6	0.002	0.0350 - 0.0352
R	0.6 - 0.8	0.0002	0.03512 - 0.03516
E	0.1 - 0.2	0.00004	0.035124 - 0.035128
S	0.8 - 1.0	0.000004	0.0351272 - 0.0351280
S	0.8 - 1.0	0.0000008	0.03512784 - 0.03512800
O	0.3 - 0.5	0.00000016	0.035127888 - 0.035127920
R	0.6 - 0.8	0.000000032	0.0351279072 - 0.0351279136

Figure 4.4   Nonadaptive arithmetic coding example.

the message will be a single, high-precision number (a decimal number in this example) between 0 and 1. As encoding proceeds and more symbols are encountered, the message interval width decreases and more bits (or digits) are needed in the output number; that is, before any symbols are encoded, the possible range of numbers—the message interval—covers all values between 0 and 1. As each symbol is encoded, the message interval narrows and the encoder output is restricted to a narrower and narrow range of values. To encode each new symbol, we compute a new message interval by doing the following: First, the interval width for this symbol is set equal to the previous message interval width. Then a new message interval is computed by multiplying the interval width by, respectively, the upper and lower bounds of the symbol range and adding to each result the lower bound of the previous message interval. In this example, because the first symbol is "C," the most significant digit of the encoder output will be a number between 0 and 0.1. As encoding progresses, the message interval continues to be subdivided within this range until all symbols have been encoded.

The final output of the arithmetic encoder may be any single value within the final message interval, as any number within this interval uniquely defines the message to the decoder. Upon receiving the number, the decoder uses the same probabilities and symbol ranges to reverse the encoding process. Decoding begins with the first symbol of the message. In this example, the first digit of the encoded message is 0, allowing the decoder to decide that "C," whose symbol range is 0–0.1, is the message's first symbol. The decoder uses subtraction to remove the appropriate symbol value from the encoded number and division by the symbol range to rescale the encoded number. The decoder continues extracting symbols from the number in left-to-right order. Because a residual value may be present when all symbols of the message have been decoded, a special end-of-message symbol may be added to the encoded message, signaling the decoder to stop.

Although arithmetic coding is not terribly complex, it can be difficult to explain, and many simplifications were made to present this example.[3] One question most practitioners will have about arithmetic coding is how can long messages be encoded because the number of digits in the encoded number will grow arbitrarily large. Real computers represent numbers with a finite number of digits, creating an overflow after a few digits have been encoded. The solution is to incrementally encode the message. When the leftmost digits of the upper and lower bounds of the message interval become equal, they will not change as additional symbols are encoded. These digits may be stored or transmitting, allowing the remaining digits in the fraction to be shifted left to fill the vacated positions so that encoding can continue.

Adaptive compression—more correctly, adaptive modeling—is a strength of arithmetic coding. Adaptive compression has several advantages: First, it allows the coding process to remain optimal by tracking changes in symbol statistics. Second, unlike Huffman coding and other static techniques, there is no need to prescan the data to decide how it should be coded, which leads to the third advantage. There is no need to send the symbol statistics to the decompressor, for it will create them on the fly, just as did the compressor, by analyzing the symbols it decodes. After encoding a symbol, the compressor updates its model, which will be used to encode the next symbol. After decoding the same symbol, the decompressor makes identical adjustments to its copy of the model, allowing it and the compressor to stay in step throughout the encoding and decoding process. Adaption for arithmetic coding is a simple process—simple at least when compared to Huffman coding where the decoding tree must be updated. As our example in Figure 4.4 showed, the model for arithmetic coding is nothing more than a list of symbol probabilities from which symbol ranges are derived. All that is needed to make arithmetic coding be adaptive is to maintain counts of the symbols encountered during coding and make adjustments to the symbol ranges when the symbol probabilities change.

Adaption was made even simpler by a real breakthrough in arithmetic coding, the development of *binary* arithmetic coding [Lang81A, Lang81B]. The main

---

[3] For in-depth treatments of arithmetic coding see [Bell90, Nels92, Penn93, Witt94].

idea of binary arithmetic coding is to treat every message as a stream of binary digits—0s and 1s—and encode them bit by bit. This may not seem a wise choice, but it is. First, as learned earlier, arithmetic coding merges the probabilities of all symbols in a message and encodes them as a single number. Consequently, there is no significant loss of coding efficiency when the symbols are binary digits—a fractional number of bits can be assigned to each symbol—and a string of 0's and 1's can be encoded as efficiently as a string of characters, or whatever symbols we choose. Second, with binary arithmetic coding, the only symbols encountered are 0 and 1. Thus, the model for binary arithmetic compression is reduced to a single statistic—an estimate of the probability for whichever symbol occurs least frequently. (The probability of the other symbol is simply 1 minus that value.) A further additional simplification results by approximating the probability estimate. Early adaptive binary coders restricted the approximation to be of the form 2^{-K} (½, ¼ . . .) which, unfortunately, resulted in a loss in coding efficiency (perhaps 10% or more). More recently, this limitation has been overcome by using a probability estimate state machine to refine the approximation [Penn88, Penn93]. The big advantage of approximating the probability estimate is that arithmetic coding can be carried out exclusively with add, subtract, and shift operations, eliminating the need for multiplication and division and making encoding and decoding much faster.

Arithmetic coding has many advantages—optimum coding, applicable to any data that can be represented as strings of 0's and 1's, adaptive—but there are disadvantages, and execution speed is one of them. When compared to nonadaptive Huffman coding, where characters can be encoded by table lookup operations, character-based adaptive arithmetic coding, which requires adds and multiplies for encoding plus more operations for adaption, is slower. Also, adaptive binary arithmetic coding, which operates bit by bit—not a good choice for software— is best suited for hardware implementation [Arps88]. Hardware is available and is used by IBM and other manufacturers of high-performance computer tape drives that provide IDRC (Improved Data Recording Capability), a binary arithmetic coding algorithm originally developed by IBM [IBM1].

Today, the key adaptive compression algorithms for symbolic data use binary arithmetic coding or some variant of Lempel-Ziv dictionary coding. Lempel-Ziv coders operate on bytes or characters. Therefore, Lempel-Ziv techniques hold sway for symbolic data in situations where processing speed and ease of implementation (particularly in software) is important. Lempel-Ziv coding is explored next.

4.6　Dictionary Compression

The main idea of *dictionary* compression is to eliminate the redundancy of storing repetitive strings for words and phrases repeated within a text stream. A string-matching front end selects strings, and the information needed for compression and decompression is stored in a dictionary, a copy of which is maintained by both the compressor and decompressor. Whereas statistical coding techniques replace each symbol by a codeword, dictionary compression replaces an entire string of symbols by a single token.[4] This approach is extremely effective for compressing text where strings of characters representing words (or phrases) occur frequently. All that is needed for compression is to look up a word in the dictionary and replace it by a token specifying the word length and an index into the dictionary. (The index is an ordinal number specifying the position of the word in the dictionary.) The token, most likely, will use far fewer bits than the word itself. Not only is dictionary compression effective but usually it is fast, too, because it works with bytes and uses simple table lookup operations.

Dictionary compression for computers is not a new idea [Whit67]. Taking a cue from Braille code and its contractions, computer software, long ago, began using so-called dictionary substitution to compactly represent text: A message number replaces the message itself. A customer number replaces the customer's name and address. "January" is replaced by "01," and so on. No question, the early dictionary compression techniques were effective, but the problem was they were custom-tailored for each situation and the dictionaries were static. If the data structure or the data changed, it was time to start anew. These were not general-purpose dictionary compression techniques. In the late 1970s, the role for dictionary compression changed dramatically when Abraham Lempel and Jacob Ziv defined a pair of adaptive algorithms (techniques)—LZ77 [Ziv77] and LZ78 [Ziv78]. Their algorithms, and many derivative efforts to follow, established dictionary compression as a powerful, general-purpose technique. This section concentrates on the Lempel-Ziv algorithms

LZ77 Dictionary compression

An example of using LZ77 to compress a stream of text is shown in Figure 4.5. With LZ77, any repeated string of symbols is replaced by a token pointing

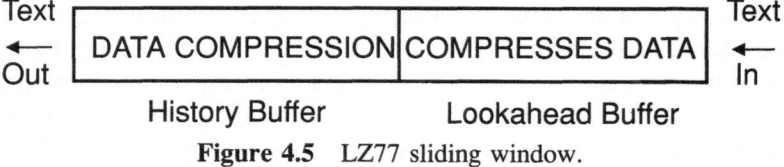

Figure 4.5   LZ77 sliding window.

to an earlier occurrence of that string. The distinguishing feature of LZ77 is the sliding window which is divided into two parts. The history buffer—the dictionary for LZ77—contains a block of recently encoded text; the lookahead buffer con-

---

[4] Some references use "code" and "codeword" to describe the output of dictionary compression; others use "token." Here, "token" will be used because the output contains multiple components.

tains symbols not yet encoded. The history buffer typically contains a few thousand symbols; the lookahead buffer is much smaller, containing perhaps 10–20 symbols. The sizes of both buffers are important parameters: If the history buffer is too small, finding string matches is less likely. If it is too large, the compression ratio is adversely affected because pointers become large when the matching string is found far back in the window and the time to search for matching strings grows large too. If the lookahead buffer is too small, longer strings will not be encoded efficiently. If it is too large, the time spent looking for long string matches, when they may not exist, will grow large.

Let us consider how the text shown in Figure 4.5 would be encoded by one of the many variants of LZ77, the QIC-122 standard for compressed ¼-inch tapes [QIC89]. (See Chapter 6 for a description of this application.) At the beginning of the encoding process, there are no previous occurrences of any strings to which to point. So each symbol in "DATA COMPRESSION" is encoded as binary 0<Raw_Byte>, where <Raw_Byte> indicates the ASCII character value. This brings us to the situation shown in Figure 4.5. The symbols "COMPRESS" and the preceding blank in the lookahead buffer form a string of length = 9 that occurred 12 symbols back in the history window. The QIC-122 algorithm encodes strings as binary 1<Offset><Length> using 7-or 11-bit offsets and 2-, 4-, 8-, 12-, or 16-bit lengths. The bit pattern in this instance is binary 1<0001100> <11110001>. The window now may slide forward nine symbols. The QIC-122 algorithm will output binary 0<Raw_Byte> for "E" and "S" and the blank preceding "DATA," which will be encoded as a string of length 4 that occurred 28 symbols back in the history buffer. The bit pattern assigned to "DATA" by QIC-122 is binary 1<0011100><10>. The original message contains 32 bytes (256 bits), whereas the encoded message contains 197 bits.

For this example, the compression ratio is an unspectacular 1.3:1. The reason it is not greater is that the history buffer was not primed with the words and phrases "DATA" and "DATA COMPRESSION" and "COMPRESSES," as it surely would have been had we encoded a few thousand symbols from this book. This illustrates an important feature of adaptive algorithms—they have a startup time. During startup there will not be much compression until the history buffer is filled. In fact, expansion occurred in the early part of this example. The results of a study that measured the effect of startup time on compression ratio are shown in Table 4.2. This data was obtained by compressing a suite of 44 test files with IBMLZ1, an LZ77-type compression algorithm [Chen95]. The files were broken into small blocks, and, beginning with an empty history buffer, each block was compressed independently. In Chapter 6, applications will be encountered where even smaller blocks of data must be compressed, and the startup time for adaptive algorithms will give us pause to consider whether they are always the right choice.

Another important characteristic of LZ77-type algorithms is the encoding time, which is dependent on how rapidly the history buffer can be searched for string matches. LZ77 is an asymmetric algorithm in that encoding can be much slower

Table 4.2   Compression ratio versus data block size for IBMLZ1. (Data courtesy of J. M. Cheng, IBM SDD, San Jose, CA.)

Block Size (Bytes)	History Buffer Size (Bytes)		
	512	1024	2048
512	2.37	2.29	2.23
1024	2.60	2.56	2.48
2048	2.74	2.77	2.72
4096	2.81	2.88	2.91
8192	2.85	2.95	3.03
No blocking	2.88	3.00	3.13

than decoding. LZ77 decompression only needs to read in a token, index into the history buffer, output the character or string it specifies, and move along to the next token; scanning or searching the history buffer is not required. To be most effective, the LZ77 compression algorithm needs a history buffer of substantial size; QIC-122 specifies 2048 bytes. But large history buffers cannot be searched in reasonable times with simple shift-and-compare techniques. Many modifications to the original LZ77 algorithm have been done in the name of efficiency—more compact encoding, to be sure—but definitely faster encoding. Therefore, most implementations augment the history buffer with data structures that make searching for matching strings more efficient—for software—binary trees, tries, and hash tables [Bell90, Nels92], and—for hardware—content-addressable memories [Wils94B, Chen95].

LZ78 Dictionary compression

LZ78 and its many variants provide an alternative for adaptive dictionary compression quite different from LZ77. LZ78-type algorithms dispense with the sliding window in favor of a separate dictionary containing previously seen phrases (i.e., symbol strings). The result is that LZ78 has two important operating differences from LZ77: First, whereas symbol strings are no longer usable when they pass out of the LZ77 history buffer, phrases can be retained in the LZ78 dictionary for as long as they are needed, independent of where they were found in the data stream. Second, with LZ78 there is no lookahead buffer and no need to constrain the length for string matches because the dictionary, which can contain long strings, can be efficiently searched.

An example of using LZW [Welc84], an LZ78 derivative, to compress a stream

Table 4.3   LZW compression example.

Input Symbol	Encoder Dictionary Update	Encoder Output	Decoder Dictionary Update	Decoder Output
D	256 = DA	D		D
A	257 = AT	A	256 = DA	A
T	258 = TA	T	257 = AT	T
A	259 = Aspace	A	258 = TA	A
space	260 = spaceC	sp	259 = Aspace	space
C	261 = CO	C	260 = spaceC	C
O	262 = OM	O	261 = CO	O
M	263 = MP	M	262 = OM	M
P	264 = PR	P	263 = MP	P
R	265 = RE	R	264 = PR	R
E	266 = ES	E	265 = RE	E
S	267 = SS	S	266 = ES	S
S	268 = SI	S	267 = SS	S
I	269 = IO	I	268 = SI	I
O	270 = ON	O	269 = IO	O
N	271 = Nspace	N	270 = ON	N
space	272 = spaceCO	260	271 = Nspace	space
C	—	—	—	C
O	273 = OMP	262	272 = spaceCO	O
M	—	—	—	M
P	274 = PRE	264	273 = OMP	P
R	—	—	—	R
E	275 = ESS	266	274 = PRE	E
S	—	—	—	S
S	276 = SE	S	275 = ESS	S
E	277 = ESspace	266	276 = SE	E
S	—	—	—	S
space	278 = spaceD	space	277 = ESspace	space
D	279 = DAT	256	278 = spaceD	D
A	—	—	—	A
T	280 = TAspace	258	279 = DAT	T
A	—	—	—	A
space		space	280 = TAspace	space

of text is shown in Table 4.3. With LZW, all symbols are replaced by tokens pointing to entries in the dictionary. The first 256 dictionary entries (not shown in Table 4.3) are preloaded with the regular symbols in the 8-bit ASCII code. The remaining dictionary entries are used to extend the alphabet with the strings of symbols encountered in the message being compressed. The compression algorithm begins with a null string. The first symbol ("D") is read in and appended to the string. If the string matches one in the dictionary, which it does here, the algorithm reads the next symbol and appends it to the string. This process continues until it finds a string that does not match one in the dictionary. In this instance, when the next character ("A") is appended, the string "DA" is not found in the dictionary. This triggers the following actions: The token for the last matching string is outputted (in this instance, the ASCII value for "D"). A new dictionary entry is created for the unmatched string and assigned to the next available token (256). The compression process restarts by building a new string beginning with the symbol that caused string matching to fail. Reading, outputting symbols, and updating the dictionary continues until all input has been read.

Decompression, like compression, begins with a dictionary preloaded only with tokens for the 256 regular symbols in the 8-bit ASCII code and builds its dictionary using nothing more than the symbols found in the compressed data stream. The decompressor begins by reading the first token from the compressed input. It outputs the symbol for this token (a "D") and retains the token, waiting for the next token from the compressed input. For each token read after the first, the decompressor does the following: It outputs the symbol(s) that the token specifies. It generates a string by appending the first symbol of the most recent input to the end of the retained token. If that string is not in the dictionary, a new token is selected, and the string is added to the dictionary. The most recent input is made the retained token, and processing continues.

Notice that updating the decompressor dictionary lags one step behind, always waiting for the first symbol in the new token. This creates a special-case situation where strings of the form "XandXandX" ("X" is any symbol; "and" is any string of symbols) cause the compressor to output a token before the decompressor has it in its dictionary. In this case, if the compressor has a token for "Xand" in its dictionary, it will send that token and add a new token for "XandX" to its dictionary. It will then move on to encode "XandX" using the token it just created. When the decompressor receives this token, it has a decoding problem because it has no dictionary entry for "XandX" and will not until the first character specified by *this* token can be appended to "Xand." Fortunately, the special case is easily recognized and there is a simple solution (create a new dictionary entry by appending the first symbol of "Xand" to itself and continue processing).

Table 4.3 is not exactly a sterling example for showing the efficiency of LZ78-type compression algorithms. In this example, 33 (8-bit) input symbols are compressed to 26 output tokens, but expansion will occur if each token requires more than 10 bits, as happens when the dictionary contains more than 1024 entries. However, Table 4.3 does highlight one characteristic of these algorithms—their startup time is long, adapting slowly when beginning with an empty dictionary. Near the end of the example, 3-symbol tokens are being added to the dictionary and the algorithm will use them the next time words such as "data" and "compression" are encountered. Unfortunately, many encounters are needed to load the dictionary with strings that can encode long words in a single token.

The most difficult part of implementing LZ78-type algorithms is designing and managing the dictionary. There are three important issues: The first is how to store a variable number of variable-length symbol strings. The most commonly used solution is to use a trie, a multiway digital search tree, where variable-length strings are stored as fixed-length tokens made up of a prefix token and a suffix token identifying a single symbol [Welc84]. For example, in Table 4.3

the token for the symbol string "ESS" would be stored as 266S, where token 266 represents the symbol string "ES" and S is the token identifying the symbol "S." In this way, long strings can be realized by tracing a path through the trie. The second issue is how large the dictionary should be. Larger dictionaries can contain more tokens, which will improve compression, but they require more bits to address each token, which will decrease compression. The simple solution is to use a fixed number of bits to address each token (the original LZW algorithm specified 12 bits for 4096 entries), but more complex schemes increase the number of bits as more tokens are added to the dictionary [Welc84, Bell90]. The third and most critical issue is what to do when the dictionary is full. One solution is to stop adaption when the dictionary fills. The dictionary then becomes static and new data will be compressed efficiently—if it has the same characteristics as the data used to fill the dictionary. Another solution is to dump the dictionary when it becomes full and begin building it anew, accepting the startup problems discussed in this section. Yet another solution is to replace tokens in the dictionary based on LRU (least recently used) or other usage criteria. However, this strategy has complications too, as there must be some means for identifying the tokens that are LRU candidates, which entails somehow adding token usage information to the basic LZ78-type algorithms. When replacing tokens in directory structures, such as the trie described above, special care must be exercised to assure they are not on the path of other tokens [Apik91].

LZ77 Versus LZ78

Obviously, LZ77 and LZ78 are two distinctly different dictionary compression algorithms with some similarities and many differences, including the following:

- Both use string-matching front ends but use different internal data structures for the dictionary.
- Both are adaptive, but only LZ78 also allows static or semiadaptive operation, an important choice especially when only small amounts of data are available for adaption.
- LZ77 starts up with fewer symbols and adapts more quickly than LZ78. In practice, neither characteristic is particularly important when large bodies of data are encoded.
- LZ78, in theory, yields more compression when the input contains very long strings. In practice, there is very little difference.
- LZ78 is a more symmetric algorithm; its compression and decompression speeds are more nearly equal. When compared to LZ77, compression can be faster because buffer searches are not required; decompression is slower because the LZ78 dictionary must be updated.

4.7   State-of-the-Art Symbolic Data Compression and Beyond

This chapter has described the principles of lossless data compression and introduced several approaches for compressing symbolic data. When faced with a real-world application, practitioners must ask two "simple" questions: How much will *my* data compress and, given so many choices, which algorithm is "best" for *my* application? The questions may be simple, but the answers are not. Selecting an algorithm for most symbolic data compression applications is a major decision, and it is one that practitioners must make. Unlike diffuse data compression applications, where usually there is a standard that must be followed, few standards exist for symbolic data compression applications. Why this is true will become clearer beginning in Chapter 6 when applications are explored.

Selecting an algorithm can be a complex task. Most algorithms have many interacting parameters, and, after all, data compression is a statistical process. So, short of applying a specific algorithm to the data in question, there is no way to say exactly what the results will be. However, general information is available, as many types of lossless algorithms have been tested on symbolic data gathered from a variety of sources. References include [Bell 89, Bell90, Will91, Fran92, Venb92, Greh93, Witt94] and many others.[5] This section will provide some guidelines for how much compression and performance to expect from each of the various data compression approaches described in this chapter. The reader is forewarned that these are general trends compiled from many sources. To obtain specific results, consult the references or, better yet, try your favorite algorithm on your own data.

First, given a particular type of symbolic data, how much compression should one expect—from *any* algorithm? Figure 4.6(a) shows the answer is "it depends." Different types of symbolic data compress by different amounts. Factors include the data structure and how or if repetition occurs. For instance, executable programs are composed of highly encoded computer instructions where pattern repetition is not obvious—a situation with little redundancy and not highly conducive to compression. In contrast, some (but not all) database files contain sequences of fixed-length records where short fields are padded with strings of identical characters and record-to-record collating sequences are observed—a situation ripe with redundancy and ready-made for compression. Another factor that defines how much compression one should expect is the compression algorithm itself. Some algorithms are better than others, perhaps consistently, perhaps not. For example, run-length coding, the least powerful of all the approaches, is hard to beat if runs are abundant but comes in dead last if they are not. Other algorithms work more consistently.

So, how do the algorithms stack up? Figure 4.6(b) provides general guidelines for comparing the algorithms described in Sections 4.3–4.6. The (author's) rankings are based on the power of the algorithms to remove redundancy and how

---

[5] Note that most studies found in the literature only measure the compression ratio and, sometimes, the compression speed—but only on large data files. Other characteristics of interest such as performance versus memory consumed by the algorithm and adaption speed are less well covered, except in [Bell90].

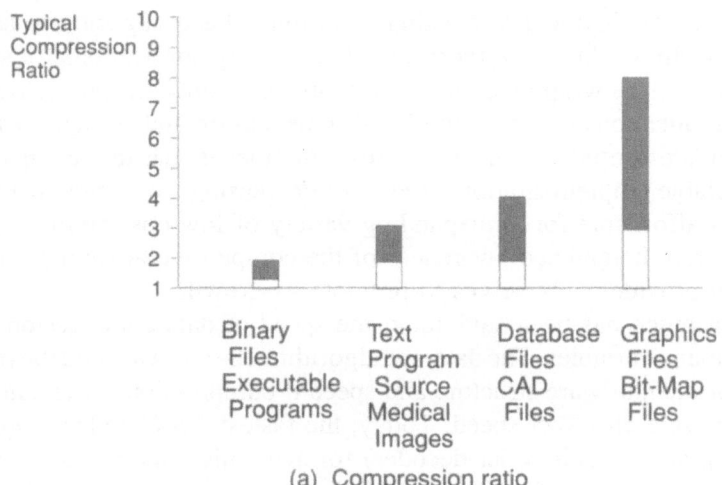

(a) Compression ratio

	Run-Length Coding	Huffman Coding	Arithmetic Coding	LZ77 / LZ78 Dictionary Compression
Compression Ratio	1	3	5	4
Encoding Speed	5	2	1	4
Decoding Speed	5	3	1	4

Low=1 High=5   (b) Algorithm performance

Figure 4.6   Symbolic data compression summary.

efficiently they process symbols or bits. Run-length coding removes only one kind of redundancy, but it is simple and fast. Huffman coding is more powerful, but encoding requires two passes, and although encoding works symbol by symbol, decoding works bit by bit. Arithmetic coding is the most powerful of all, but also the slowest because its most effective implementations work bit by bit. The Lempel-Ziv dictionary algorithms are nearly as powerful and work on entire strings of symbols.

Studies of live data have repeatedly shown there is no easy answer for which algorithm is best—because no one algorithm is superior in every respect. There are trade-offs to be made—not just in compression ratio and speed of compression or decompression—but also whether software or hardware is needed for efficient execution, and many other factors. As previously noted, an additional complicating factor is that a particular algorithm may provide outstanding compression on one data type but not do well on others.

Looking to the future, advances in symbolic data compression can be expected, including wider deployment of existing algorithms, faster algorithms, and more effective algorithms. Although there already are many applications for symbolic data compression, new applications will continue to appear. One reason is the number of applications that rely on digital transmission and storage, where data compression is essential, continues to grow. Another is that less complex, more readily available implementations and ever-decreasing costs are making data compression affordable for an expanding variety of low-cost products and services. Then, too, heightened awareness of the competitive advantages that data compression provides only serves to promote its growth.

So far not much has been said about the speed of data compression because there are so many variables. The data, the algorithm, the software and the processor it runs on, or the hardware structure and speed if compression is done in special-purpose hardware all affect speed. Today, the fastest ASIC codec (application-specific integrated circuit coder-decoder) for symbolic data executes an LZ77-type algorithm, one of the fastest, at 40 MBS (megabytes per second) [Wils94B]; various other algorithms and software implementations are slower. Now, sheerly through improvements in VLSI, the compression speed for existing algorithms will go up by perhaps tenfold, or more, in the next decade, which is good news for both software and special-purpose hardware data compression implementations. But, wait, there is more, especially for special-purpose hardware: Increases in circuit density mean existing algorithm implementations can be improved through, for example, larger dictionaries, or better methods for storing them that make searching faster, or whatever additional circuits can do to make the algorithm more effective and faster. More extensive use of lookaside buffers, content-addressable memories, parallel execution, or any of the speedup tricks digital circuit designers have at their disposal are possible. Thus, the compression speed of existing algorithms can be increased by perhaps 10 times, even 100 times, or more—if the marketplace demand for greater speed warrants the development cost. When it comes to symbolic data compression, there is ample opportunity to go faster.

Can more effective compression algorithms be found (i.e., algorithms that use fewer bits per symbol to encode data)? As Figure 4.6 shows, on text data the best algorithms achieve compression ratios of 2:1 or 3:1 and higher or lower values on other data types. There are special situations where higher compression ratios may be obtained, such as when text data is padded with trailing blanks to fit in fixed-size record formats. But for general text data a 4:1 compression ratio is rarely achieved. What is the limit? According to one study, it is estimated that with little training ordinary people can achieve 1.3 bits per symbol (6:1 compression ratio) when predicting English text [Cove78]. If true, how can computer systems achieve similar results? Improved implementations of existing algorithms may help, but more powerful models with capabilities beyond those for current algorithms are a safer bet. Context-based or knowledge-based models specialized for natural language compression and other techniques that are being researched may provide the answers [Bell89].

4.8 Summary

In this chapter, the general operating characteristics of data compression algorithms were introduced and some important lossless algorithms for compressing symbolic data were studied. We learned the following:

- Data compression algorithms transform a stream of symbols into a stream of codewords in a finite number of steps.
- Symbolic data compression algorithms use only lossless compression, whereas algorithms for diffuse data compression use combinations of lossless and lossy compression.
- Important building blocks for all data compression algorithms include the model for describing the structure of the data, the coder for producing a compressed bit stream, and the adaptor for adjusting the model and coder to match the data. Some algorithms do not make adjustments during operation; they are called static algorithms, as opposed to adaptive algorithms that do change.
- Symbolic data compression algorithms process input data symbols and provide variable-to-fixed-length encoding, fixed-to-variable-length encoding, or, by combining both, variable-to-variable-length encoding.
- Run-length coding is a variable-to-fixed-length, static encoding technique where sequences of consecutive identical symbols are replaced with three elements: a single symbol, a run-length count, and an indicator that signifies how the symbol and count are to be interpreted. It applies to both sequences of bytes, such as characters in text, and to sequences of bits, such as black-and-white pixels in an image.
- Huffman coding, a fixed-to-variable-length encoding technique, is called a statistical coder because the number of bits assigned to each symbol is determined by the frequency of occurrence of the symbol. It may be either static or adaptive, but most implementations of Huffman coding are static; adaptive Huffman coding can be complex to implement, and other adaptive algorithms generally outperform it.
- Arithmetic coding, like Huffman coding, is a fixed-to-variable-length statistical encoding technique, but individual symbols are encoded as a part of a fractional number according to their frequency of occurrence. Arithmetic coding provides improved coding efficiency by allowing infrequently occurring symbols to be represented as less than 1 bit, and the symbols need not be characters. In fact, binary arithmetic coding, which operates on bits, is one of the more popular, best performing, more implementable versions. Arithmetic coding can be either static or adaptive, but adaption, which is not difficult to implement, makes it more effective.
- Lempel-Ziv algorithms are examples of variable-to-fixed-length dictionary encoding techniques, where entire strings of symbols are replaced by a single token that identifies a dictionary entry containing the symbol string. The encoder and decoder maintain identical copies of the dictionary, which may be static, semistatic, or adaptively updated.
- How much a collection of symbolic data will compress depends on the data itself and the compression algorithm chosen. Generally, compression ratios for symbolic data range from less than 2 : 1 to as much as 8 : 1.

- Selecting an algorithm for compressing symbolic data involves many factors including compression ratio, speed of encoding and decoding, and implementation-related issues.
- There are few de facto or official standards for symbolic data compression, unlike diffuse data compression, where there are many.
- In the future, expect wider deployment of existing algorithms and faster, more effective implementations of these algorithms for symbolic data compression.

5

Compression Algorithms
for Diffuse Data

In this chapter, the introduction to data compression algorithms continues with discussions of those algorithms selected as the official standards (or, in some cases, de facto standards) for compressing diffuse data—speech, audio, image, and video. Marketplace forces tremendously influence which compression algorithms become standards, and this is most evident for diffuse data compression standards. The algorithms described in this chapter were selected as standards—first, because they can provide good quality compressed speech, audio, image, and video at reasonable data rates. Second, they can be economically implemented in VLSI hardware (or software, sometimes). Third, they can deliver data in real time— a requirement for speech, audio, and video applications. However, diffuse data compression—particularly video compression—is still new, with a plethora of compression techniques to pick from and still more—and likely better ones— waiting to be discovered. This, coupled with the continuing discovery of new applications for diffuse data compression, means the process of creating standards is hardly finished. In fact, it may have just begun. Throughout the chapter, we will be describing the evolution leading up to today's standards, pointing out those standards in decline and areas where new standards are likely to emerge. As with our discussion of symbolic data compression algorithms, the simplest, most general algorithms for each data type are described first, followed by more powerful or more specialized algorithms.

5.1 Diffuse Data Compression

Diffuse data is compressed by applying lossy compression, which throws away nonessential information, in combination with lossless compression for efficient coding. Many advances in compressing diffuse data have been made by exploiting the limitations of human auditory and visual systems. Humans, who usually are the end receivers of diffuse data, do not need—or cannot use—all the information captured during digitization. Powerful and complex models for speech, audio, image, and video data have been created using what is described as *perceptual coding* techniques that exploit the limitations of human ears and eyes. These are also called psychoacoustic and psychovisual coding techniques because they are based on the principles of human hearing and vision. A perceptual coding model followed by an entropy coder, which uses one or more techniques of the type examined in Chapter 4, produces effective compression. However, a unique model (and entropy coder) is needed for each type of diffuse data because the requirements are so different. The state of the art in compressing and decompressing diffuse data using lossy perceptual coding and lossless entropy coding is described in forthcoming sections of this chapter. Examples are drawn from products and the official standards for speech, audio, image, and video data.

5.2 Speech Coding

The objective of speech coding[1] is to represent speech using as few bits as possible while preserving its perceptual quality. Speech coding began over five decades ago with research and development of coders for analog telephone transmissions, and it has continued to grow and expand with digital telephony. Beyond the realm of telephony, speech coding is used by other communications and storage applications that demand high-quality speech reproduction. There has been continual upgrading of speech quality for telephone systems and other voice communications channels and for storing voice messages. As Table 5.1 shows, wideband speech, a class of service beyond telephone-quality speech but stopping short of wideband audio, has emerged for applications that require higher quality.

There are two classes of speech coders. *Waveform coders* attempt to preserve the input signal waveform in the sense that the decoded speech signal they produce is a close approximation of the original speech signal. In contrast, *vocoders* (voice coders, which are also called parametric or source coders) attempt to produce a decoded signal that sounds like the input speech signal. Vocoders incorporate vocal-tract models specially tuned for speech signals, unlike waveform coders that rely solely on exploiting the perceptual limitations of the human ear for compression. As a result, vocoders achieve greater compression—but only on speech. Waveform coders may need up to 32 Kbps for telephone-quality

---

[1] The term *speech coding* is used rather than speech compression, which in speech research and development is sometimes reserved for time-scale modification of the speech signal. For example, as a learning aid, speech may be speeded up during playback.

Table 5.1   Speech and audio signals.

Audio Channel	Frequency Range (Hz)	Sampling Rate (KHz)	Bits per Sample	PCM[1] Bit Rate (Kbps)	Encoded Bit Rate (Kbps)
Telephone speech	200 - 3,200	8	8	64	4 - 32
Wideband speech	50 - 7,000	16	8 (or more)	128 (or more)	32 - 64
Wideband audio	10 - 20,000	32 / 44.1 / 48	16	512 -768	64 -192

Notes:
[1] See Figure 1.1 for an example of PCM (pulse code modulation).

speech, and still more for wideband speech, whereas vocoders can produce perceptually intelligible speech at bit rates reaching down to 2 Kbps. There also are modern hybrid speech coders that—by combining elements of both waveform coders and vocoders—exploit models of speech production and auditory perception. They offer telephone-quality speech at 4–16 Kbps and wideband speech at less than 64 Kbps.

Throughout its long, rich history, speech coding has made significant contributions, not only to speech but also to audio coding. For instance, subband and transform coding (to be described in Section 5.3) were first used for speech coding. However, the main thrust of speech coding research and development has been focused on techniques suitable for just one application—telephone systems. One consequence is that many speech coders operate at a constant bit rate, sampling at regular, fixed intervals like the speech digitization example shown in Figure 1.1. They take no advantage of the pauses and silent intervals that occur in conversational speech, nor do they attempt to code different speech segments at different rates while maintaining a given reproduction quality. Variable bit-rate coders may be more efficient, but, until recently, there was no demand for them because most analog telephone and telecommunications channels operated at fixed rates. With the availability of digital, packet-oriented broadband communications services, like ATM (asynchronous transfer mode), this has changed, and variable-rate speech coders are beginning to appear. Another constraint imposed on the design of most speech encoders (and decoders) is that they must operate in real-time, two-way communications systems. In this environment, encoding and decoding times must be nearly equal, and neither can introduce much delay because delaying the signal disrupts voice communications. A third constraint is that speech encoders and decoders must operate when nonspeech signals are present on the communications channel, whether those signals are channel control signals or just channel noise.

The point to be made is that other applications for speech coding such as broadcasting and voice messaging do not have these constraints. For some of these applications, more complex algorithms that use more processing power may provide higher-quality speech at lower bit rates (while incurring longer delays). For others, simpler algorithms having different design parameters and requiring less processing power may be more appropriate.

Another influence on speech coding has been the technology available for its implementation. Vocoders, which first appeared in 1939, were constrained by the limitations of analog (telephone) signals and analog signal processing. Later, when the telephone network went digital, new signal processing opportunities developed but speech coding was still constrained by the speed (and cost) of digital circuitry. Only applications such as military communications could afford to use the low-bit-rate speech coders that researchers knew how to build. Today, with advances in VLSI technology, along with advances in the theory of digital signal processing, the selection of affordable speech coding algorithms is wider than ever.

Although a tremendous variety of speech coders have been developed and standards created for them, some have quietly passed into history, having been replaced by improved techniques. Some currently popular, widely used, standardized techniques for telephone-quality and wideband speech are examined in this section. For a more thorough treatment of speech coding techniques, the reader is directed to surveys by [Gers94, Span94, Noll95] and many references cited by those surveys.

ADPCM coders

Adaptive differential pulse code modulation (ADPCM) was formalized as a standard in 1984 by the ITU-T G.721 recommendation (a standard since replaced by the ITU-T G.726 recommendation). ADPCM operates by encoding and transmitting the difference between the original speech signal and its predicted value. As shown in Figure 5.1, the encoding process begins by breaking digitized, time-continuous speech into a series of discrete frames, each containing the PCM (pulse code modulation) samples for a few milliseconds of speech, and processing each frame. Then, the difference between a frame of the (8-bit, 64 Kbps) PCM input speech signal and a prediction of that signal is fed to a quantizer. By exploiting the correlation between adjacent samples, the quantizer constructs a 16-level (4 bit, 32 Kbps) representation of the difference signal. This coded difference or prediction error signal is sent to the decoder. Meanwhile, within the encoder, the same coded difference signal is used by the inverse (quantizer) function to reconstruct the original difference signal. The inverse function supplies the reconstructed difference signal to the predictor, which attempts to predict the original speech signal. Both the quantizer and the inverse function are adaptive in that the quantization levels are not fixed, as in standard PCM, but change with the signal. The predictor is adaptive too. It operates in two modes as determined by the characteristics of the difference signal: In the fast mode, the original signal

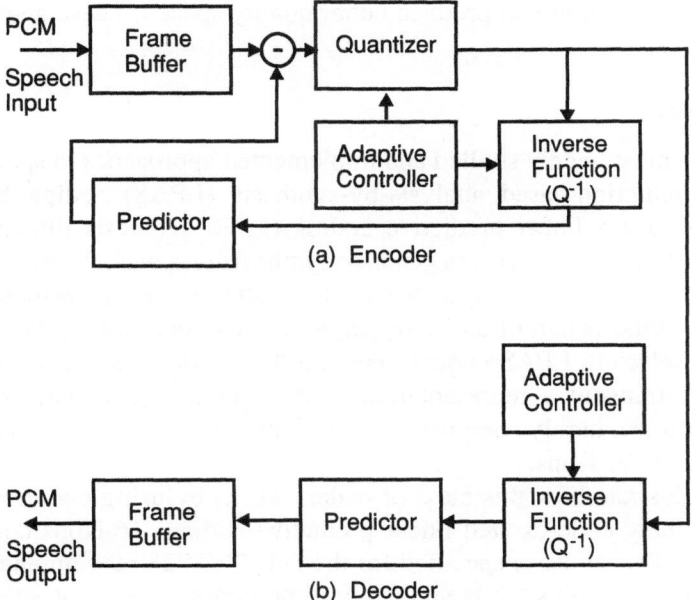

Figure 5.1　ADPCM coder.

is assumed to be speech, whereas in the slow mode, it assumed to be nonspeech, network signaling or voiceband data. Two different modes are required because speech and modem-generated signals have different statistical characteristics.

The decoder receives only the difference signal and uses it to reconstruct an approximation of the original speech signal. The decoder has a copy of the inverse function and the predictor, both of which operate and adapt identically to the corresponding encoder functions. Therefore, if the predicted signal really is a good estimate of the original speech signal, the encoder output will be too.

It is important to note that, like most speech encoders designed for communications applications, the ADPCM encoder operates in a "backward adaptive" mode. Backward adaptive means that the encoder uses only previously seen samples of the difference signal to generate its output. It does not buffer large blocks of the input speech signal (nor does the decoder). Thus, the encoder avoids delaying the signal while looking forward for information to adapt its output. This provides the low delay needed for real-time, two-way voice communications.

Beyond the ITU-T G.721 recommendation, which operated at 32 Kbps, the basic ADPCM algorithm has been extended to operate at higher and lower rates in systems with variable bit rates. The ITU-T G.726 and ITU-T G.727 recommendations operate at 16, 24, 32, and 40 Kbps.[2] However, at 16 Kbps (or

---

[2] ITU-T G.726 replaces ITU-T G.721 and another recommendation pertaining to ADPCM, ITU-T G.723 [Sayo95]. Later, ITU-T reused the G.723 designation for a new recommendation discussed later.

lower), other algorithms can produce better quality speech. These algorithms are considered next.

LPAS coders

Today, the most widely studied and implemented approaches to speech coding use linear prediction-based analysis-by-synthesis (LPAS) coding techniques. LPAS coders use a linear predictive coding (LPC) synthesis filter (the linear predictive part of the acronym) to generate synthesized speech from stored excitation signals. Analyzing the speech signal by attempting to synthesize it (the analysis-by-synthesis part of the acronym) allows the most appropriate excitation signal to be selected. LPAS coders, like ADPCM coders, are waveform coders because they transmit a representation of the speech signal waveform to the decoder. But it is a highly compressed representation, and these coders can work effectively at 4–16 Kbps.

We will illustrate how this class of coders works by using one type, the LD-CELP (low-delay code-excited linear predictive coding) 16-Kbps coder shown in Figure 5.2. This coder is specified for the ITU-T G.728 recommendation. The encoding process begins by breaking the time-continuous input speech signal into a series of frames, each containing the PCM samples for a few milliseconds

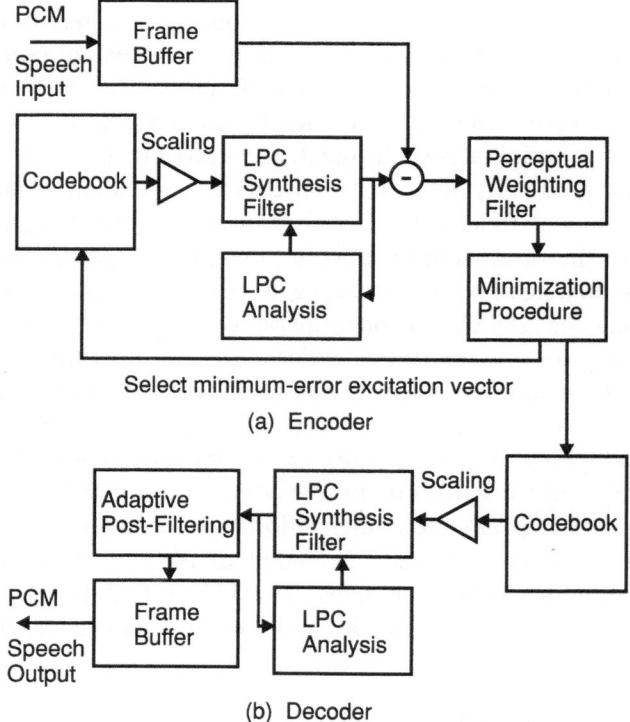

Figure 5.2   Low-delay CELP coder.

of speech, and processing each frame. Here, we see the difference between a frame of the (8-bit, 64 Kbps) PCM input signal and a synthesized speech signal is fed to a perceptually weighting filter that computes a "score" for the frequency-weighted difference of the two signals. The result is provided to the minimization procedure whose job is to cycle through all the excitation signals stored in the codebook and find the one that will generate a synthesized speech signal that achieves the best score—the one most closely matching the input speech signal. When the match is found, the codebook address for that excitation signal is transmitted to the decoder. Because the codebook address is much smaller than the segment of speech it represents, compression results.

An identical codebook is maintained at the decoder. From it, a copy of the same excitation signal is selected and is used to regenerate the synthesized speech representation most closely matching the input signal. After the synthesized speech signal is filtering to reduce the perceptual effects of quantization noise (at the expense of signal distortion), it becomes the output speech signal.

Let us look more closely at the heart of LPAS coders—the excitation signals and the codebook that contains them. Excitation signals are vectors of numbers representing common phonetic sounds. These signals are generated according to voice-production models that imitate the human vocal tract. Excitation refers to how the human vocal tract is stimulated to generate sounds. There are numerous models for excitation signals. The one for LD-CELP uses a complete sequence of impulses to represent each excitation. The representation is stored as a code in a codebook (the CE part of the LD-CELP acronym). Incidentally, LD means low delay because backward adaption, a small frame buffer, and short (five-sample) excitation signals are used.

Creating and managing the codebook is a major challenge for LPAS coders. A typical CELP codebook may contain 1024 excitation vectors, each of which may be up to 40 samples in length. Because each sample is 8 bits in size, 40 KB of storage is required for the codebook. Advances in VLSI capacity no longer make storage capacity the important factor it was when CELP algorithms were first proposed, but searching the storage—efficiently—was and still is an issue. Indeed, many variations and improvements on CELP algorithms have been directed to finding ways to locate the one excitation vector which best matches the input speech signal while avoiding the time and computation overhead incurred by a complete search of the codebook. Another issue, beyond the scope of this discussion, relates to finding the best excitation signals to place in the codebook: If the codebook is not adaptive, then the initial excitation signals are critical. If the codebook is adaptive (which the LP-CELP codebook is not) and the excitation signals are frequently changed to track changes in the input speech signal, the overhead for codebook adaption may be great.

Vocoders

The basic idea of vocoders is that the encoder can analyze speech in terms of a model and the model parameters can be extracted and transmitted to the decoder. The available bit rate for some communications channels, particularly for military and cellular telephone applications, is lower than for regular telephone lines; yet, intelligible speech communications are required. As bit rates fall below 4 Kbps, the speech produced by the best available waveform coders exhibits noticeable noise and distortion causing both speech quality and intelligibility to markedly degrade. The reason this happens is that not enough bits are available to transmit even a highly compact representation of the original waveform. For very low bit-rate speech coding, vocoders are solutions because they do not try to reproduce a waveform similar to the original. Instead, vocoders rely on reproducing a signal that sounds perceptually similar to the original, using only parameters obtained from models of human speech. Consequently, they obtain lower bit rates; but, as noted earlier, they work only on speech signals.

Vocoders were the earliest type of speech coders but fell into disuse because the speech they produced was unnatural, machinelike, and not particularly intelligible. However, interest in vocoders has revived. Speech quality has improved thanks to advances in speech models and technology that allows more complex, more powerful algorithms to be implemented. Indeed, many of the adaptive techniques used in LPAS coders are also used in vocoders (or perhaps LPAS coders borrowed them from vocoders; the distinction between the two is not always clear).

While the search for still better vocoder algorithms continues, one known as LPC-10 has been standardized as (U.S.) Federal Standard FS-1015 for speech coding at 2.4 Kbps. The LPC-10 algorithm uses a 10th-order linear predictor to estimate the vocal tract parameters which are sent to the decoder without sending bits that describe the excitation waveform. The decoder uses a linear prediction filter to synthesize speech from an excitation signal that it generates using only the passed parameters. Further details can be found in [Gers94, Span94].

Another vocoder based on a multipulse maximum likelihood quantization (MP-MLQ) linear predictive coding (LPC) technique has recently been standardized by ITU-T as part of their G.723 recommendation.[3] The G.723 recommendation, which specifies operation at 6.3, 5.3, and 4.8 Kbps, is intended for use in visual telephony over the public telephone network [Dspg95]. This technology was first offered by the DSP Group, Inc. in their Truespeech™ family of speech compression algorithms and software. Truespeech has become a widely used de facto standard for digital speech in personal computer and computer telephony applications.

Wideband speech coding

Wideband speech is an important part of computer-generated speech, videoconferencing, and other new applications that use ISDN (Integrated Services Digital Network) telecommunications. We shall consider two of the many approaches

---

[3] This is a new ITU-T G.723 recommendation. An earlier ITU-T G.723 recommendation pertaining to ADPCM coding was replaced by ITU-T G.726 [Sayo95].

for wideband speech coding. One is provided by the MPEG-2 audio standard which will be examined in Section 5.3: It uses subband and adaptive transform hybrid coding techniques developed for MPEG-1 audio coding. MPEG-2 extended the MPEG-1 audio standard to include lower sampling rates at 16, 22.05, and 24 KHz. This allows wideband speech signals with bandwidths of 7.5, 10.3, and 11.25 KHz, respectively, to be coded at bit rates of 32 Kbps or higher.

Another approach is provided by the ITU-T G.722 recommendation for wideband speech coding. This standard uses a sampling rate of 16 KHz and 14-bit PCM samples, allowing wideband speech signals with a 7 KHz bandwidth to be coded at bit rates of 48, 56, and 64 Kbps. This coder is a hybrid too; it uses two subband filters followed by ADPCM coders. Both subbands are subsampled to 8 KHz. The low (frequency) subband signal is roughly equivalent to telephone-quality speech; it is coded with a 6-bits-per-sample quantizer. The high subband contains less information and is coded with a 2-bit per sample quantizer. The 48- and 56-Kbps bit rates are achieved by reducing the low subband quantizer resolution to 4 and 5 bits per sample, respectively, with a reduction of speech quality.

State-of-the-art speech coding and beyond

Among the speech coders examined in this section, those intended for communications over telephone lines achieve compression ratios in the 2:1 to 4:1 range. For applications such as military communications, cellular telephones, and personal communications systems, where channel bandwidth is more restricted or more expensive, higher compression ratios (and lower bit rates) are required. These applications also demand improved coding techniques because their communications channels have higher error rates, and more background audio noise is present in mobile environments. In computer-based speech applications, the requirements for speech coding are different too. There, reducing the amount of storage consumed by speech files (really low-bit-rate coding in disguise) and ease of coding are equally important as speech intelligibility itself. Then, too, speech and audio (music) are mixed for many applications where lower bit-rate coding would be welcome.

Progress in speech coding continues in all these areas. One can expect that lower bit rates will be achieved for higher-quality speech by using ever-more-complex algorithms based on improved models of speech production and better understanding of the human auditory system. Continued advances in faster and more highly integrated VLSI signal processing devices will make real-time implementation of more powerful speech coding algorithms possible. Meanwhile, many standards have been set for speech coding. Some of today's most important speech coding standards are listed in Table 5.2. More information about the speech coding algorithms they use can be found in the references cited in Table 5.2.

Table 5.2(a)   Telephone-quality speech coding standards.

Organization Standard[1]	Algorithm[2]	Encoded Bit Rate (Kbps)[3]	Application
ITU-T G.711	PCM	64	General telephony [Port94, Trow94]
ITU-T G.726	ADPCM	16 / 24 / 32 / 40	General telephony and digital circuit multiplication equipment, an extension of G.721 [Gers94, Span94, Noll95]
ITU-T G.727	Embedded-ADPCM	16 / 24 / 32 / 40	Speech transmission over packet-oriented networks [Noll95]
ITU-T G.728	LPAS (LD-CELP)	16	General telephony [Gers94, Port94, Span94, Trow94, Noll95]
ITU-T G.729	LPAS (CELP)	13	Cellular telephony [Noll95]
GSM	LPAS (RPE-LTP)	13	European cellular telephony [Gers94, Span94, Noll95]
JDC TDMA	LPAS (PSI-CELP)	11.2	Japanese cellular telephony [Gers94, Span94, Noll95]
BTI Skyphone Service	LPAS (MPLP)	9.6	Aeronautical telephone service [Span94]
TIA IS54	LPAS (VSELP)	7.95	TDMA cellular telephony [Gers94, Span94, Noll95]
TIA IS95	LPAS (QSELP)	< 8 (variable)	CDMA cellular telephony [Gers94]
ITU-T G.723	MP-MLQ LPC (Vocoder)	4.8 / 5.3 / 6.3	Visual telephony and computer-generated speech, based on an industry wide de facto standard —Truespeech™ [Dspg95]
FS 1016	LPAS (CELP)	4.8	Secure voice transmission [Gers94, Span94, Noll95]
ITU-T SG 15/2 (Future proposal)	na	4	Videotelephone [Port94]
FS 1015	LPC (Vocoder)	2.4	Secure voice communications [Gers94, Span94]

Table 5.2(b)   Wideband speech coding standards.

Organization Standard[1]	Algorithm[2]	Encoded Bit Rate (Kbps)[3]	Application
ITU-T G.722	Subband-ADPCM	48 / 56 / 64	Videoconferencing [Gers94, Noll95, Port94, Trow94]
MPEG-2	Subband-adaptive transform	32 / 48 / 64 or higher	General voice communications [Noll95]

Notes:
[1] Standards groups:

BTI	British Telecom International
FS	U.S. Government Federal Standards
GSM	Groupe Spéciale Mobile
ITU-T	International Telecommunication Union - Transmission
JDC	Japanese Digital Cellular
MPEG	Motion Picture Experts Group
TIA	(North American) Telephone Industry Association

[2] Algorithms:
    Acronym names are provided in the Acronyms and Abbreviations section of this book.
    Descriptions are found in the preceding text and the references listed in this table.
[3] Input bit rate is 64 Kbps (8 bits per sample x 8 KHz sampling rate) except:

G.723	128 Kbps (16 bits per sample x 8 KHz sampling rate)
G.722	224 Kbps (14 bits per sample x 16 KHz sampling rate)
MPEG-2	256 / 353 / 384 Kbps (16 bits per sample x 16 / 22.05 / 24 KHz sampling rate)

5.3 Audio Coding

There is an ever-growing demand for high-quality audio—sometimes called wideband audio—for communications, consumer-electronics products, and entertainment applications. The marketplace trends for audio continue unabated— provide more fidelity and more channels, often together with video, over communications channels where bandwidth is limited, using ever-smaller storage devices where capacity is limited. All these factors provide the motivation for efficient audio coding.[4]

Audio perceptual coding takes advantage of the inability of humans to hear every sound that impinges upon their ears. Two psychoacoustic principles are

---

[4] The terms *audio coding*, rather than data compression, and *audio coder*, rather than data compression algorithm, are used, following the conventions of literature in this field.

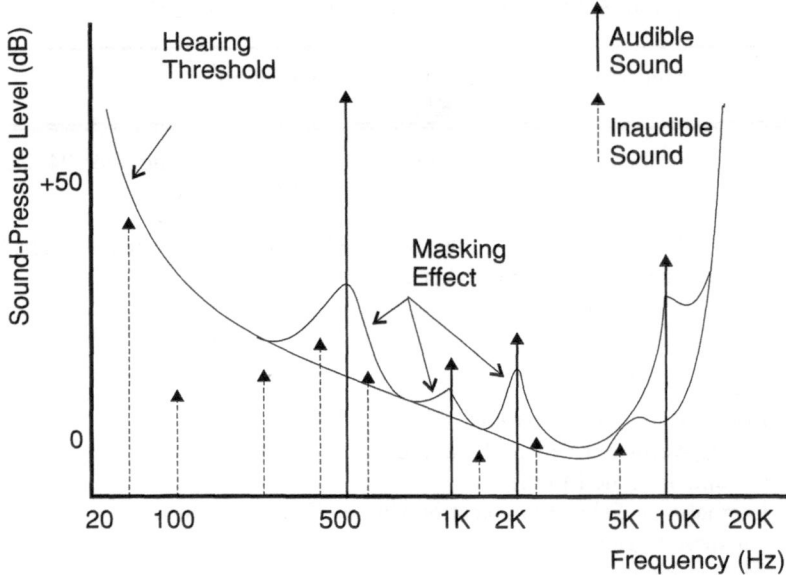

Figure 5.3   Audio thresholding and masking.

involved: thresholding and masking. These concepts are illustrated in Figure 5.3. Thresholding simply means there are sounds too soft for humans to hear because they fall below the threshold of audibility, the hearing threshold. Masking means there are sounds that cannot be heard because—temporarily—they are masked by nearby louder sounds that raise the threshold of audibility. When two sounds with a small difference in frequency are present simultaneously, *frequency-domain masking* (the effect shown in Figure 5.3) occurs and the stronger sound masks the weaker. This is one type of masking exhibited by the human ear. Another type is *temporal masking,* which occurs when a weaker sound of similar frequency appears within a small interval of time, before or after (or simultaneously with) a stronger sound. In either case, the stronger one masks the weaker one.

Thresholding and masking lay the groundwork for state-of-the-art audio coders. Some compression is achieved by simply ignoring sounds that are too soft—those that fall below the threshold of audibility. Further reduction is achieved by recording audible sounds with only the degree of digital resolution necessary for high-fidelity reproduction. The most effective audio coders continuously vary the number of bits used to record each component of a complex sound. Adaptively, they assign bits according to the audibility of that component, the potential audibility of the playback noise generated by the encoding (quantization) process itself, and the number of bits available for storing or transmitting the compressed data.

Another characteristic of the human ear is used in designing effective audio coders: The human auditory system can be thought of as bandpass filter bank covering the frequency range of 10–20,000 Hz. Within this range, the bandpass filters strongly overlap each other, and their bandwidth, which may be as narrow as 100 Hz at low frequencies, becomes increasingly wider, growing to 5000 Hz for the highest frequencies. This characterization of the human ear, along with thresholding and masking, becomes the basis for designed effective *frequency-domain audio coders*. These coders achieve compression by splitting the audio spectrum into frequency bands that can be individually quantized and coded according to the rules for perceptual coding.

Audio coding basics

The encoding and decoding processes for audio data are shown in Figure 5.4. They begin with a source signal that has been time sampled and digitally coded

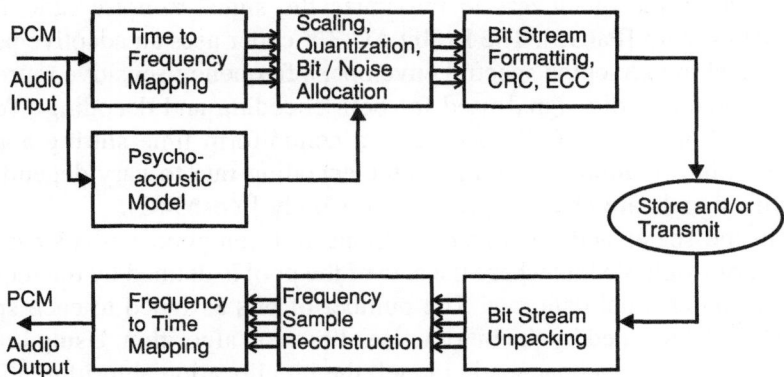

Figure 5.4   Audio encoding and decoding.

using PCM. For high-quality audio, 16-bit PCM samples are used and sampling rates range up to 48 KHz. The first step of encoding is a time-to-frequency transformation that breaks the audio frequency spectrum down into many narrow spectral components arranged according to the ear's sensitivity characteristics. The number of spectral components varies with different designs; current applications of *subband coders* use as few as 32 subbands whereas those for *adaptive transform coders* use up to 576 spectral components or transform coefficients. Generally, more spectral components allow greater compression at the expense of more complexity. To generate the spectral components, subband coders feed the source signal into a set of bandpass filters arranged contiguously in frequency. Adaptive transform coders process the input signal using a discrete transform— either a discrete Fourier transform (DFT) or a modified discrete cosine transform (MDCT). There also are *hybrid coders* that combine subband and adaptive transform coding techniques. This allows the characteristics of the human ear to be matched more closely, providing higher frequency resolution at the lower frequencies where it is needed, and lower resolution at higher frequencies.

The spectral components are fed to a scaler and quantizer along with the output from a psychoacoustic model which provides the information needed for deciding how many bits to allocate each spectral component. The complexity and details of psychoacoustic models vary, but the general idea is to analyze each spectral component for the masking and thresholding characteristics of the signals it contains. Simple ideas are involved: If a spectral component is not audible, or contains no energy at all, then it should receive no bits. The closer the signal is to being audible, the more bits it should receive. There are no rules for setting up psychoacoustic models—other than the audio coder must provide a certain compression ratio for specific applications—and different coders take different approaches: A technique used by the MPEG-1 audio standard and Philips PASC™ coders is to measure the distance from the peak value of the signal to the masking level, the SMR (signal-to-mask ratio), to find the number of bits needed to record each component of a complex sound [Pan94, Hoog94]. An adaptive noise allocation scheme is used for the MPEG-2 audio standard where the encoder iteratively varies the quantizers to maximize the signal-to-noise ratio for the encoded data stream [Pan95]. The Dolby AC-3™ coder uses an adaptive psycho-acoustic model to extract the spectral envelope, a frequency-sensitive representation of the overall audio signal used for both encoding and decoding [Todd94, Noll95]. The Sony ATRAC™ coder uses a nonuniform time slitting approach that provides information which allows the encoding rate to vary depending on whether the signals are changing rapidly or slowly [Yosh94C].

Next, in the scaler and quantizer, each spectral component is allocated bits from a pool of available bits where the size of the pool is defined by the recording or transmission channel data rate. The number of bits assigned to each spectral component is determined by the bit or noise allocation algorithm. Using informa-tion supplied by the psychoacoustic model, the bit allocation algorithm allocates bits so as to use the minimum number, whereas a noise allocation algorithm does the same thing but attempts to minimize the audible noise in the encoded output. Each spectral component is coded as a quantization value and a scale-factor value (called mantissa and exponent in floating-point number notation), allowing the signal to cover a wide dynamic range.

There are no standards for representing spectral components, and different algorithms have chosen different schemes. In MPEG-1 and PASC the quantization values range from 0 to 15 bits, whereas 6 bits are used for scaling, which allows an input signal range of 120 dB [Pan94]. In Dolby AC-3, each spectral component can be quantized to a maximum resolution of 16 bits. But rather than just encoding the most significant digits, AC-3 scales and offsets the mantissa to provide zero-centered, equal-width, symmetrical quantization levels that reduce distortion and noise [Davi93, Davi95]. The exponent of each AC-3 spectral component can range in value from 0 to 24 (where a delta of 1 represents a 6-dB sound-pressure level change). But rather than sending all the bits, exponents (except the lowest-frequency term) are encoded as differential values. Changes in value of +2 to −2 from the spectral component next lower in frequency are allowed, and each is encoded by AC-3 using only slightly more than two bits [Todd94, Davi95]. In the AC-3 decoder, the mantissas and exponents are restored to their actual values.

Lossless coding, which was mentioned earlier, may be applied after all the preceding steps have taken place, but only the more sophisticated coders—that need the extra compression it provides—choose to use it. For example, Huffman entropy coding is included in the more advanced forms of MPEG-1 audio [Pan94].

The last step of encoding is to pack the encoded spectral components into blocks of data for storage or transmission. In this step, depending on the needs of the storage or transmission channel, CRC (cyclic redundancy check) error-detecting code or ECC (error-correcting code) may be added.

The decoding process reverses what was done during encoding. Most audio decoders provide a straightforward inversion of the encoding process, but there is no provision for psychoacoustic modeling in the decoder—with the exception of Dolby AC-3 [Noll95].

Multichannel audio coding

The audio encoding and decoding processes shown in Figure 5.4 apply to one audio channel. Multiple audio channels can be coded by duplicating the encoder and decoder for each channel. However, for the predominant multichannel audio systems—two-channel stereo and 5.1-channel surround sound—this is wasteful for there is considerable correlation between individual channels. In stereophonic audio, the left and right channels are not totally independent. In addition, the human ear has yet another perceptual weakness when it comes to stereo imaging that allows interchannel masking effects to be exploited. The net result is that much of the data in stereophonic audio does not contribute to the localization of sound sources, allowing some spectral components of the individual channels to be combined and coded as single values.

There is even more potential for combining multiple channels with surround sound, an audio reproduction technique that provides realistic lifelike three-dimensional spatial acoustics. Surround sound was originally developed for motion pictures and soon will be applied to HDTV. It uses left, center, and right main channels, left and right surround channels, and a low-frequency enhancement subwoofer channel. The subwoofer channel is band limited (15–120 Hz), resulting in surround sound being designated as a 5.1-channel system. State-of-the-art MPEG-2 and AC-3 multichannel coders compress the 5.1 channels and provide satisfactory performance using a total bit rate of only 320 or 384 Kbps. This is about the same bit rate as for compressed two-channel audio and one-fourth that of ordinary (uncompressed) two-channel CD-quality audio.

State-of-the-art audio
coding and beyond

The characteristics of today's perceptual audio coders are that they achieve 4:1 or 5:1 compression ratios on CD-quality audio, and up to 12:1 compression for multichannel applications. They are almost symmetrical (decoding is about 2 times faster than encoding), somewhat computational intense, and quite readily implemented in DSPs (digital signal processors). Table 5.3 summaries key attributes of the audio coders discussed in this chapter. The simplest applications require audio coders for two channels of CD-quality audio. The more complex MPEG-2 and Dolby AC-3 audio coders provide multichannel coding for 5.1 audio channels. In addition, the MPEG-2 audio standard supports a wide range of data rates and bandwidths from studio quality to telephone toll-line quality.

Table 5.3 Perceptual audio coders.

	ATRAC	MPEG-1[1] & PASC	MPEG-2	Dolby AC-3[2]
Audio sampling rate (KHz)	44.1	32, 44.1, 48[3]	16, 22.05, 24, 32, 44.1, 48	32, 44.1, 48
Audio channels	2	2	5.1	5.1
Compression ratio	5:1	Varies (4:1 PASC)	Varies	Varies
Encoded bit rate (Kbps)	292 (stereo)	32-224 (mono) 384 (stereo)	384 (5.1)	32-640 (mono) 320/384 (5.1)
Coding	Hybrid	Subband	Hybrid	Transform
Subband filters	3	32	32	-
Spectral components	512	32	192 / 576 (dynamic)	64 / 128 / 256 (dynamic)
Psychoacoustic model	Adaptive transform block size using signal change rate	Signal-mask-ratio	Signal-mask ratio	Log-domain spectral envelope encoding and decoding
Bit or noise allocation scheme	Implementation dependent	Mask-to-noise ratio	Adaptive noise allocation	Mask-to-signal ratio
Quantization bits per component	na	0 -15	0 - 15	≤ 16
Scale factor bits per component	na	6	6	< 5[4]
Entropy coding	No	No	Yes	No

Notes:
[1] MPEG-1 has three layers of coders: Layer I is described. The Layer II coder is similar to Layer I. The Layer III coder is similar to MPEG-2.
[2] AC-3 is specified for HDTV and DVD as an alternative to the MPEG-2 audio standard coder.
[3] PASC operates only at 44.1 KHz.
[4] Differential encoding assigns about 2.3 bits per exponent. See text.

A variety of applications are anticipated for MPEG-2 audio, not only in consumer audiophile products but also for cellular phones, digital radios, conferencing gear, and just about anywhere high-quality audio is needed.

Perceptual audio coding is a relatively new application of data compression and, as is apparent, there are several approaches. In the future, there may be new solutions for audio coding based on improved psychoacoustic models. Many applications, particularly multichannel audio coding, are also new, and there remains much to be learned. Perhaps the algorithms described in this section provide audio of sufficient quality, at acceptably low data rates, for costs that will spur mass-produced products—perhaps not; audiophile experts are still debating the merits of these psychoacoustic coding techniques [Mitc95, Taki95B]. This issue will be examined in more detail in Section 9.2. Interesting new applications for audio are emerging too. Some require coding at much lower bit rates, and others use audio to support low-bit-rate video coding where speech information can be used to enhance picture quality. These applications will require extensions of existing designs, or they may result in completely new approaches [Noll95].

5.4 Image Compression

In this section, compression techniques for still images are examined; in the next section, moving images (video) will be examined. The applications for digitized still images are many and varied—the now familiar FAX machine, commercial imaging systems for paperless offices, medical imaging, satellite imaging for remote sensing of earth and space, filmless electronic cameras, computer-generated images, and more. All digital image systems represent a two-dimensional picture as a string of bits, which, as learned in Chapter 1, is accomplished by scanning the image in a regular pattern (say left to right, top to bottom) and collecting samples at prespecified points. As shown in Figure 5.5, usually these points are arranged as an equally spaced rectangular grid on the image. Each sample is called a pixel (picture element). The digital value(s) of each pixel represents some measure of the brightness, color, or spectral attributes sensed at that point in the image. This data may be stored (typically as a row-column matrix that corresponds to the image grid), processed by computer, transmitted, and used to reproduce a likeness of the original image. How faithful the reproduction will be depends on many factors, one of the most important being the sampling resolution that determines how many pixels represent the image. Using more pixels allows more image detail to be captured; it also means larger capacities for storing images and larger bandwidths for transmitting them (and more expensive, complex imaging systems for collecting them too).

The adage "A picture is worth a thousand words" may be true for human communications, but digital pictures, especially large-format, high-resolution color images, are worth far more—in the realm of digital words (or bits). Digital imaging systems generate huge amounts of data. For example, a color image

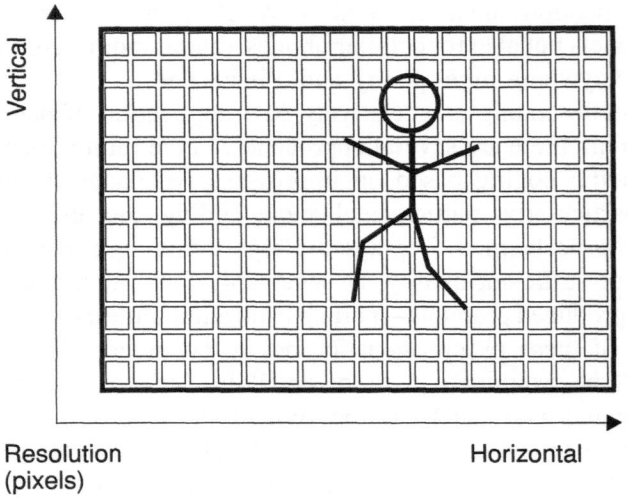

Resolution   Horizontal
(pixels)

Figure 5.5   Digital image representation.

digitized at 24 bits per pixel and displayed at VGA resolution (a 640 × 480 pixel computer screen format) requires nearly a megabyte of storage; transmitting this image via telephone, even over the fastest lines, would take several minutes. Luckily, digitized images are highly compressible because (1) when an image is digitized, the pixels in any region of the image are similar and (2) many imaging systems capture information the human eye cannot see. Image compression algorithms take advantage of these redundancies and reduce the number of bits required to represent images. Compression ratios range from as little as 2:1 or 3:1 to 100:1 or more depending on the characteristics of the image and whether the application can tolerate the use of lossy compression. However, as learned in Chapter 2, even compressed images still use a lot of bits, several times more than the proverbial thousand words.

There are many different types of images, and each demands different compression techniques. This section examines the standardized compression algorithms for bi-level images and for continuous-tone, gray-scale and color, photographic-quality images. The pixel representations for bi-level, gray-scale, and color images are shown in Figure 5.6. These types of images arise in the following situations:

Bi-level or binary images are captured by scanners that use only two intensity levels, one for "information" and another for the "background." Therefore, each pixel is a single bit whose value is either 1 or 0. One-bit pixels are appropriate for human-created documents containing text, line drawings, or illustrations. The best known example of bi-level imaging is transmitting black-and-white documents via FAX. Photographs, too, are sometimes captured as bi-level images with a digital halftoning process. This is similar to the technique newspapers use to reproduce photographs where black dots of varying sizes, spaced closer or further apart, are used to simulate shading, creating the effect of continuous tones.

Gray-scale images are captured by scanners that use multiple intensity levels

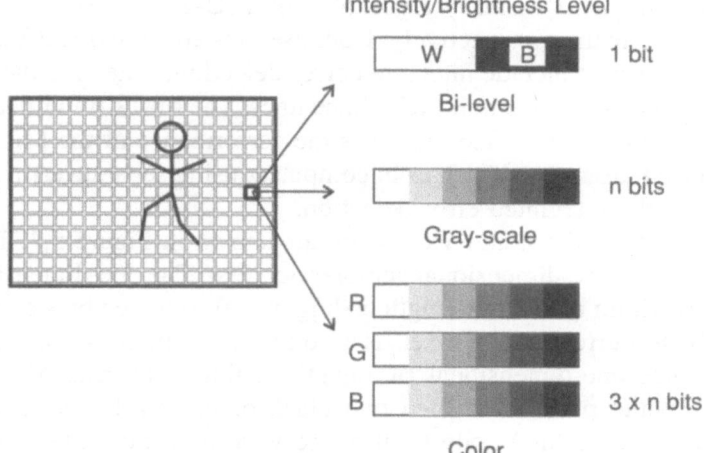

Figure 5.6 Pixel representation.

to record shadings between black and white. Typically, each pixel is represented by N bits—8–12 bits, or more. Gray-scale imaging techniques are appropriate for monochrome photographs and medical images where accurate representation of shading is important.

Color, photographic-quality images are captured by scanners that use multiple intensity levels and filtering to capture the brightness level for each of the three primary colors in visible light—red, green, and blue.[5] Here, each pixel is represented by three values, one for each of the primary color intensities, requiring up to 24 bits or more. This imaging technique is appropriate for images of natural scenes or even human-created images where it important to capture continuous tones.

There are also multispectral images that include information which lies outside the visible-light spectrum. For instance, satellite imaging systems for remote sensing of earth and space may capture infrared radiation. Multispectral images will not be specifically addressed in this book, except to remark that either the JBIG or JPEG algorithm can be used to compress them.

ITU-T T.4 and T.6 recommendations

The ITU-T T.4 and T.6 recommendations (standards) for Group 3 and Group 4 facsimile machines contain algorithms that losslessly compress bi-level FAX images. They provide compression ratios that vary widely for different documents but can easily approach 15:1 or more. Their algorithms use spatially nearby neighbor pixels to compress successive image pixels. The MH and MR (modified

---

[5] Red, green, and blue are the *additive* primary colors for light-emitting systems such as computer displays and scanners. Cyan (a blue-green), magenta, and yellow are the *subtractive* primary colors that, in combination with black, are used in printing, a light-absorbing process [Penn93, Trow94].

Huffman and modified READ[6]) algorithms of ITU-T T.4 use one- and two-dimensional information, respectively. Both use run-length and Huffman coding. These algorithms also include integrated error detection, reflecting their application to communications over noisy telephone lines. The MMR (modified modified READ) algorithm in ITU-T T.6 improves the performance of the MR algorithm for noise-free environments (such as in computers using separate error detection) by eliminating the integrated error detection.

Examples of ITU-T T.4 and T.6 coding are shown in Figure 5.7. The ITU-T committee defined one-dimensional compression first. The one-dimensional ITU-T T.4 MH algorithm uses a run-length coding model followed by static Huffman coding. Only the current line of pixels is used for one-dimensional coding. Figure 5.7(a) illustrates one-dimensional run-length coding with runs of three black pixels, three white pixels, and then two black pixels. Each line is terminated with an EOL (end of line) code to allow resynchronization after transmission errors. Additional details of modified Huffman coding are provided in Section 4.4.

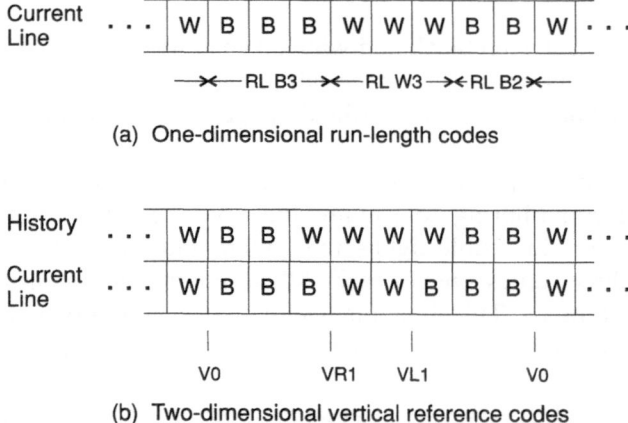

(a) One-dimensional run-length codes

(b) Two-dimensional vertical reference codes

Figure 5.7   ITU-T T.4 and T.6 bi-level image coding.

One-dimensional coding of a page containing dense text did not give enough compression to achieve subminute page transmission over 4800 bits/second communication lines. So the ITU-T T.4 committee also defined an optional two-dimensional MR coding technique in which some lines are coded using one-dimensional MH coding while others are coded relative to the previous line using vertical relationships (to be explained momentarily). Each line is terminated with an EOL code followed by a bit to specify whether the next line is coded one or two dimensionally. Error recovery from transmission errors is possible at the one-dimensionally coded lines (which are forced to occur at least every four lines to minimize possible error propagation). The two-dimensional MR algorithm

---

[6] READ is an acronym standing for Relative Element Address Designate.

begins by applying MH coding to a line of pixels. It then goes on to code the next several lines by finding matching pairs of black-white and white-black transitions in consecutive lines and coding the vertical relationships between them. Figure 5.7(b) shows a section of a current line in which the first white-black transition is vertically aligned with that in the previous (history) line; it is coded as "V0." The next black-white transition is vertically offset right one position from the history line; it is coded as "VR1." The next white-black transition is vertically offset left one position; it is coded as "VL1," and so on. This vertical mode of coding is used only when a transition occurs within ±3 pixels of an identical transition in the history scan line. When this condition is not met, one of two alternative coding modes applies: If the history line contains a run of black or white pixels that are not in the current line, the pass mode is used; the coder outputs a special code to indicate this run has been skipped and should not be used during decoding. If the current line contains a run that is not in the history line, the horizontal mode is used; the coder outputs yet another special code and codes the next two runs of the current line using one-dimensional MH coding. Additional details of both MH and MR coding can be found in [Mcco92, Witt94].

For digital transmission environments where transmissions can be guaranteed to be error free, the MR algorithm was further modified to create the ITU-T T.6 MMR coding technique. In MMR, every line is coded two dimensionally and no EOL codes are used. By eliminating the MR provision for error detection, compression is maximized. According to one source, if MR compresses a simple text document by 20:1, MMR will increase compression about 30% [Penn93]. However, compression results for individual documents may vary widely.

JBIG—ITU-T T.82 recommendation

More recent developments in bi-level image coding are incorporated in the ITU-T T.82 recommendation known as JBIG. In 1988, JBIG, the Joint Bi-level Image Group, was chartered to establish an improved standard for lossless coding of bi-level images. The JBIG algorithm they defined introduced adaptivity and new capabilities, including the following:

- Adaptive modeling using two-dimensional prediction to achieve higher compression in images with periodicity (i.e., halftone images)
- Adaptive arithmetic coding to replace static Huffman coding, allowing robust compression of more data types
- Hierarchical coding, allowing the same image to be decompressed at progressively higher spatial resolutions from a compressed data stream
- Scalability to amplitude precision greater than one bit per pixel for lossless compression of gray-scale or color images

JBIG uses neighboring pixels as a template to statistically predict the current pixel X. As shown in Figure 5.8, JBIG uses a two-dimensional, three-line template

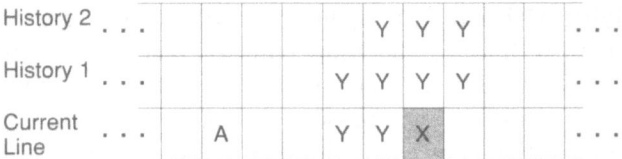

Figure 5.8   JBIG two-dimensional, three-line prediction template.

that includes neighboring *context* pixels (Y)—two from the current line, four from the history line, and three from the previous history line. It also uses an *adaptive* template pixel (A) whose position can vary, depending on the image being coded. As to function, the context pixels control the arithmetic coder decision probabilities and the adaptive template pixel provides more effective coding of halftoned images.

JBIG allows both sequential (nonprogressive) and progressive modes of operation. The sequential mode captures an image and codes it at full resolution. Besides providing slightly better compression than the progressive mode, the sequential mode can be somewhat faster because a simplified two-line template is a coding option. The progressive mode captures a low-resolution rendition image and, with a sequence of encodings, progressively doubles the vertical and horizontal resolution. Progressive coding can be advantageous for displaying images, such as situations where different displays have differing resolution capabilities. It is also useful for browsing a collection of images, where a low-resolution rendition is sufficient to screen out unwanted images, and for transmitting images over noisy channels, where part of the image may be corrupted.

Although the main objective of JBIG was to improve bi-level image coding, it can also be used to losslessly code (multilevel or multitonal) gray-scale and color images. This is accomplished by compressing the "bit planes" used to describe multitonal images coded with multiple bits per pixel. For instance, a gray-scale image composed of 8-bit pixels would be compressed by repetitively applying the JBIG algorithm, once to each of the 8 bits. For a color image, the JBIG algorithm would be applied to each bit of each color component.

JBIG compression performance, according to one source, improves bi-level image compression about 30% when compared to the MMR algorithm; on gray-scale images, JBIG is about equal to the JPEG algorithm (in lossless mode with arithmetic coding) [Penn93]. The results of extensive tests of the JBIG algorithm on both bi-level and multitonal images are provided by another source, where, on color images, very little difference was observed between JBIG and JPEG (again, in lossless mode with arithmetic coding) [Arps94]. However, compression results for individual documents may vary widely.

JPEG—ITU-T T.81 recommendation

JPEG is an international standard for compressing gray-scale and color, photographic-quality (continuous-tone) images. The JPEG acronym stands for the Joint

Photographic Experts Group.[7] The intent of JPEG is to provide algorithms and tools for a variety of image compression applications. Implementations are flexible too; the JPEG algorithms are symmetric and they allow for software-hardware cost-performance trade-offs. Very quickly, JPEG has become the image coding standard by which all others are judged, and many of its compression techniques have found their way into standards for compressing video data (which will be examined in Section 5.5).

A motivation for developing JPEG was to promote the usage of color, photographic-quality images as commercially viable media. When uncompressed, they simply are too expensive to transmit or store. Consider the following: A typical digitized color image may use 24 bits per pixel—8 bits each for RGB (red, green, blue) or YC_BC_R (luminance, chrominance, chrominance) components.[8] The explosion in transmission times (and storage costs) for color, photographic-quality images is evident when compared to FAX images that use only 1 bit per pixel. Thus, the JPEG group set about developing algorithms that would offer quality image representation at 1.0 bits per pixel (a 24:1 compression ratio for the above example). JPEG accomplishes this (and more) by using both lossless and lossy compression, resulting in an image that is an approximation of the original. In fact, JPEG allows the user to select the compression ratio, with the understanding that higher compression ratios lead to poorer approximations and lower-quality images. JPEG allows compression of any continuous-tone image by as little as 2:1 with absolute visual image fidelity (using only lossless compression). It also allows these same images to be compressed by 10:1 with "visually lossless" image fidelity and by 20:1 or even 100:1 with lesser degrees of visual image fidelity (using lossless and lossy compression).

To reduce the number of bits used to represent a digitized image, JPEG takes advantage of redundancy and irrelevancy. We are familiar with *statistical redundancy*—the kind of redundancy that occurs in a sequence of symbols—that can be removed by lossless compression algorithms, such as Huffman and arithmetic entropy coding, which JPEG uses in its final stage of coding. But, in images there is another kind of rudundancy—*spatial redundancy*. Within images, neighboring elements for any one of the RGB or YC_BC_R matrices are highly correlated because all the pixels in a region of the image tend to represent the same color, luminance, or chrominance. Also, it should be noted that spatial redundancy increases with higher image resolutions (needed to capture detail)

[7] The JPEG committee was first chartered in 1986 by ISO and ITU-T. The JPEG standard is a collaborative effort of three major international standards organizations, ISO, ITU-T, and IEC. It is formally specified by the ISO Draft Information Standard 10918 | ITU-T Recommendation T.81 [Penn93].

[8] The Y luminance component provides a gray-scale version of the image. It is formed as a weighted sum of red, green, and blue color components. The C_B and C_R luminance components provide the additional information needed to convert the gray-scale image to a color image. They are formed by combinations of the luminance and color components [Penn93].

because more pixels represent each region of the image. JPEG removes this type of redundancy, too, by using transform techniques to be discussed shortly.

To understand *irrelevancy* and how, through quantization techniques, JPEG uses it for image compression, we turn to psychovisual compression techniques that result from studies of the human visual system. Psychovisual compression takes advantage of several limitations of the human eye, including imperfect response to color. The human eye is less sensitive to some image components than others. Research has shown the human eye is less sensitive to chrominance than to luminance, meaning that fewer bits are needed for chrominance information, and it can be coded more coarsely than luminance. Another trick of psychovisual compression is to take advantage of the human eye being most sensitive to mid-spatial frequencies and not so sensitive to low- and high-spatial frequencies. This allows designers to make compromises in the fidelity of edge contours where rapid transitions in brightness occur. Also, the human eye is less sensitive to quantization distortions at high luminance levels, the so-called noise-masking property. This allows more coarse quantization to save bits at high luminance levels.

These data compression concepts are embodied in the JPEG standard for still, color, photographic-quality image compression. Figure 5.9 shows the baseline system, the most basic mode of JPEG encoding and decoding. To begin the process, the components of the digitized image are placed in a frame store. The JPEG algorithm operates on each component of the image. It produces a single compressed image for gray-scale images, one for each of the RGB color components or YC_BC_R luminance-chrominance components, or an appropriate set for whatever may be the chosen image representation. JPEG does not specify how the image should be represented, so any color transformation—say from RGB to YC_BC_R, where luminance-chrominance psychovisual differences can be best exploited—must precede the steps shown in Figure 5.9.

The JPEG encoding algorithm breaks each image component into blocks of 8×8 pixels and processes each block as follows:

- Spatial redundancy within the image is removed when waveform processing techniques are applied with DCT (discrete cosine transform) coding. The objective of transform coding is to decorrelate the image pixels; that is, statistically dependent image elements are converted into independent coefficients in a transformed space, where the energy of the image is concentrated onto as few coefficients as possible. This allows removing the irrelevant components within the image during the next step.

- Irrelevancy reduction occurs when lossy compression is applied and the DCT coefficients are quantized (encoded) according to whatever rules are loaded into the quantization table. Typically, larger step sizes are used to more-coarsely quantize any coefficient representing color data whose frequencies lie above some threshold (because the eye is not so sensitive); smaller step sizes are used to quantize those below the same threshold (because the eye is more sensitive). Often different values

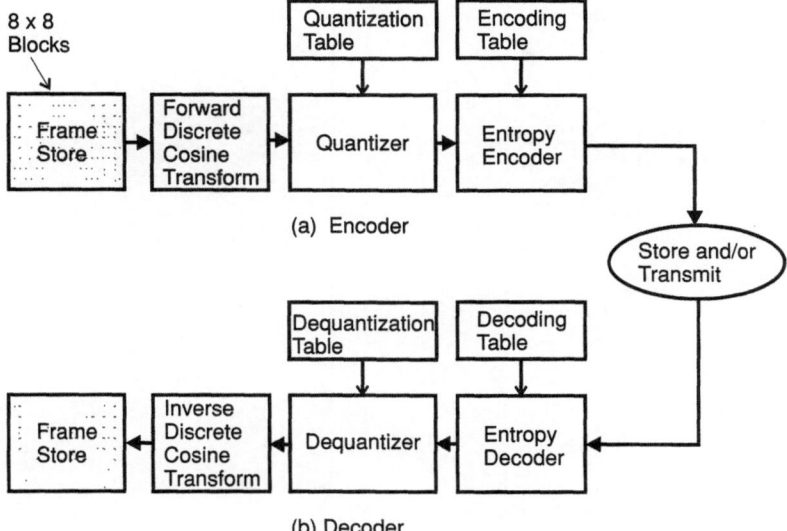

Figure 5.9   JPEG encoding and decoding.

are loaded in the quantization table for each of the RGB or YC_BC_R matrices, corresponding to the limitations of the human eye.

- Statistical redundancy reduction occurs when lossless compression is performed using run-length and Huffman entropy coding which is specified for the baseline system. Arithmetic coding may be selected for other modes of operation (to be described shortly), yielding approximately 10% more compression at the expense of execution time [Witt94].

The results from processing individual 8×8 blocks are combined to form the encoded image which may be stored or transmitted. By reversing the encoding operations, the JPEG decoder produces an approximate representation of the input image.

Figure 5.10 provides insight to how JPEG processes blocks of 8×8 pixels. The steps JPEG uses to process images reflect the state of the art in commercial image compression technology. Because these same steps appear in the video compression algorithms to be examined in Section 5.5, a closer look into their operation is warranted. For the example shown in Figure 5.10, we have chosen to transform the pixels for a small, shaded gray square set in a field of white.

The encoding process begins with the DCT step that transforms the two-dimension block of pixels from the spatial domain to a two-dimension array of frequency coefficients in the frequency domain.[9] The purpose of the DCT step

---

[9] Before the DCT step, the spatial domain pixel values are threshold shifted (by 128 for 8-bit pixels), becoming positive and negative values. Following the IDCT, this threshold shift is undone.

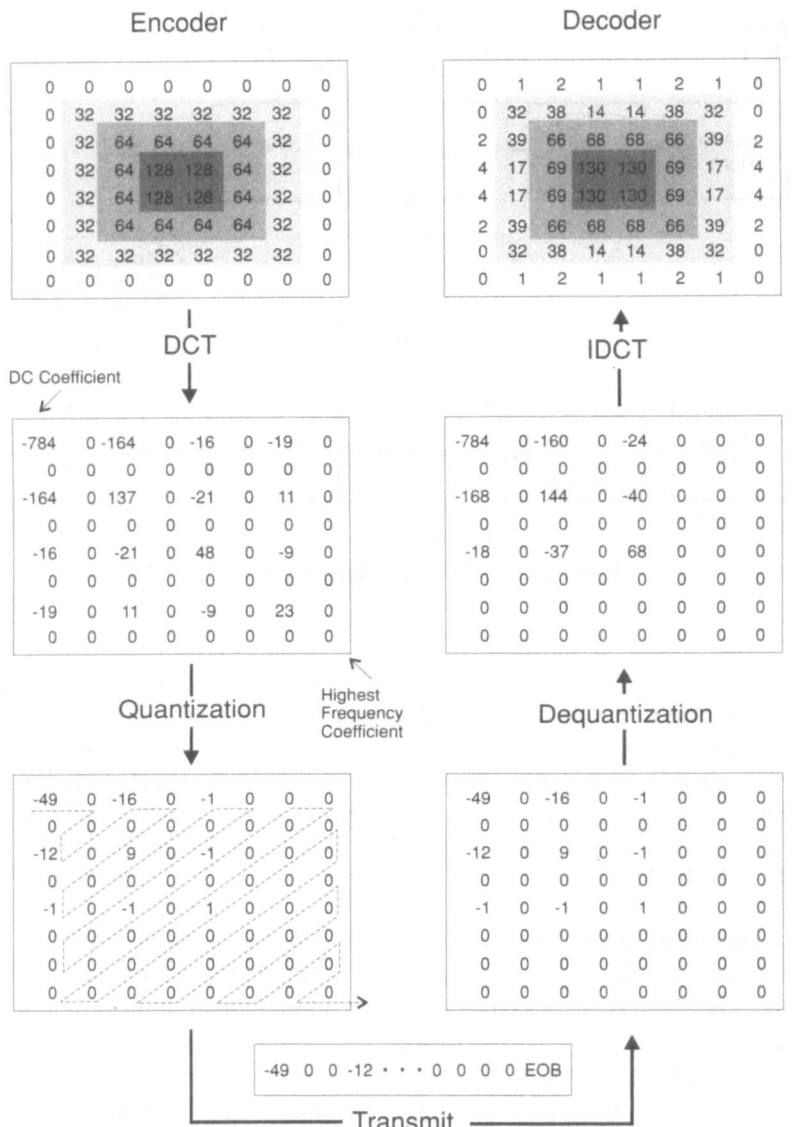

Figure 5.10   JPEG 8 × 8 pixel block coding.

is to decorrelate the 64 image pixels and concentrate most of their energy into coefficients in the top left corner of the frequency array, rendering the other coefficients to have near-zero values. Among the frequency coefficients, the "DC coefficient" represents the average intensity value (color, luminance, or chrominance) of the 64 pixels in the spatial domain. The other coefficients represent spatial features occurring at different frequencies in the 8 × 8 block of pixels. Within the frequency coefficient array, the lowest frequency coefficients are located up and left; the highest are down and right. Moving down the array one finds coefficients representing higher vertical frequencies; moving right in the array, one finds coefficients representing higher horizontal frequencies. The terms "vertical frequency" and "horizontal frequency" refer to patterns found within the 8 × 8 block of pixels in the spatial domain—variations of intensity in the vertical and horizontal dimensions. It should be noted that DCT is a lossless operation because, if the coefficients are represented with sufficient accuracy, the 8 × 8 block of pixels can be recovered exactly.

The next step, quantization, is a lossy operation, after which only an approximation of the 8 × 8 block of pixels can be recovered. Quantization is designed to drive small, nonessential frequency components to zero by scaling each coefficient to the nearest multiple of a value found in a quantization table. To produce the quantized two-dimensional array of frequency components shown in Figure 5.10, a quantization table provided as an example by the ISO JPEG standard was used.[10] JPEG allows the user to decide what is nonessential by making the 64-element quantization table loadable. In general, quantization tables are constructed so that the quantization step size varies with frequency and image component. Low frequencies are more important than high, luminance is more important than chrominance, and nonessential elements are quantized with larger step sizes (i.e., quantized more coarsely). The zigzag sequence shown in the lower left corner of Figure 5.10 is used to read out the quantized frequency coefficients into a one-dimension array in preparation for transmission. This orders the frequency coefficients from lowest to highest, allowing run-length and Huffman or arithmetic entropy coding (not shown) to be applied for efficient transmission to the decoder.

In the decoder, using the same quantization table, the quantized coefficients are dequantized. Then, an inverse discrete cosine transform (IDCT) is applied, which allows an approximate representation of the 8 × 8 block of pixels to be reconstructed. The effects of quantizing the original small, shaded gray square are clearly visible in the reconstituted 8 × 8 block of pixels, shown in the upper right corner of Figure 5.10.

The baseline system, which all JPEG decoder implementations must support, is only one option that may be selected. The JPEG standard describes the following modes of operation:

- Sequential DCT based: This mode (which includes the baseline system) encodes each image component in a single left-to-right, top-to-bottom scan.
- Progressive DCT based: This mode encodes the image in multiple scans. It is appropriate for applications in which transmission time is long and the viewer prefers to see the image build up in multiple coarse-to-fine passes.
- Sequential lossless: This mode allows the decoder output to bit-identically match

---

[10] In the ISO JPEG standard, see "Table K.1 Luminance quantization table," as reproduced on page 503 of [Penn93].

the encoder input, supporting applications where no loss can be tolerated. Predictive coding techniques are used.

- Hierarchical: This mode provides progressive coding with increased spatial resolution between successive stages. (Note: JBIG defines this to be its progressive coding mode of operation.) The image is encoded at multiple resolutions so that lower-resolution versions may be accessed without first having to decompress the image at its full resolution. The JPEG hierarchical mode allows DCT-based (lossy) coding, lossless coding, or both in combination.

The JPEG standard encompasses a diversity of techniques for compressing color, photographic-quality images and offers immense flexibility: Images may range in size from 1×1 to $65,535 \times 65,535$ active pixels. Each pixel may have from 1 to 255 color components or spectral bands (except the progressive mode where only 1 to 4 are allowed). Pixels can have 8 or 12 bits of precision for DCT-based coding and any value between 2 and 16 bits for the sequential lossless coding mode. The JPEG standard allows for interleaved data supporting, for example, still images captured from television. Besides defining the algorithms for image compression and decompression, the standard defines the compressed image data stream, including an interchange format for storage and transmission. More detailed descriptions of the JPEG standard and its many options can be found in several sources, including [Wall91], [Arav93], and [Witt94], and [Penn93], where the complete JPEG specification can be found.

State-of-the-art image coding and beyond

The image coding techniques examined in this section are in various stages of deployment. For bi-level images, the MH, MR, and MMR coding techniques specified by the ITU-T T.4 and T.6 recommendations are ubiquitous, being used in all FAX equipment. JBIG, which applies to bi-level images, too, and allows for coding multilevel, multitonal images, has not yet been widely deployed. Although these standards may not be end-all solutions for bi-level image coding, they are highly effective, and they achieve lossless coding results that are near optimum.

JPEG is *the* standard for coding still, photographic-quality (continuous-tone) images. Although there are *many* other image compression techniques, some of which offer superior compression ratios in some situations, none yet provide the balance of coding efficiency, implementability, and breadth of applications that JPEG provides. None has the widespread acceptance that JPEG does. Algorithms other than JPEG have been and will continue to be used for niche image compression applications. However, they do not appear destined to become new image compression standards, at least not until they are more than the equal of JPEG in all respects. Meanwhile, JPEG image coding is not stagnant; it is an extendable standard. Many advancements in continuous-tone, still-photographic image coding can be made through compatible extensions to the current JPEG standard.

Improved coding techniques for greater coding efficiency, wider ranges of image types, wider ranges of image quality, including handling noisy images, preprocessing and postprocessing—all are possible under the JPEG umbrella. A list of some proposed extensions can be found in [Penn93]. More recently, the JPEG committee is now defining new lossless algorithms to be included in future versions of the standard [Mitc96].

5.5   Video Compression

During the 1980s and early 1990s, compressed digital video made the transition from research topic to commercial products. Among all types of data, video is without question the most difficult to compress, and finding techniques that meet all the challenges of compressing video has not been quick or easy. Real-time operation, very high data rates, stringent transmission channel bandwidth limitations, compatibility with existing standards for television broadcasting and telecommunications transmission, a marketplace with an ever-increasing demand for higher picture resolution—all set high barriers for success. Today, thanks to advances in microelectronics and improved compression techniques, we have ITU-T H.261 and ISO MPEG, the first generation of video compression standards containing algorithms that are practical and effective for videoconferencing and television applications, respectively. We will examine these standards in this section, realizing that additional applications for compressed video are still being discovered, too, and some of these applications demand improved (or totally new) compression algorithms to support them. Without a doubt, new video compression standards will emerge in coming years, and this section will conclude with a glimpse of what to expect.

At first thought, video compression might not seem much more difficult than image compression. In one sense, the distinction between compression techniques for still and moving images—video—is thin: A sequence of video frames can be treated as a sequence of still images to be coded individually but displayed sequentially at a video rate. Actually, this is what some applications do—the ones that use the so-called M-JPEG (motion-JPEG) video compression algorithm. The only problem with M-JPEG is that although the video quality can be very high, compression is not. In contrast, H.261 and MPEG are specifically designed for low-bit-rate video coding. They exploit the characteristics of video to maximum advantage and do produce highly compressed video—but not without additional complexity. One of the things they do differently is to exploit the *temporal redundancy* (or temporal correlation) that all video sequences contain because persons or objects in the scene do not move very much from frame to frame. By extracting frame-to-frame temporal redundancy, H.261 and MPEG compress the video data stream an additional three times (three times more than M-JPEG)—at the same quality level.

The H.261 and MPEG standards, and the systems that use them, employ temporal redundancy and many other techniques to compress video. Techniques to be discussed later in this section include the following:

- Color-space transformations, say from RGB to YC_BC_R where luminance-chrominance psychovisual differences can be exploited
- Picture resolution reduction (for applications where less than broadcast-quality pictures are acceptable)
- Frame rate reduction (for applications where less than full-motion video is acceptable)
- Intraframe coding using JPEG-like techniques to remove spatial redundancy (except the video algorithms allow for variable quantization)
- Interframe coding using temporal redundancy removal techniques
- Entropy coding techniques similar to those of JPEG

Analog video basics

To understand digital video, we need to look at how analog video systems operate. Consider television: A video camera captures a sequence of still pictures displayed one after the other as images on a television receiver. As shown in Figure 5.11, each picture is captured and converted to an electronic signal by a raster scanning process. Starting at the upper left corner and moving downward, picture information is captured in a sequence of scan lines that form a field. When the bottom of the picture is reached, scanning resumes at the top of the picture to form a second field, interleaved (interlaced) with the first. The two

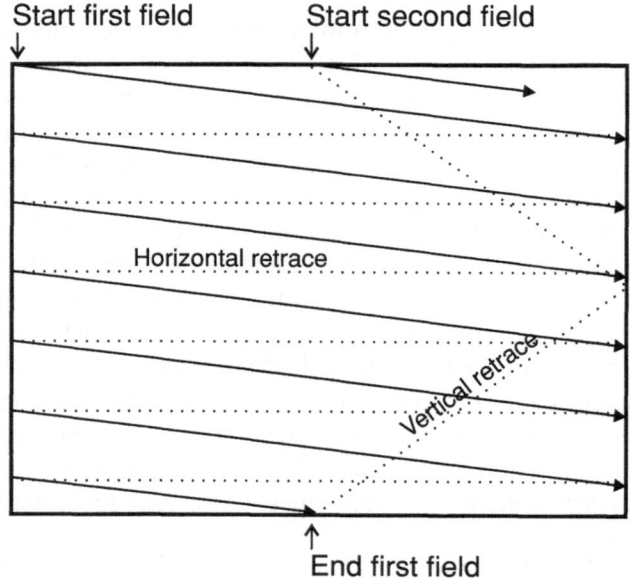

Figure 5.11 Interlaced TV raster scan.

fields, together, make up the picture and are called a frame.[11] There also are video systems that progressively scan the picture, filling the frame sequentially left to right, top to bottom. Computer video monitors use this scanning method, as will some future HDTV (high-definition television) receivers. In either scanning method, using more scan lines increases the (vertical) picture resolution, whereas to increase the horizontal resolution (which in digital systems is measured by the number of pixels per scan line), more bandwidth must be used to transmit the analog video signal. The scanning process is repeated at regular intervals of time, establishing a frame rate for transmission, which is measured in frames per second (fps). The frame rate must be high enough to produce the effect of smooth motion for moving objects, but increasing the frame rate increases the transmission bandwidth too.

There are three analog television transmission standards in use throughout the world today: NTSC, PAL, and SECAM. NTSC is used in North America and Japan, whereas PAL and SECAM are used in European countries. The rest of the world shares these three standards on a country-by-country basis [Trow94]. Each standard specifies a different number of scan lines and frame rate. NTSC uses 525 scan lines and 30 fps (actually 29.97 for color), whereas PAL and SECAM use 625 scan lines and 25 fps. There are more differences, too, particularly in how the analog signals are encoded for transmission and the resulting horizontal resolution realized by these systems.[12] In the recent past, one of the challenges faced by applications such as videoconferencing—which must interoperate with these existing incompatible standards —has been to create a digital television transmission system that can bridge between them. The ITU-T H.320 suite of standards for videoconferencing, of which the ITU-T H.261 compression standard is a part, does this.

A fourth worldwide standard for television transmission—*digital* HDTV (high-definition television)—looms in the immediate future. NTSC, PAL, and SECAM provide television pictures at a resolution that in the 1990s world of digital television is called SDTV—standard-definition television. It is not clear whether there will be one standard for HDTV, another for SDTV, or even several standards for both, defined on a country-by-country basis. In any event, it (or they) will be digital, which simplifies matters somewhat.

Digital video systems

Figure 5.12 shows the elements of digital video transmission systems. Because digital systems represent picture information as a series of digital bits, the first

---

[11] Interleaving is a "trick" analog television systems use to conserve transmission bandwidth. It exploits psychovisual properties of the human eye, making the frame rate appear to be twice its actual value. This reduces the "flicker" that is visible when frames are displayed at too low a frame rate.

[12] The CCIR 601 recommendation (standard) for studio-quality, digitized NTSC television specifies 480 active lines per picture and 720 active pixels per line. Home television receivers can display

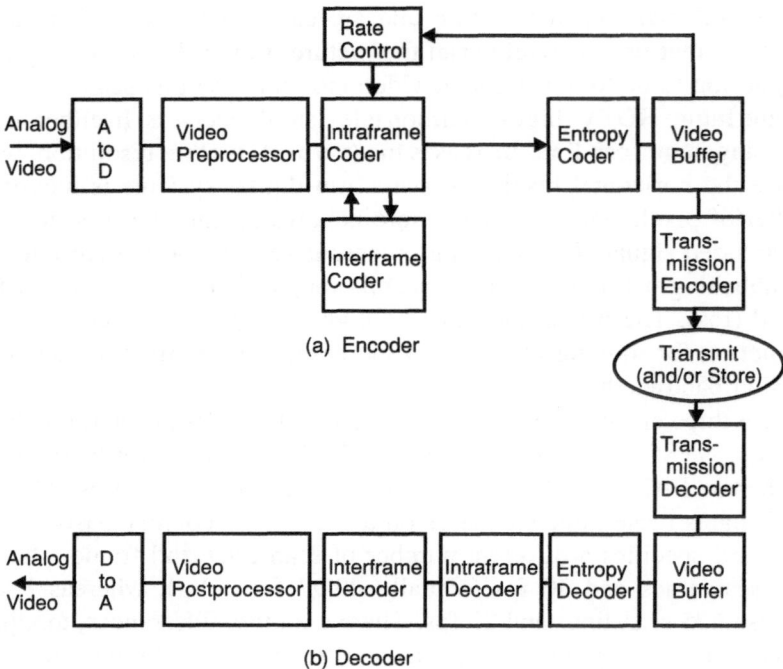

Figure 5.12   Digital video system dataflow.

step is to convert analog video signals to digital bit streams. Digital color television can be compressed most effectively when it is represented in RGB (red, green, blue) color component format or any of several luminance-chrominance component formats. These include YUV, YC_BC_R (a color coordinate system closely related to YUV), and YIQ (another luminance-chrominance format preferred for NTSC-standard video).[13] If the analog video signal arrives in one of these component formats, it can be directly converted to digital format. Or, if it arrives encoded into what is known as an analog composite format for transmission, it first must be decoded into analog component format and then converted to digital component format.

The next step is to preprocess the digital video in preparation for compression. The main purpose of preprocessing is to reduce the number of pixels to be coded and arrange the remaining pixels in a format most suitable for coding. The video preprocessor performs some or all of the following transformations:

all the lines but, thanks to the bandwidth-limited standard NTSC transmission channel, can reproduce only 300-350 pixels per line.

[13] The H.261 and MPEG standards specify YC_BC_R format. References to YUV format appear frequently in popular digital video compression literature, where the two formats are used interchangeably. For a comparison of the various color component systems, see [Penn93].

- Conversion, if needed, to the color component format best suited for compression (usually YC_BC_R)
- Removal of digital bits collected during blanking intervals[14]
- Conversion from interleaved to progressive scan format (for compression algorithms such as H.261 and MPEG-1 that work only on progressively scanned pictures)
- Conversion from analog standard picture resolution to digital standard picture resolution (by downsampling or upsampling as appropriate)
- Subsampling the chrominance components (by downsampling in the horizontal direction, the vertical direction, or both to take advantage of the human eye's insensitivity to changes in color)
- Subsampling in the temporal direction to reduce the frame rate prior to coding[15]

The H.261 and MPEG video compression algorithms operate on individual pictures (frames) and share processing methods that are common to the JPEG still-image compression standard. The intraframe coding step in these algorithms processes each picture component with DCT transforms and lossy quantization techniques. This step is followed by an entropy encoder that does run-length and Huffman coding. Both steps are similar to those described for JPEG in Section 5.4.

The new element in video compression is the interframe coder. Its objective is to reduce the number of bits to be transmitted by finding the temporal redundancy that exists between frames in the video data stream. The most extensively used intraframe coding technique is motion-compensated prediction. The concept is this: The intensity (and color) of an object will change only slightly from frame to frame. Also, if the object moves, its motion is slight. Therefore, when coding a new frame, use frames that have already been encoded to predict what the object will be and where it will be. Instead of transmitting all the pixels representing the object, transmit pixel changes resulting from object change and motion—as a prediction error and a motion vector.

Figure 5.13 shows the simplest type of motion-compensated prediction, the type used by the H.261 algorithm, where the prediction is based only on the previous frame. In H.261, each frame to be interframe coded is broken into blocks of 16×16 pixels and only blocks from the luminance component are used for motion-compensated prediction. The previous frame is examined to locate the best-matching block, which may not be in the same position because of object motion. So, nearby blocks in the previous picture are also searched. When the best-matching block is found, it and the block in the current frame are differenced, DPCM (differential pulse code modulation) is applied to predict

---

[14] Blanking intervals are those times when the scanning process is moving between lines and fields within a frame (shown as horizontal and vertical retrace in Figure 5.11). Only the digital bits that represent active parts of the picture need be coded and transmitted.

[15] Frame rate subsampling is only used for applications where the resulting jerkiness in motion can be tolerated. Often, when frame rate subsampling is used, it is done dynamically by the encoder and only if there is no other option for meeting an immutable transmission bandwidth or storage constraint.

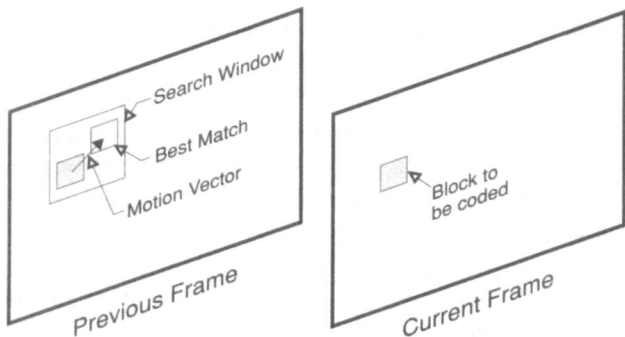

Figure 5.13 Motion-compensated prediction.

the block in the current frame, and a prediction error is generated. The prediction error along with a motion vector, which specifies the horizontal and vertical pixel-displacement of the block within the picture, are encoded for transmission.

The final elements for video coding (shown in Figure 5.12) are buffering, where the various picture components are stored while compression is in process, and a transmission encoding function, where the compressed pictures are assembled into a standard video data stream for transmission (or for storage). The decoding process, like other algorithms examined, performs inverse operations to restore an approximate representation of the original video data stream.

To date, three international standards have been defined for video compression, ITU-T H.261 and two MPEG standards by the Motion Picture Experts Group within ISO. All three are based on discrete cosine transforms, and all three support compression between frames as well as compression within each frame. The ITU-T H.261 standard is designed for videoconferencing over ISDN digital, switched circuits. ISO MPEG-1 was originally designed for playing multimedia from industry-standard CD-ROMs, with the fixed video data rate of 1.2 Mbps (1.5 Mbps total for audio and video). More recently, it has been used for direct broadcast satellite (DBS) transmissions and computer-generated video applications. ISO MPEG-2 is designed for higher-quality multimedia playback, for conferencing, and, most important, HDTV. Let us now look at these standards in more detail.

ITU-T H.261

The ITU-T H.261 recommendation is part of ITU-T H.320, a suite of recommendations for audiovisual terminals that provide videotelephone and videoconferencing services on IDSN (Integrated Services Digital Network).[16] H.320-com-

---

[16] H.320 actually is the third videoconferencing standard created by ITU-T. The first, H.120, was adopted by the ITU-T in 1984. It operated at 1.5 Mbps and could not compete with proprietary algorithms that offered better picture quality and lower data rates. The same fate afflicted N x 384, a mid-eighties effort that never became a formal standard [Port94, Halh91].

pliant products provide low-latency, jitter-free, full-duplex communication of coordinated sound, video, and data over limited-bandwidth ISDN channels. H.261, which was approved in 1990, defines a standardized video bit stream and a decoding algorithm. It provides the low-delay, real-time video decoding (and encoding too) needed for face-to-face videotelephone and videoconferencing conversations.[17] H.261 is designed for transmission of color video at bit rates of p $\times$ 64 Kbps, where p is an integer ranging from 1 to 30 (64 Kbps–1.92 Mbps). In practice, 64 or 128 Kbps ($p = 1, 2$) are appropriate for videotelephony, whereas rates of 128 Kbps and higher are needed for acceptable picture quality during videoconferencing.

Two digital image formats are defined for H.261, as shown in Table 5.4. When H.261 is used for videotelephony or videoconferencing, video signals from all equipment must be converted to one of these two formats. CIF (common intermediate format) is an optional higher-resolution format, whereas QCIF (quarter-CIF) is a standard lower-resolution format that must be supported by all H.261 implementations. The picture aspect ratio is 4:3 (horizontal:vertical). The frame rate can be 30 (actually 29.97), 15, 10, or 7.5 noninterlaced frames per second. CIF and higher frame rates apply to videoconferencing; QCIF and lower frame rates are appropriate for videotelephony.

Table 5.4 H.261 video formats.

Format	CIF		QCIF	
	Lines/Frame	Pixels/Line	Lines/Frame	Pixels/Line
Luminance (Y)	288	352	144	176
Chrominance (C_R)	144	176	72	88
Chrominance (C_B)	144	176	72	88

Selection of CIF or QCIF, and the frame rate, depends on the picture-quality objective and available channel bandwidth. When transmitted at the maximum frame rate, the uncompressed bit rates for CIF and QCIF are 36.45 and 9.115 Mbps, respectively. In practice, transporting these video signals on ISDN requires selecting the number of ISDN channels, the format, and the frame rate so that the compression ratio is 100:1 or less to retain reasonable picture quality—with available encoders. Table 5.5 shows various combinations of channels, formats, frame rates, and compression ratios.

---

[17] H.261 restricts encoding delay to be 150 milliseconds so as not to disrupt interactivity in two-way, face-to-face conversations. Longer delays produce effects similar to those experienced when telephone conversations are transmitted by satellite.

Table 5.5   H.261 compression ratios.

ISDN Bandwidth (Channels)	CIF				QCIF			
	30	15	10	7.5 fps	30	15	10	7.5 fps
64 Kbps (p = 1)	556:1	278:1	185:1	139:1	140:1	70:1	47:1	35:1
128 Kbps (p = 2)	278:1	139:1	93:1	70:1	70:1	35:1	23:1	18:1
384 Kbps (p = 6)	93:1	46:1	31:1	23:1	23:1	12:1	8:1	6:1

H.261 defines a data structure for encoding a sequence of pictures that allows a decoder to unambiguously decode the received bit stream. Each video frame is organized into a hierarchical block structure consisting of pictures, GOBs (groups of blocks), and macroblocks as shown in Figure 5.14. In turn, pictures are sequenced to form the compressed bit stream. The macroblock is the basic unit for encoding. It is composed of four 8×8 luminance blocks (Y) and two 8×8 chrominance blocks (C_B and C_R), where the chrominance blocks are formed by subsampling the chrominance pixels related to the corresponding luminance pixels.

Block diagrams for an H.261 encoder and decoder are shown in Figure 5.15. There are two modes of operation: intraframe coding and interframe coding. Intraframe coding is used for the first picture in a sequence; interframe coding is used for subsequent pictures in the sequence that are similar to the first picture. Intraframe coding removes redundancy within a picture. The steps for intraframe coding—DCT, quantization (Q), and entropy coding—are nearly identical to those for the JPEG algorithm, the primary difference being that the quantizer stepsize can be adjusted depending on the fullness of the encoder transmission buffer. H.261 does not specify how this should be done—it is an encoder implementation decision. In fact, only the decoding operation is completely specified by the H.261 recommendation. Encoder designers are free to make implementation decisions about when (or if) to use motion-compensated prediction, about how motion vectors are estimated, about controlling the encoder buffer rate, about controlling adaptive quantization to maintain uniform picture quality—about anything that does not corrupt the encoded bit stream or, thus, prevent the decoder from doing its job.

The second mode of operation, interframe coding, removes redundancy between similar pictures in a sequence. The technique used, motion-compensated prediction, was described in Figure 5.13 and the related discussion that appeared earlier in this section. In the H.261 implementation of motion-compensated prediction, only the previous frame is used for prediction, thus reducing the encoding delay. The previous frame is recovered (by Q^{-1} and DCT^{-1}) and stored in the motion-compensated prediction (MCP) memory. Also, during motion-compen-

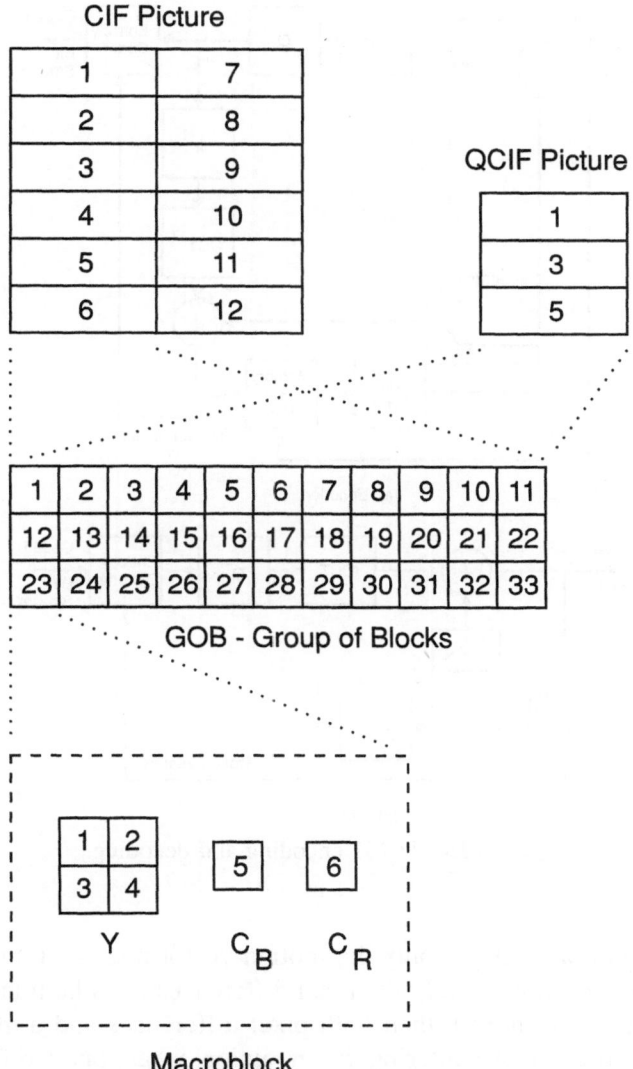

Figure 5.14   H.261 picture structure.

sated prediction, a loop filter may be used to improve picture quality by removing any high-frequency noise present in the picture. The encoder switches on the filter as needed. [To simply the encoder depicted in Figure 5.15(a), loop filter switching is not shown.]

The encoder chooses which mode of operation to use, intraframe or interframe coding, based on which will produce the fewest encoded bits. When the picture is changing rapidly, intraframe coding may give the best result, whereas for sequences of nearly similar pictures, interframe coding is preferred. Actually, there are several options the encoder may choose for interframe coding: If a macroblock has not changed or moved, no information need be transmitted. If

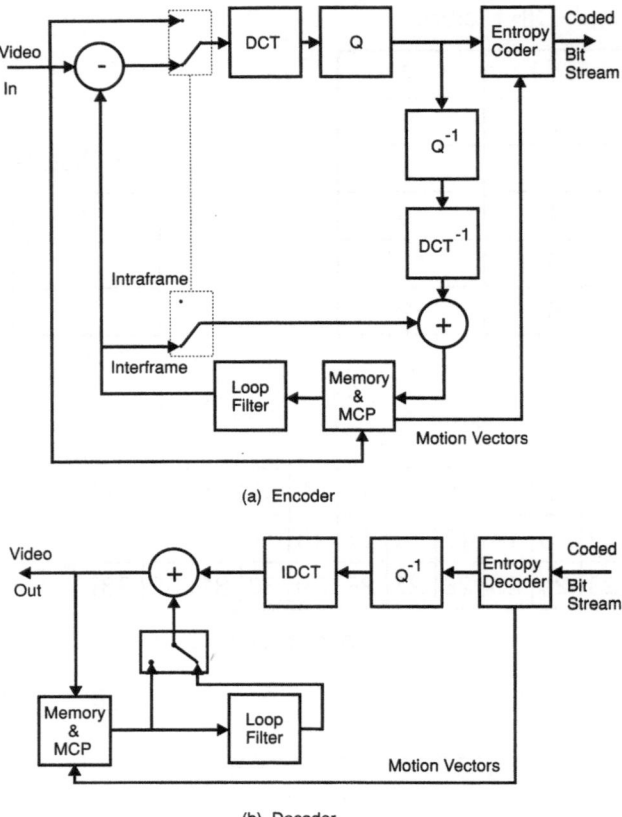

(a) Encoder

(b) Decoder

Figure 5.15   H.261 encoding and decoding.

it has moved but not changed, only the motion vector need be transmitted. If it has changed but not moved, only the pixel differences need be transmitted. If it has both changed and moved, then both pixel differences and a motion vector must be transmitted. Loop filtering is an option when pixel differences are transmitted and picture noise is present.

Although H.261 allows the encoder design to be flexible, there are requirements it must satisfy to assure the transmitted bit stream meets the standards set for decoding. To control error propagation, every macroblock must be intraframe coded at least once within every 132 transmitted picture frames. No more than 256 Kbps can be used to transmit each CIF frame (64 Kbps for QCIF). Thus, roughly 8 kilobits (2 kilobits) are the maximum allowed for each frame. As a result, the quantization step size may need to be increased during intraframe coding (or interframe coding be used). If neither can meet the transmission bandwidth constraint, then frame dropping is allowed.

H.261 is the most fully developed and widely deployed of today's digital video compression standards. Almost all room-size videoconferencing systems provide H.261 as an option, allowing them to interoperate with other manufacturer's products. H.261 is also specified for some desktop videoconferencing products. The H.261 compression algorithm, as should be apparent from our discussion, is somewhat complex, and when first available, it was expensive to implement. For several years after its introduction, manufacturers interested in low-cost, one-on-one desktop videoconferencing sought to find lower-cost solutions. However, advances in VLSI have made the cost of H.261 less formidable and the lure of interoperation with an established market for room-sized systems has brought many desktop videoconferencing equipment manufacturers around to H.261.

Although H.261 has established itself as a standard for videoconferencing, it has known limitations: One is picture quality at low transmission bandwidth. Some proprietary algorithms from manufacturers of room-size videoconferencing equipment provide higher-quality video at 128 Kbps or less [Trow94]. Interestingly enough, as noted in Chapter 3, H.261 allows parties with the same proprietary algorithm to negotiate and use it, retaining the H.261 compression algorithm as a fallback mode while operating completely within the standard [Port94, Trow94]. Another limitation is picture quality at higher transmission bandwidth, where proprietary algorithms for large room-size videoconferencing systems offer more resolution [Trow94]. In response, a new ITU-T standard (H.262, which specifies MPEG-2 video) will allow high-resolution videoconferencing over ATM (asynchronous transfer mode) networks, where increased bandwidth is available [Schä95].

MPEG

In 1988 the Moving Picture Experts Group (MPEG) began working to develop international standards for digital audio and video transmission and storage. The outcome of this joint effort by ISO/IEC has produced MPEG-1 and (together with ITU-T) MPEG-2. Soon, these standards will be joined by a third, MPEG-4. Just as H.261 is designed for particular applications and transmission media, the MPEG standards, as shown in Table 5.6, are too. MPEG-1 was designed for playback of stored multimedia and, by performing significant between-frame compression on limited-resolution pictures, aimed to get visually acceptable picture quality at the 1.2 Mbps video data rate provided by CD-ROM. MPEG-1 has also proved useful in other applications, such as for early DBS (direct broadcast satellite) transmissions and for computer-generated video, where transmission bandwidth and storage capacity are limited or expensive. In contrast, MPEG-2 is intended for both playback and conferencing, providing considerable flexibility in the amount of between-frame processing and the use of much higher-resolution pictures—at higher data rates. MPEG-2 can produce the video quality needed for multimedia entertainment piped to the home and for more demanding business and scientific applications too. MPEG-2 also supports the picture resolution and quality needed for HDTV. MPEG-4, a standard still in the making, has

Table 5.6 MPEG Parameters.

	MPEG-1	MPEG-2	MPEG-4
Final draft	1992	1995	1998
Data rate	≤ 1.86 Mbps[1]	≥ 4 Mbps	≤ 64 Kbps
Resolution - maximum	720 x 576[1]	1920 x 1152	na
- typical	352 x 240	Varies by application	na
Scanning method	Progressive	Progressive / interlaced	na
Frame rate - maximum	30 fps[1]	60 fps	na
Coding methods	DCT and BMCP[2]	DCT and BMCP	DCT and BMCP ? Object oriented ?
Applications	< SDTV-quality video storage on CD-ROM Computer-generated video < SDTV-quality video transmission	SDTV → HDTV-quality storage and transmission	Video on PSTN and mobile networks Video on low-capacity storage devices

Notes:
[1] MPEG-1 constrained parameter set maximum values [Chia95].
[2] Discrete cosine transform and bidirectional motion-compensated prediction.

a different set of objectives—to provide video on low-bandwidth transmission links or for low-capacity storage devices where no existing standardized video compression algorithm has proved satisfactory.

Each MPEG standard defines the syntax of an audio-video bit stream for storage or transmission and specifies both audio and video decoding algorithms.[18] Very much like H.261, but for different reasons, the video encoding approach is not completely specified. This allows trade-offs to be made between encoding time and compression efficiency or image quality. Asymmetric algorithms (complex, slow encoding and simple, fast decoding) are highly appropriate for most MPEG applications, which involve one-way communications—broadcasting or storage for delayed presentation. Here real-time encoding is not always needed, whereas improved compression ratios and improved image quality always are, and increasing the encoding time delay (and complexity too) may be a wise choice. From an economic viewpoint, asymmetric algorithms make sense because there are few encoders but many decoders for most one-way communications applications.

---

[18] MPEG audio was described in Section 5.3.

The MPEG standards (excluding MPEG-4 which is still in development and whose details are not finalized) can be considered the outgrowth of H.261, and JPEG too. The MPEG standards use variations of the same data compression techniques, and the details will not be repeated here. Instead, let us concentrate on the major innovations MPEG introduces beginning with the interframe compression technique.

Interframe coding and how compression is achieved through temporal redundancy removal are shown in the MPEG model for interframe coding depicted in Figure 5.16. MPEG-1 images are organized in groups of pictures (GOPs) that may be transmitted in an order different than the display order. GOP is an option for MPEG-2. Within a GOP, there are three types of pictures: intraframe pictures (I), predicted pictures (P), and bi-directional pictures (B). Intraframe pictures are complete pictures coded in isolation with DCT and quantization techniques similar to those used by H.261 and JPEG to remove spatial redundancy. Intraframe pictures provide random access points into the video stream, but they lead to only moderate compression. Predicted pictures are interframe coded with reference to the closest past I or P pictures. Like H.261, motion-compensated prediction is used for interframe coding. Predicted pictures provide more compression and serve as references for bi-directional pictures. MPEG departs from H.261 in using motion-compensated interpolation technique to perform bidirectional prediction for coding B pictures (those between I and P pictures). B pictures are coded using both past and future pictures as reference. They provide the most compression and, because they are never used as a reference, they do not propagate errors. B pictures allow MPEG to improve the quality of the compressed picture stream and to increase compression beyond that provided with H.261.

The MPEG standard allows the encoder to choose the frequency of occurrence

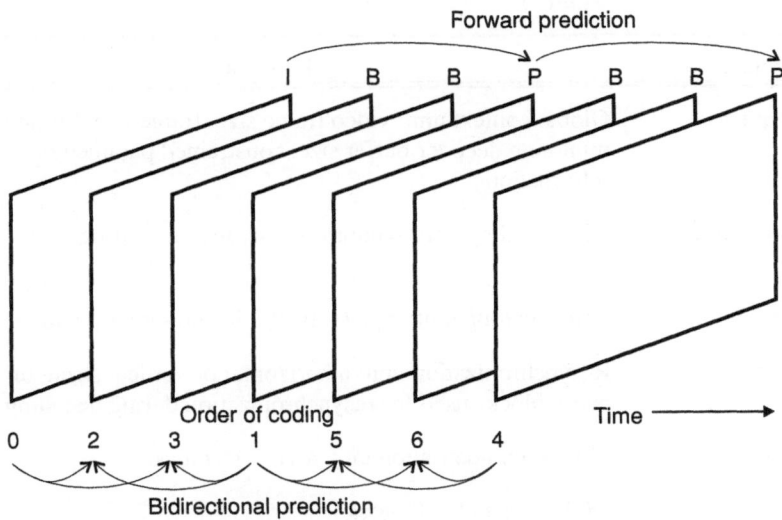

Figure 5.16 MPEG group of pictures.

of I, P, and B pictures based on application-specific needs for random accessibility, coding delay, visual image fidelity, and—most important for video transmission and storage applications—compressed video stream bit rates [Schä95]. Coding the bit stream with only I pictures improves random accessibility and editibility but achieves low compression. Coding with only I and P pictures achieves moderate compression while still allowing random access and fast-forward/fast-reverse searches through the encoded bit stream. Using I, P, and B pictures provides the most compression, as B pictures can be coded in very few bits, leaving more bits for I or P pictures. It is advantageous to use more B pictures but, as can be deduced from Figure 5.16, there is a downside. When the number of B pictures in a GOP is increased, the random access points into the video stream grow further apart and the encoding (and decoding, too) delay time grows longer, characteristics that many applications cannot tolerate. An implementation detail is that an entire GOP must be buffered to allow I, B, and P pictures to be resequenced and played back in the correct order; increasing the number of B pictures in a GOP increases the buffer size, a characteristic that many applications cannot afford. Movement within the video scene also affects the number of B pictures that can be used, necessitating the use of adaptive techniques to vary how many B pictures can be coded between I and P pictures [Chal95].

The MPEG bit-stream syntax is more flexible than that of H.261, reflecting the wider variety of applications anticipated for MPEG. As shown in Table 5.7, it is constructed in several hierarchical layers. Further details can be found in [Arav93, Chen93].

MPEG-2 is an algorithms toolset and also a set of performance specifications for various operating environments. MPEG-2 is a superset of MPEG-1 with the

Table 5.7 MPEG bit-stream syntax.

Syntax	Function
Video sequence layer	Global context unit: video frame size, frame rate, bit rate, minimum decoder buffer size, constrained parameters information
Group-of-pictures layer	Video coding unit: random access, search, editing
Picture layer	Frame coding unit: type (I, B, P), display-order position
Slice layer	Resynchronization unit: a horizontal or vertical string of macroblocks used for resynchronization during decoding
Macroblock layer	Motion compensation unit: a 16 x 16 block
Block layer	DCT unit: an 8 x 8 block

requirement that every MPEG-2 compatible decoder must also decode valid MPEG-1 bit streams. MPEG-2 introduces new coding features not found in MPEG-1 to accommodate the functionality and quality of an expanded range of applications. Enhancements include [Chia95, Schä95] the following:

- A choice of picture scanning methods, interlace and progressive scan, to fit television-oriented and computer-oriented applications
- A choice of chrominance signal encoding methods
- Two bit streams are defined, transport and program, to support transmission and storage media applications
- Spatial and temporal scalability is supported

The macroblock is the basic unit for MPEG-2 encoding. Each frame is composed of nonoverlapping macroblocks. Each macroblock is made up of four 8 × 8 luminance blocks (Y), one, two, or four 8 × 8 C_B chrominance blocks, and an equal number of C_R chrominance blocks. The chrominance blocks are formed by subsampling the C_B and C_R pixels related to the corresponding Y pixels. This results in the three different MPEG-2 chrominance signal encoding methods shown in Figure 5.17. The 4:2:0 format provides MPEG-1 and H.261 compatibility. The 4:2:2 and 4:4:4 formats are provided for future higher-resolution applications such as studio video coding [Anas94, Schä95].

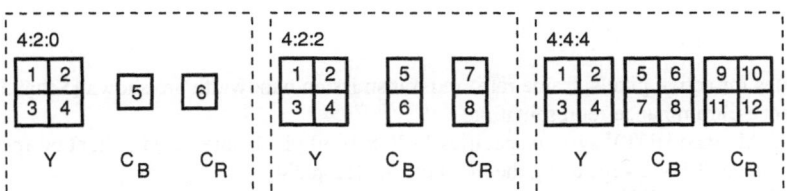

Figure 5.17   MPEG-2 macroblock structure.

The most expansive addition is support for spatial and temporal scalability through a set of "profiles" and "levels" which are shown in Table 5.8. In the spirit of "one size does not fit all," the intent is to allow equipment to be designed for interoperation at the profile and level that best matches an application. The profiles define the degree of functionality from no B frames (simple profile) to fully scalable video (high profile), with the main profile considered the most important profile having immediate application for cable, DBS, and SDTV/HDTV broadcasting. In general, moving left to right in Table 5.8, each successive profile includes new algorithms that build on those found in less functional profiles. Each profile is further divided into four levels which define various image resolutions. Within a profile, at any level, an MPEG-2 compatible decoder must decode bit streams from lower levels. As indicated in Table 5.8, only some profile-level combinations are expected to be used for known, practical applications.

If we take a closer look at the MPEG-2 profiles, we find that the simple profile

Table 5.8   MPEG-2 profiles and levels.

Level[1]	Profiles				
	Simple (No B Pictures) (4:2:0)[2]	Main (Nonscalable) (4:2:0)	SNR-Scalable (4:2:0)	Spatially-Scalable (4:2:0)	High (Fully Scalable) (4:2:2)
High - HDTV[3] 1920 x 1080 60 fps 80 Mbps	—	✓	—	—	✓
High - HDTV[4] 1440 x 1080 60 fps 60 Mbps	—	✓	—	✓	✓
Main - SDTV[5] 720 x 480 30 fps 15 Mbps	✓	✓	✓	—	✓
Low - SIF[6] 352 x 240 30 fps 4 Mbps	—	✓	✓	—	—

Notes:
[1] Maximum values for active pixels, frame rate, and transmission bandwidth are shown [Schä95].
[2] YC_BC_R luminance-chrominance representation.
[3] The U.S. Grand Alliance HDTV system specifies 1920 x 1080 pixels interlaced scan at 60 fps and progressive scan at 30 or 24 fps using the main profile [Hopk94].
[4] The U.S. Grand Alliance HDTV system specifies 1280 x 720 pixels progressive scan at 60, 30, and 24 fps using the main profile [Hopk94].
[5] SDTV (standard definition television) CCIR 601 studio standard compatible - 4:3 (and 16:9) aspect ratio.
[6] SIF (source input format) MPEG-1 compatible - 4:3 aspect ratio.

is a subset of the main profile where there are no B pictures. The main profile is an extension of MPEG-1 to include fields and frame pictures for interlaced video. The remaining three profiles (SNR scalable, spatially scalable, and high) deal with interoperation between video services and products where different bandwidth, spatial resolution, or temporal resolution capabilities must be bridged. The SNR scalable profile provides tools for quality scalability allowing, for example, recognizable video to be transmitted over limited-bandwidth channels. The spatially scalable profile addresses supporting displays with various resolutions. For instance, there would be no point in displaying an HDTV signal at full resolution on a small-screen receiver used for casual viewing. Here, SDTV resolution would be appropriate. The high profile supports full scalability, including temporal scalability where different frame rates can be bridged. Further details of MPEG-2 scalability can be found in [Chia94].

Together MPEG-1 and MPEG-2 are *the* video coding standards for television-based applications in the 1990's. The original application for MPEG-1 (storing movies for playback from CD-ROM) had but a brief moment in the limelight, and in its second application (DBS compression), it was quickly replaced by MPEG-2. But MPEG-1 has moved on, proving its merit for a variety of multimedia computer applications where quality video at moderate resolution is acceptable, low data rates are desirable, and inexpensive encoders and decoders are essential. And, thanks to both hardware and software implementations, MPEG-1 is available to all who choose to use it. For entertainment television, MPEG-2 has widespread endorsement, both from the standards-dominated communications industry and from the consumer-electronics industry that will build receivers for SDTV and HDTV applications. Mass production will assure a variety of low-cost MPEG-2 decoders, but it is unclear whether MPEG-2 encoders will be mass marketed or remain rare and expensive, as they will if MPEG-2 is used only for broadcast applications.

State-of-the-art video coding and beyond

Real-time video compression is leading-edge technology today. Although H.261 is a mature standard, widely deployed in commercial videoconferencing products, there is need for extending videoconferencing to networks other than ISDN. For general digital video applications, the MPEG algorithms and the MPEG standards are new and they are still being refined (or defined) to fit the products that use them, which are new too. Thus, there are opportunities and a need to advance video coding beyond the level set by H.261, MPEG-1, and MPEG-2. Here are some examples:

- Simplified encoding is needed for multimedia computing, digital VCRs, and other applications doing low-cost video source production. For these applications, symmetrical real-time compression is essential. M-JPEG and H.261 are more symmetrical (than MPEG) but do not always provide sufficient compression. Nonstandard, proprietary compression algorithms, some widely acclaimed as solutions for multimedia computing, may be more symmetric and may provide sufficient compression. But the problem is that they are not recognized as standards outside the multimedia-computing industry, particularly by industries that control the production of video source material.

- Economical frame-accurate random access is needed for digital VCRs. MPEG provides this function but at the cost of extensive buffering for groups of pictures.

- Preprocessing is needed to adjust the image before compression, not only to scale the image resolution but also to remove noise and provide whatever data-filter operations are necessary to make the compression process operate more efficiently.

- Postprocessing is needed to reduce the undesirable aesthetic effects of artifacts introduced by compression. This can be as important as the compression process itself, but it has received little attention.

- Better performance is needed at low bit rates. When operated at their lower design limits, today's DCT-based algorithms provide a picture with noticeable "blockiness." When an inadequate number of bits are available for transmitting DCT coefficients, blockiness artifacts make the discontinuities in gray-scale values between 8×8 blocks highly visible.

Of these, the most pressing need is for improved picture quality at lower bit rates because many "hot" applications for video have bandwidth or storage limitations far more restrictive than what current standards can deal with. In the brief history of video coding, the quest for ever-lower bit rates has been never-ending, as Figure 5.18 illustrates for the oldest, best-developed digital video application, videoconferencing. The progress in video coding for moderate-quality videoconferencing (QCIF resolution—176×144 pixels) has been nothing short of remarkable. Initially, intraframe coding and, later, the combination of intra-frame and interframe coding reduced the coding bit rate by nearly 30 times. But videoconferencing products and videoconferencing standards have been stuck at 112/128 Kbps for several years. With renewed interest in the most personal of all videoconferencing applications, videotelephony over analog telephone lines, and new interest in transmitting all kinds of video over mobile radio communications networks, it is clear there exists a class of applications that H.261 (or

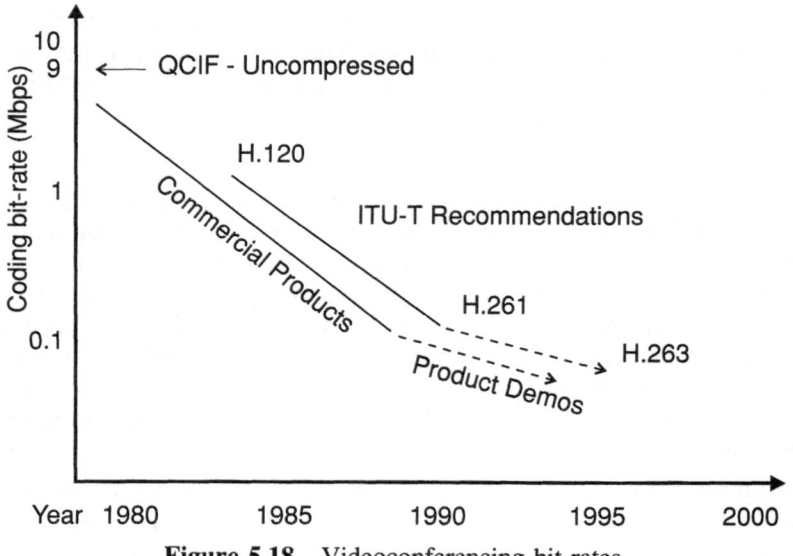

Figure 5.18   Videoconferencing bit rates.

MPEG-1 or MPEG-2) cannot serve. H.261 simply is not applicable to analog PSTN (public switched telephone service, i.e., POTS—plain old telephone service), where even 64 Kbps is problematical, and mobile radio communications networks—they are digital but offer even less bandwidth.

Recognizing a demand for this service, ITU-T has initiated efforts to develop new standards for video coding at rates of 64 Kbps or less. The first result of their efforts is the H.324 suite of recommendations that includes H.263, a new video compression algorithm designed to outperform but interoperate with H.261 [Port94, Mess95B]. The purpose of H.324 is to provide an international standard for interoperation of videotelephones connected to the PSTN, where, today, several noncompatible products exist. It also applies to interoperation of desktop videoconferencing computers connected to the PSTN. ITU-T is also working on a yet-unnamed standard, to be introduced in the 1998 time frame, that will provide for video transmission via mobile radio networks as well as the PSTN and provide more advanced performance [Scha94]. ISO is also focusing on a new standard for the 1998 time frame. ISO MPEG-4 will operate in these same environments and serve a wide range of applications, including videotelephone via PSTN and mobile radio. It will also address telecommunications, computer multimedia, and remote sensing applications that require a high degree of interactivity, interoperability, and flexibility. Included are communications with mobile experts, emergency crew communications, educational networks for remote areas, interactive editing and playback of audiovisual material, networked games, security and surveillance systems monitoring, and more [Scha94, Schä95].

All these new standards will employ "low-bit-rate video coding" techniques. The definition of what constitutes a low bit rate is a moving target, usually meaning any value lower than what existing algorithms can provide. In 1980, 1.5 Mbps was low-bit-rate video; today, it is 64 Kbps with mention of 10 Kbps as a future target. To reach 64 Kbps, or even lower, new approaches are required. Picture resolution and frame rates can be decreased, giving fewer pixels to process, but the negative impact on applications is severe; therefore, this is not a general solution.[19] The direction that H.263 will take is to improve upon existing inter/intraframe techniques: Smaller motion vector search windows for more precise prediction and refined motion vector quantization will reduce the number of bits to be transmitted. Optimizing entropy coding will help too. But long-range solutions mean moving beyond coding techniques based on blocks of pixels and their motion. To improve coding rates by an order of magnitude, which is what must happen to go below 64 Kbps, a new generation of coding techniques is required. These coding techniques most likely will deal with video content as

---

[19] Experience with current video coding algorithms teaches that about 25K luminance pixels per frame and about one-fourth this value for the chrominance pixels (i.e., QCIF resolution) at frame rates that approach 30 progressively-scanned frames per second are needed to achieve acceptable quality video for general applications [Ebra95].

something humans would recognize, rather than treating it as blocks of pixels. In Chapter 15, we will return to this subject and learn more about the coding techniques that future video compression algorithms will use.

5.6   Alternative Image and Video Compression Methods

Our introduction to compression algorithms for diffuse data has concentrated on the coding techniques used by the official standards. Many real-world applications do not use these coding techniques and standards, and no discussion would be complete without considering some of the alternatives. In today's marketplace, there are situations where nonstandard, proprietary compression algorithms are *the* de facto standards. This is most evident for image and video compression where the alternatives to official standard compression algorithms are numerous. There are many reasons this situation exists. The proprietary algorithms may have been there first. There may be marketing advantage in using them. They may be easier to implement, faster, and of lower cost. Most important, they genuinely may work better than the official standards. In this section, let us briefly consider three of the coding techniques frequently used by de facto standard compression algorithms. All are lossy compression methods that apply to images and video and, sometimes, other diffuse data types.

Vector quantization

Vector quantization compresses an image by replacing each block of pixels with an index into a codebook (or dictionary). Usually, the blocks do not overlap and all are the same size and shape, but they need not be. Within each block of pixels, each pixel value is treated as a component of a multidimension vector for reasons that will be discussed momentarily. To compress the image, as shown in Figure 5.19, the encoder cycles through its codebook and finds the stored

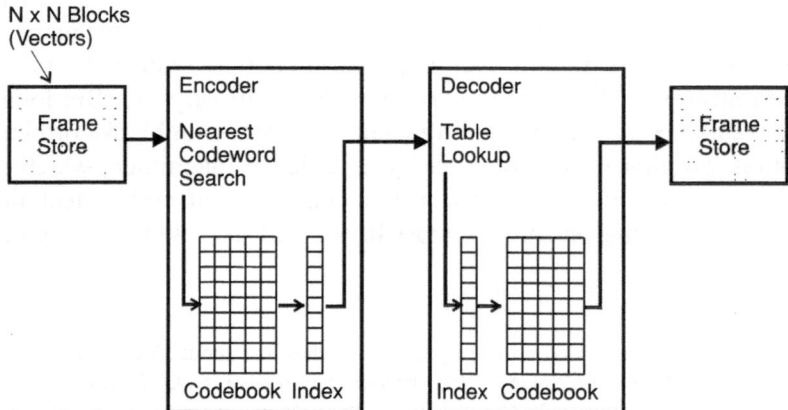

Figure 5.19   Vector quantization encoding and decoding.

codeword (or code vector) that best approximates each input block. The elements of this code vector are the quantized values of the pixels. When the match is found, the encoder transmits the corresponding index (codebook address) to the decoder. To decompress the image, the decoder maintains an identical codebook. The decoder reconstructs the image by looking up each index in its codebook and outputting the corresponding codeword. Because the compressed image is represented by indices, the compressed representation requires fewer bits. For example, assume each input block contains 4 × 4, 8-bit pixels and there are 16 codewords in the codebook. Because each codeword requires a 4-bit index, the compression ratio is 32:1.[20]

Does this process seem familiar? It should, because LPAS speech codecs use the same technique. (See Figure 5.2 and related discussion in Section 5.2.) Also, just as with speech coding, the difficult part of using vector quantization for image (and video) coding is finding efficient ways to search the codebook and deciding what codewords should be stored in the codebook. These issues are beyond the scope of this discussion, but extensive treatments can be found in several sources, including [Nasr88, Cosm93, Sayo95].

Vector quantization offers several advantages: The obvious one is that decoding is extremely simple, requiring only a table lookup operation. This makes vector quantization a favorite technique for software decoding and all applications where limited resources and time is available for decoding. Another advantage of vector quantization is that the quantization operation is more efficient than scalar quantization. All the previously described algorithms use scalar quantization, working on one component at a time. Vector quantization groups several components and encodes them as a single block. To appreciate why this is more efficient, consider that lossless Huffman coding is less efficient than arithmetic coding which groups symbols and encodes them as a single number. The same principle applies to lossy quantization, where, for a given bit rate, the result will be higher-quality images or video.

The illustration of vector quantization in Figure 5.19 indicates that it operates directly on the image pixels. Although this is how vector quantization is often used—because it is simple and effective—vector quantization can be combined with other signal processing techniques [Nasr88]. For example, one could use DCT or another form of transform coding and then quantize the transformed coefficients more efficiently with vector quantization. The result is better picture quality at lower bit rates. Another example is applying vector quantization for efficient video compression, a technique employed by several PC software video compression algorithms described in Section 9.6. When interframe coding is required, it is possible to develop vector quantizers that work in three dimensions on both intraframe and interframe components.

---

[20] In most vector quantization applications, the compression ratio is further increased by applying entropy coding to the codewords before transmission.

Wavelet coding

Basically, wavelet coding is a variant on DCT-based transform coding that reduces or eliminates some of its limitations. The name "wavelet" comes from the special localized *basis functions* used to break down an image (or other data) into its essential details. By using bursts of short-duration waves, rather than the continuous sinusoids used by the DCT, wavelet coding can more efficiently represent small features in an image such as the rapid transitions that occur at object edges. Another advantage is that rather than working with 8×8 blocks of pixels, as do JPEG and other block-based DCT techniques, wavelet coding can simultaneously compress the entire image. Thus, a wavelet-compressed image never suffers from the blocking artifacts apparent when block-based DCT techniques are pushed to high compression ratios. Taken in combination, these factors allow wavelet coding to offer higher compression ratios for a given image quality level. In some image compression applications, compression ratios as high as 300:1 are possible, several times greater than for JPEG and other DCT-based algorithms [Edge95A].

A two-dimensional spatial discrete wavelet transform (DWT) is used for coding digital images. Most often, this transform is used for coding video (as a sequence of images), but there also are three-dimensional DWTs. Essentially, DWTs are subband coding systems [Sayo95]. Therefore, as shown in Figure 5.20(a), the first step for compression is to process the entire image with a bank of filters conceptually similar to those used by the audio subband coders described in Section 5.3. The wavelet filters separate the image into a series of subbands of logarithmically increasing spatial frequency. The filter outputs create a set of transformed images at different resolutions that can be efficiently coded. The lowest-frequency subband contains a reduced-resolution, blurred copy of the

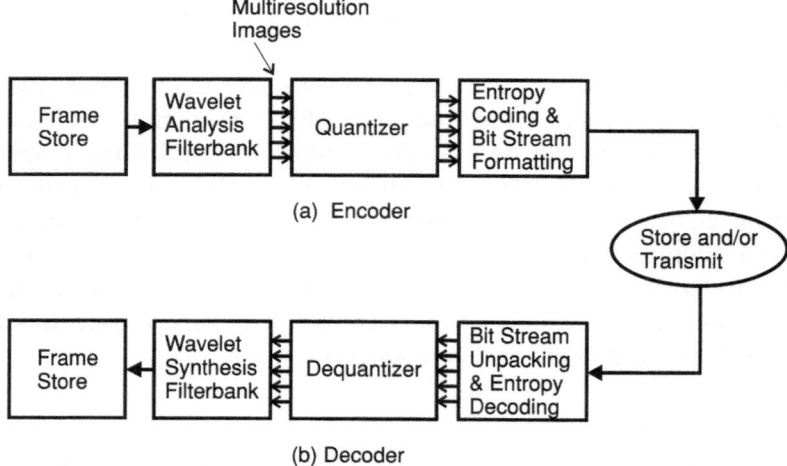

Figure 5.20 Wavelet encoding and decoding.

original image. The higher-frequency subbands contain edge information needed to reproduce the fine detail of the original image at successively larger resolutions. Because of the way humans perceive spatial detail, the wavelet coefficients for consecutively higher-frequency subbands can be quantized more coarsely. Either scalar or vector quantization can be used [Anto92]. The final step is to combine the quantized coefficients from all subbands and then entropy code them with run-length and Huffman or arithmetic coding. By reversing the encoding operations, the wavelet decoder shown in Figure 5.20(b) produces an approximate representation of the input image.

One of the advantages of wavelet coding is that it quite naturally supports progressive transmission and decompression of images; that is, by simply ordering the compressed image file, an image can first be displayed at low resolution and fine detail can be added as more image subbands are transmitted. The multiresolution characteristics of wavelet-compressed images can also used to advantage for wavelet-compressed video. When storage or transmission limits are encountered, image resolution can be temporarily reduced to produce slightly "softer" images. This, a form of quality-level scaling, is easily accomplished by dropping one of more of the subbanded images. In contrast, under the same conditions, those DCT-based compression techniques which do not use progressive transmission may deliver images with blocky artifacts or must resort to more drastic measures such as frame dropping.

Another advantage is that wavelet coding is a symmetrical coding technique which can be implemented either in software or hardware. Although often judged superior to DCT-based techniques in this and many other ways, wavelet coding is not a standardized technique. As such, it has found its way into only a few applications. These include PC software video compression (described in Section 9.6) and law enforcement applications including a fingerprint identification system implemented by the FBI (U.S. Federal Bureau of Investigation) [Hunt93].

Fractal coding

Fractal coding provides yet another alternative to DCT-based transform coding, one that can provide resolution-independent decoding and higher compression ratios at the expense of far more complex encoding. The term "fractal" comes from a Latin word meaning broken or irregular fragments. Fractals are shapes or pieces of images that can be described by mathematical formulas. Historically, fractals were first used to generate natural-looking images having the interesting property that they can be shrunk or magnified without loss of detail. The same mathematics is used to analyze an image and create a compressed representation that can be decompressed into resolutions which are both lower and higher than the original image. Fractal coding is a block-based technique, and although fractal-coded images may display blocking artifacts, in practice the compression ratio can be pushed to higher values that for images coded with block-based DCT coding. Although, in some situations, fractal coding can achieve compression ratios up to 10,000:1, results on real-world images suggest it is about three times more efficient than traditional block-based DCT (or vector quantization) algorithms at comparable quality levels [Jacq93, Boyd95].

The basic idea of fractal image compression is to exploit the self-similarity in an image by modeling a picture as several smaller pictures of itself. As shown in Figure 5.21, block-based fractal image coding accomplishes this in the following way: To compress an image, first, a pool of domain (D) blocks is created. These blocks will act as prototypes to represent the entire image. Then the image is broken into a set of nonoverlapping range (R) blocks. Typically, domain block sizes are 16 × 16 pixels and range blocks are 8 × 8 pixels. The block sizes are chosen to efficiently compress large, smoothly varying regions of the image. Also, each range block may be split into up to four nonoverlapping subblocks to capture fine detail in complex areas such as at object edges. For each range block, one by one, domain blocks are selected from the pool and through a series of transformations, known as affine transformations, are mapped to the range block. These transformations scale, translate, and transform pixels within the domain block (through luminance shifts, rotations, and so on). This process continues until a transformed domain block is found that closely approximates the range block. The list of block transformation parameters, known as the fractal code, is then transmitted to the decoder.

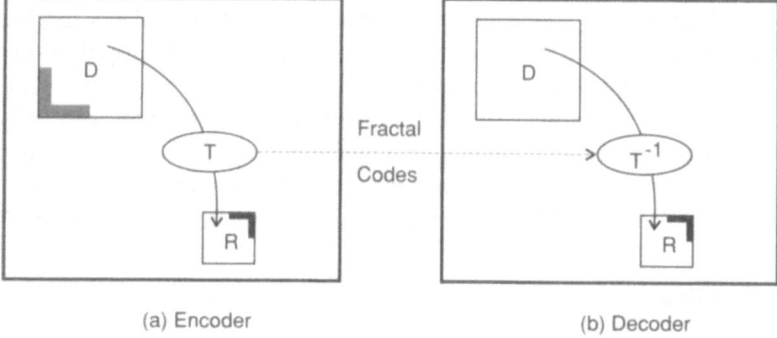

(a) Encoder   (b) Decoder

Figure 5.21   Fractal encoding and decoding.

Decoding is accomplished by iteratively applying inverse transformations. An interesting feature of fractal coding is that the domain blocks need not be transmitted because any arbitrary image can be used to start the reconstruction process. The pixels in this image can have any value—black, white, random, even pixels from another picture—for, iteratively, they will be changed to closely match those in the original image. The first application of the transformations generates an image containing rough approximations of the range blocks. Then, the transformations are applied to that image to better approximate the range blocks and so on. Usually, only a few iterations are required to create an image that closely resembles the original [Sayo95].

A limitation of fractal coding is that it is highly asymmetric because the process of searching for the best-matching domain blocks is computation intensive. Smart encoding strategies can reduce the workload, as there are classes of blocks whose similarity can be recognized (do they contain an edge, for instance) before applying the transformations. Also, most often, the best-matching domain block is found nearby the range block being coded. Decoding is far less complex, even less complex that DCT-based techniques, and most current implementations for both image and video coding are in software. Block-based fractal coding can be extended to three dimensions for coding image sequences, but this technique has not yet proven practical [Jacq93]. Therefore, current implementations for video coding, including those described in Section 9.11, operate on one frame at a time.

5.7 Summary

This chapter continued our introduction to data compression algorithms, examining some important algorithms for compressing diffuse data—algorithms incorporated in standards for speech, audio, image, and video. We learned the following:

- The algorithms described in this chapter were selected as standards because they meet the needs of the marketplace: They provide good quality compressed speech, audio, image, and video at reasonable data rates. They can be economically implemented in VLSI hardware (or, sometimes, software). Also, they can deliver speech, audio, and video data in real time.

- Diffuse data compression, particularly video compression, is still new, and although there already are many compression techniques to pick from, still more and likely better ones are possible. This, coupled with the continuing discovery of new applications for diffuse data compression, means the process of creating standards is hardly finished. In fact, the next generation of standards is already being defined.

- Powerful and complex models have been created for speech, audio, image, and video data. These models, based on the principles of human hearing and vision, use psychoacoustic and psychovisual perceptual coding techniques to exploit the limitations of human ears and eyes.

- Diffuse data is compressed by applying lossy compression, which throws away nonessential information, in combination with lossless compression for efficient coding.

- Speech coders represent speech using as few bits as possible while preserving its perceptual quality. Historically, they were developed for telephone transmissions, and, more recently, speech coders have been developed for new communications and storage applications that demand high-quality speech reproduction.

- Speech coders either use perceptual, waveform coding techniques related to audio coders or incorporate a model of the human vocal tract that achieves greater compression but only on speech.

- Many speech coding standards exist; some were abandoned when techniques offering improved quality at lower data rates emerged. Thanks to research, more complex, more powerful algorithms have been developed, and advances in VLSI technology (and software) support them.

- Audio coders exploit two psychoacoustic principles, thresholding and masking, to achieve compression. Some sounds are too soft for humans to hear; those that fall below the threshold of audibility can simply be ignored. Other sounds either are audible or are masked by louder sounds that temporarily raise the threshold of hearing; by adaptively assigning bits to audible and partially masked sounds, they may be recorded with only the degree of digital resolution necessary for high-fidelity reproduction.

- Multichannel audio coders achieve additional compression by exploiting the correlation between individual channels. Thus, state-of-the-art audio coders can deliver CD-quality audio using 64 Kbps per channel, reflecting a compression ratio of 12:1.

- Standards for audio compression exist as MPEG-1 and MPEG-2 audio, which are applicable to a variety of applications, and Dolby AC-3, which has been selected for transmitting HDTV audio and for a variety of other applications.

- Future applications will require that high-quality audio be coded at much lower bit rates, allowing it to be delivered along with low-bit-rate video.

- Image systems represent two-dimensional pictures as arrays of pixels, samples collected at regularly spaced points in the image. Compression is obtained by exploiting the correlation that exists between pixels and by exploiting psychovisual properties.

- There are many different types of images including bi-level, gray-scale, and color images, each demanding different compression techniques.

- Some image applications use only lossless compression, affording compression ratios as low as 2:1 or 3:1; others use combinations of lossless and lossy compression, affording compression ratios that can approach 100:1, or more.

- Lossless image compression exploits both spatial redundancy, the kind that exists between pixels in a region of the picture, and symbol redundancy, the kind found in the output bit stream produced by the coder. Lossy compression exploits irrelevancy to remove information from the picture that is unimportant to the human eye.

- Standards for image coding exist as ITU-T T.4 and T.6 for bi-level FAX images, JBIG also for but not limited to bi-level images, and JPEG for photographic-quality (continuous-tone) gray-scale and color still images.

- The coding techniques used by JPEG—DCT (discrete cosine transform), quantization, and entropy coding—also are basic to video coding.

- Among all types of diffuse data, image compression has the fewest, most-encompassing, extendable standards. Ignoring breakthroughs in image compression technology, which are always possible, future requirements are likely to be addressed by extensions to existing standards.

- Video systems represent video as a time-ordered sequence of pictures (frames).

- Video systems require compression that operates in real time at very high data rates, meets stringent transmission channel bandwidth limitations, provides compatibility with existing television broadcast and telecommunications transmission standards, and satisfies a marketplace with an ever-increasing demand for higher picture resolution.

- Video coding algorithms use a variety of techniques to reduce the number of bits to be coded plus interframe coding to remove temporal redundancy between frames, intraframe coding to remove spatial redundancy within frames, and (statistical) entropy coding to remove symbol redundancy in the output bit stream.

- Video coding algorithms that use interframe coding obtain compression ratios which typically are three times greater than when the video sequence is compressed with JPEG-like intraframe coding—at the same quality level.

- ITU-T H.261 and ISO MPEG are the first generation of video compression standards containing algorithms that are practical and effective for videoconferencing and television applications, respectively.

- The most pressing need continues to be finding new video coding algorithms that can operate at lower bit rates. Standards that will operate at 64 Kbps or lower are emerging or are in development.

- Vector quantization, wavelet coding, and fractal coding are alternative image and video coding techniques used by de facto standard compression algorithms.

Part III—Applications

This third part of the book provides a comprehensive guide to applications for data compression. For each application, we will examine the marketplace factors, including the role data compression plays in bringing the application to market, and consider the technical issues relating to data compression. We will show which data compression standards are applicable and provide a glimpse of future requirements.

An industry-by-industry overview of data compression applications is provided, beginning in Chapter 6 with computer applications. Communications applications are described in the next two chapters, network applications in Chapter 7 and broadcasting communications applications in Chapter 8. Consumer-electronics applications are described in Chapter 9, publishing applications in Chapter 10, and entertainment applications in Chapter 11. A healthcare industry application is described in Chapter 12.

Part III—Applications

6

Computer Applications

In this chapter, we examine applications in digital computers, where data compression is used for efficient storage of data and programs. Data compression is also used to conserve bandwidth in computer data communications networks, and those applications will be examined in Chapter 7. Most applications described in this chapter deal with symbolic data, the predominant data type found in traditional digital computers, and lossless compression techniques are needed. Where appropriate, we will examine how lossless techniques apply when these applications encounter diffuse data. Section 6.13 will explore multimedia computer applications. Here, diffuse data predominates and combinations of lossless and lossy compression are needed to compress speech, audio, image, and video data.

6.1 Industry Overview

Digital computers come in many sizes and configurations. The simplest are the microprocessors buried in many noncomputer products. Among products that the computer industry labels as *computer systems*, the smallest are portable, battery-operated mobile computers. Larger desktop and server computers are definitely not portable, but, generally, they are more powerful and offer greater storage capacity and communications capability. Distributed computers, really a collection of network-connected computers, are yet another type of computer system. Each of these computers have unique needs for data compression, which will be examined momentarily. The software needed to run computer systems realizes a competitive advantage by incorporating data compression too. Therefore, later in this chapter we will examine several computer software applications where data compression improves function, increases performance, and lowers cost.

In the computing industry, standards for data compression are problematical. Some computer applications for data compression are closed processes in the sense that compressed data is not shared or exchanged with other applications or with other computers. Computer disk storage compression is one such application. As a result, the computer industry has been free to develop and deploy a variety of algorithms for compressing data, particularly, symbolic data. Whereas within a particular application there may be widespread voluntary compliance with a single standard for compressing symbolic data, different standards often apply when the same data is compressed by other applications. Standards for compressing diffuse data pose problems too. The speech, audio, image, and video data compression standards developed for communications and other industries have proven to be difficult to adapt to computers. This has given rise to many efforts for creating new data compression standards to meet the needs of multimedia computing.

The computer industry was founded on symbolic data—text and numbers—and, therefore, many of its data compression applications involve compressing text and numbers. The addition of diffuse data—speech, audio, image, and video—is a relatively new phenomenon, producing new applications and a new definition of computing, *multimedia computing*. Today, multimedia computers are created by adding hardware and software—including compression technology—to existing computer systems as the need arises. Looking to the future, we explore how the practice of treating multimedia as an add-on may give way to new integrated designs. Another characteristic of today's multimedia computers is that the application programs mostly just compress diffuse data, then store and move it about with, for the most part, very little actual computing taking place. Later in this chapter we will examine how future multimedia computing applications may actually process diffuse data, sometimes transforming it to symbolic data.

Computer system organization

All digital computer systems are organized as shown in Figure 6.1.[1] The processor controls the entire system by executing programs stored in main storage. The main storage contains both programs and data. Programs contain instructions that the processor fetches, examines, and executes. Each instruction that the processor fetches from main storage specifies arithmetic or logical operations to be performed on data and specifies whether a result is to be stored back into main storage. Before any of this can happen, the computer must execute instructions to receive the programs and data from "the outside world," and when the computation

---

[1] Technically, only *stored-program* digital computers have this system organization.

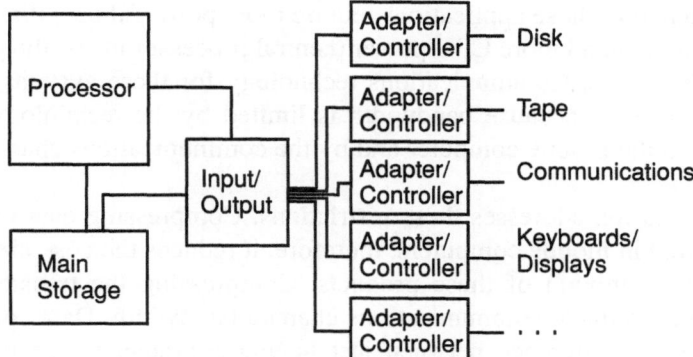

Figure 6.1 Digital computer system organization.

is completed, the results must be given to whomever posed the problem. Input/ output provides this function; via adapter/controllers, it connects the computer to I/O devices for creating, storing, transmitting, and displaying data.

Every digital computer presents many opportunities for compressing programs and data to use main storage, input/output data paths, and I/O devices more efficiently. In the sections that follow, we will examine these opportunities. First, let us consider the special needs for data compression in some important classes of digital computers.

Mobile computers

In the early 1990s, two of the hottest growth areas in the computer industry were portable PCs and multimedia computers. Mobile computers combine the best of both in one product. There are many types of mobile computers, including notebooks, laptops, palmtops, personal digital assistants, and wireless computers. They may operate standalone or be networked—wired or wireless. Products that recognize voice commands, allow input of handprinted data, provide image and interactive video display, and offer all that multimedia can promise are what is needed. The question is, How can all these functions be provided within the extraordinary limitations of mobile computers, including the following:

- Low cost
- Small size
- Light weight
- Low power consumption
- Limited communications bandwidth?

Mobile computer system designers are faced with finding processing and storage technology that will result in acceptable battery life and that will offer enough capacity to handle the high-function applications that the marketplace demands. Then, too, those applications require more powerful operating systems, which, in turn, demand more CPU power (central processor unit—the processor) and more disk space. Communications technology for these systems is just as much of a challenge because bandwidth is limited by the technology that can be packaged in the mobile computer and by the communications channels themselves.

Data compression addresses these restrictions. Compressing data reduces the storage required in mobile computers; therefore, it reduces the cost, size, weight, and power consumption of these products. Compressing the transmitted data maximizes the available communications channel bandwidth. Data compression can represent the difference between just having *a* system in the market and being there with the right system at the right price—and having the applications to sell that system.

There are many problems with enabling these products for multimedia—problems that data compression cannot address. Microphones, speakers, cameras, and CD-ROM drives must be miniaturized and their power dissipation must be reduced. Many innovations are required to package these components in mobile computers, along with the storage and processing logic necessary for multimedia. Clearly, highly integrated designs are required. To do data compression most effectively, a key element is a centralized compression facility—probably in CPU software or DSP technology.

Desktop computers

Desktop computers include both personal computers and workstations, their high-function cousins. The marketplace for both is defined by modular hardware platforms that allow users to tailor their systems with processor performance and storage capacity options. Another important feature is that a wide range of I/O devices can be connected to these systems. Desktop computers are built around a motherboard that contains the CPU and the main storage. They also include several adapter cards, each of which contains the control and processing logic and the storage needed to connect the various types of I/O devices.

There is a price to be paid for this modular flexibility, and nowhere is this more evident than in how desktop computers handle data compression. Some data compression is done in CPU software. It is a popular, low-cost solution for data compression of disks, tapes, and communications links lacking compression facilities on their adapter cards. The real advantage of software compression is that by trading idle CPU instruction cycles for reading and writing fewer bytes, it provides essentially transparent performance with essentially zero additional cost. Software compression works well with single-user, single-tasking operating systems like DOS, where CPU instruction cycles often go unused; it also performs well with multitasking operating systems like OS/2™ and UNIX if there are idle CPU instruction cycles. However, in the desktop system world, if software data compression performance is a problem, usually a processor upgrade is a low-cost option.

CPU software data compression is cheap and easy to provide, but it is not always the right answer. In the past even the fastest microprocessors were not fast enough to execute the data compression algorithms for speech, audio, image, and video data. This fact, coupled with the current highly modular and eclectic approach to enabling desktop computers for multimedia, creates a situation where some desktop products include unique data compression facilities for each source of speech, audio, image, or video data. A system may use several adapter cards, perhaps one for each I/O device type. Each adapter card may include hardware (or software) data compression that does the same thing, or nearly the same thing, as functions found on other adapter cards. Multimedia contributes to the price of a desktop computer, and one reason is duplication of functions, including data compression.

In a more integrated, low-cost approach to multimedia desktop computer design, one can envision how data compression could be centralized in the CPU. As discussed in Chapter 2, there is some movement today toward providing data compression functions in more powerful microprocessors, a design equally applicable to both mobile and desktop computers. Further discussion of the issues surrounding computer system design trends and where to do compression can be found later in this book in Part IV (Digital Systems).

Large computers—servers

There are many different products that can be rightly called large computers including PC and workstation servers, midrange or minicomputers, mainframes, parallel computers, and supercomputers. In the client-server computing world, these are the large computers that manage files and databases for client computers and control the interconnecting networks. They execute application programs too. Many companies offer a broad range of servers. For example, IBM server products include PS/2™, RISC System/6000™, AS/400™, ES/9000™, and the SP1™ and SP2™ Scalable POWERparallel Systems™.

Although it is convenient to label all these products as servers, because that is what they do, they are a diverse lot. Hardware configurations range from highly integrated, small deskside boxes to highly modular, room-filling systems. Their computation capabilities differ too. Most are general-purpose computers; super-computers and some parallel computers, which were once highly specialized for numerical computation, are also emerging as servers. Software is just as diverse too. In systems like AS/400, the operating system is highly integrated and is provided by one manufacturer. In other systems, including those based on UNIX, the operating system is highly modular, allowing the user to select database managers and other software components from various sources. Operating system structure, as we will learn, affects how effectively data compression can be applied and utilized.

Great diversity is also apparent in how data compression is used in large computers. Symbolic data compression is widely deployed in large computers.

Hardware-assisted compression facilities are available in CPUs, including the IBM ES/9000, and they are found in a variety of I/O control units for tape drives and disk subsystems from various manufacturers. Software compression is provided in a diversity of products, including database managers, communications network managers, and I/O device managers for tapes and other I/O devices. It is not surprising that symbolic data compression is widely used in large computers, as text and numbers are the "stuff" of digital computing and large computers were the first engines for doing digital data compression decades ago. In contrast, data compression for diffuse speech, audio, image, and video data in large server computers is still evolving. We will examine how in Section 6.13.

Distributed computers

Some computing problems are too geographically distributed, too large, or too complex for any single computer system. In these situations, as shown in Figure 6.2, connecting several systems through high-speed communication links to form a coupled, distributed computer can be an effective solution. Some examples are UNIX workstations running the CONDOR software package [Litz88] and PS/2-class systems running the ARCADE distributed environment [Cohn91]. This software allows LAN-connected workstations and PCs to distributively execute compute-intensive applications in parallel. Midrange systems, including DEC™ VAX™, IBM AS/400, and IBM RISC System/6000 systems, can be coupled (clustered) via high-speed, local communications links to take on commercial workloads once reserved for mainframe systems. Mainframe systems, the ES/9000 Sysplex™, for example, can be coupled via high-speed channels to provide affordable solutions for problems that are too large for any single system.

The success of any distributed computer depends on high-bandwidth, low-latency communications and quickly moving data—sometimes lots of data—and control messages between systems. So, typically, the fastest hardware links and

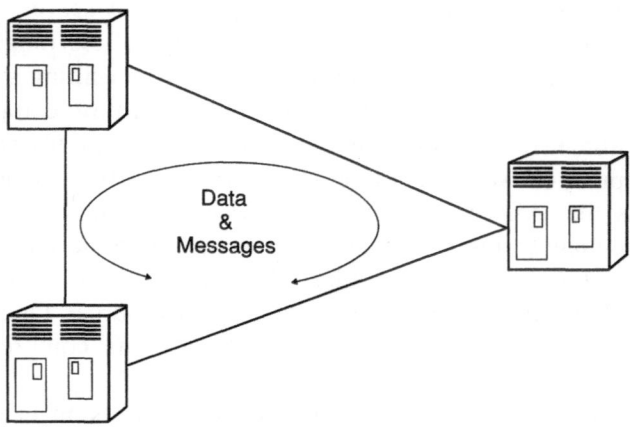

Figure 6.2   Distributed computers.

custom fast-path software are used. Noticeably missing from the distributed computers that have reached the marketplace is data compression on the interconnect links, and for good reasons. First, data compression usually is done in CPU software for the products cited above. Using the CPU to compress interconnect link-bound data improves the apparent bandwidth of the link, but it adds latency. It also steals CPU cycles, when making more CPU cycles available for computation is the reason for interconnecting systems in the first place. Second, all kinds of data are passed on system interconnect links. Contemporary data compression algorithms usually operate effectively on certain data types (text, for example) and not on others (images or video, for example).

In the future, perhaps data compression will prove useful for improving the performance of interconnected systems. In Section 6.12, we will learn how data compression is beginning to appear on chip-to-chip interconnections and, conceivably, variations of the same technology can be adapted to interconnection links. True, it adds latency, but hardware can reduce the latency, and the cost of data compression hardware is coming down. Furthermore, if data compression hardware is fast enough, it can reduce the total latency of the system because fewer bytes (bits) are transmitted over the interconnection links. Whether data compression will improve the overall performance depends on the speed of compression and the speed of the links. Granted, the 1990s is an era when finding system links that provide more bandwidth is perceived not to be a problem; just widen the bus or add another fiber. But there are situations where cost is a constraint or where systems must be interconnected over installed, low-bandwidth links, and, here, even software data compression makes sense. For instance, the balance between data compression and communications link speed/latency is likely to favor using data compression when distributed workstations or personal computers are interconnected via a low-speed LAN. Finally, data compression technology continues to advance and compressing a general data stream, selecting from a diversity of algorithms suitable to all types of data, may become an acceptable and affordable practice.

6.2   Computer Storage Hierarchy

Most computer systems employ a variety of technologies for storing programs and data. Computer storage is organized into a hierarchy of levels as shown in Figure 6.3. However, not all levels are used by all computers. Most modern processors (CPUs) operate on programs and data stored in a cache backed up by main storage, which, in turn, is backed up by the lower levels in the hierarchy. When information that is not in the cache is needed, the CPU hardware looks in the main storage and moves what it needs to the cache. The cache is small, it is fast, and each bit of storage is expensive; the main storage is larger, it is slower, and each bit is less expensive. This same relationship exists between all consecutive levels. Moving down the hierarchy, the storage capacity increases,

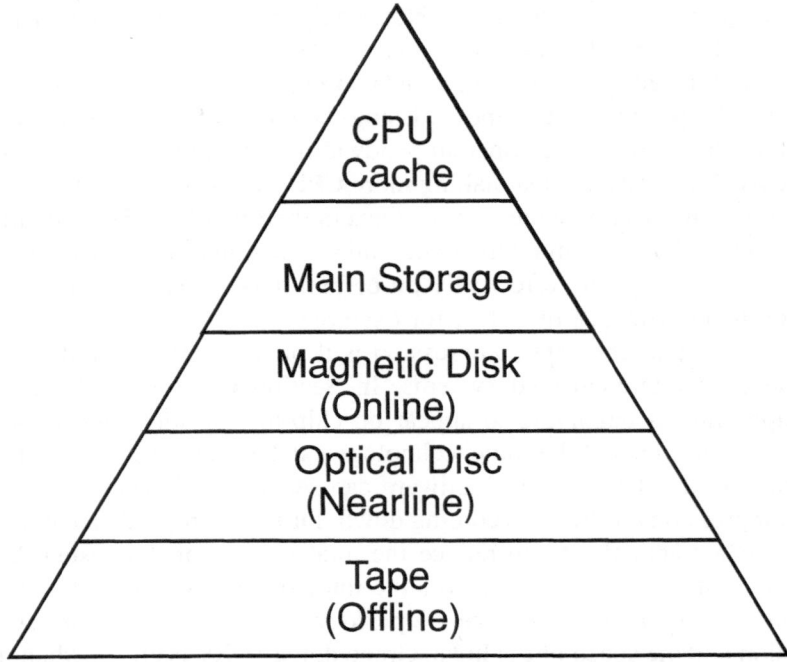

Figure 6.3 Computer storage hierarchy.

as do the storage block sizes and access times, while cost per bit decreases—all by orders of magnitude. It is common that lower levels of the hierarchy are designated by unique terms—online, nearline, and offline—referring to how quickly the storage can be accessed, with access time ranging from milliseconds for online magnetic disk to minutes for offline tapes.

The storage at each level is an expensive resource in terms of dollars, physical space, and power consumption. Therefore, intensive storage management strategies for data fetching, placement, and replacement are employed to make the best possible use of each level. By intelligently managing this hierarchy, locality of reference can be used to advantage; that is, processor storage reference patterns tend to be nonuniform and highly localized. Recently used data is likely to be reused soon, and data that is logically close to recently used data is likely to be referenced soon [Deit83, Pete85, Tane92]. By dynamically moving data between levels to anticipate processor needs, computer hardware and operating system software can make the computer system storage appear to have the capacity of the largest levels while having the access time of the fastest. Data compression is applicable too, allowing more information to be contained in each level of the hierarchy. In the immediately following sections of this chapter, we will examine how data compression improves the storage efficiency for each level of the hierarchy.

6.3   Tape Storage Devices

In the early 1970s, 3M™ and other manufacturers began producing ¼-inch cartridge tape systems for computer storage. Low data transfer rates and modest cartridge storage capacities limited their application to the least-demanding computer systems of that era. Data transfer rates and cartridge capacities gradually improved; yet, by the mid-1980s ¼-inch cartridge tapes were still unable to address the growing demand for archival (backup) storage, an opportunity presented by the then-booming market for workstations and midrange computers. True, ½-inch cartridge tape systems had become available, and they met the performance-capacity requirements of these systems, but they were too large and too expensive. Enter data compression. Since 1989, with the introduction of data compression, the market for ¼-inch cartridge tape has expanded greatly. Also, new cartridge formats (8-mm and 4-mm DAT) have been added. Today, almost every cartridge tape drive from almost every manufacturer has data compression, making compressed cartridge tape the archival media of choice for all small computer systems, including personal computers.

Actually, using data compression for tape storage devices preceded the introduction of compressed ¼-inch cartridges by nearly a decade. By 1970, nonremovable disk storage was becoming predominant, and online databases, although still relatively new, were growing rapidly. Consequently, the users of large computers begin spending more time copying data from disk to tape—moving older or infrequently used data into an offline archive, creating copies of active online data for offsite disaster recovery, or just creating backup copies. It was well known that data compression could improve the process—cutting the running time nearly in half—and software utility programs for compressing archival data soon appeared. By the 1980s, the need for compressing data to support archival *save/restore* operations for backup and recovery had spread to all sizes of computers. All types of tape storage devices were involved including ½-inch reel-to-reel, ½-inch cartridge, and the above-cited ¼-inch cartridge devices. Performance became an issue because software data compression was no longer fast enough for the tape storage devices used on large, multiuser systems. Therefore, the tape adapters and control units for large-system tape storage devices began incorporating data compression hardware.

When compared to other data compression applications, the tape compression/decompression process for data save/restore is uncomplicated. As shown in Figure 6.4, the save operation reads data from disk storage to a buffer in main storage. The data is blocked into records that contain hundreds to thousands of bytes and is then passed record by record to a compression function. This can be either a CPU software program or hardware logic in the tape I/O adapter or control unit. Each compressed record is buffered before being written to tape. The restore operation reverses the process. There are three important points to note: First, only lossless compression is appropriate because the restore operation must

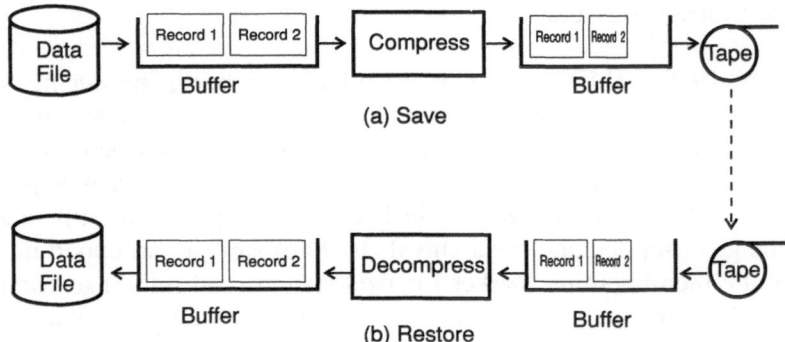

Figure 6.4   Compressed tape save/restore.

produce an exact, bit-identical copy of the original data. Second, when fixed-length records are compressed, variable-length records are produced; the number of bytes in each compressed record depends on the data. However, storage and retrieval of data from tape are unaffected when variable-length records are produced by compression because data is always stored on tape in variable-length records, whether uncompressed or compressed. Third, compression/decompression proceeds record by record, with variable-length records written to and read from tape one after the other. Sequential processing greatly simplifies handling compressed data, allowing data to be efficiently stored on tape with no wasted space and to be efficiently retrieved. In contrast, disk compression, which we will examine in the next section, requires random access to data and is much more complex.

Standards for compressed ¼-inch tapes were first introduced in the late 1980s by QIC, the Quarter-Inch Cartridge Drive Standards, Incorporated group. Before QIC, standards for compressed tapes were not given high priority. The conventional wisdom of the time was that, because save/restore is a closed process, any effective lossless compression algorithm could be used because tapes usually were read back on the system where they were created. There was little need for interchange, thus, rendering a standard unimportant. However, with the passage of time, interchange and the needs for standards have become far more important. Not only have many software data archiving products been introduced, but the number of hardware products that include data compression has grown too. Examples include ¼-inch cartridge tape drives from various manufacturers, ½-inch reel-to-reel tape drives such as the IBM 3430 for System/38™ and AS/400, and ½-inch cartridge tape drives such as the IBM 3490 for AS/400 and ES/9000 [IBM1].

As shown in Table 6.1, the hardware products mentioned in this section use different data compression techniques. In systems that include several of these products, managing the inventory of compressed tapes becomes a challenge. For example, when an older product is replaced, the tapes it has produced may still

Table 6.1   Compression standards/algorithms for tape.

Tape Product	Compression Standard / (Algorithm)	Lossless Coding Techniques Employed
¼-in. Cartridge	QIC-122	Lempel-Ziv [Ziv77]; Stac Electronics adaptation
¼-in. Cartridge	QIC-130	Lempel-Ziv [Ziv78]; H-P™ adaptation
¼-in. Cartridge	QIC-154	Lempel-Ziv [Ziv77]; IBM adaptation
½-in. IBM 3430 Reel-to-reel	(HDC)	Run-length encoding; IBM adaptation
½-in. IBM 3490 Cartridge	(IDRC)	Adaptive binary arithmetic coding; IBM adaptation

be important. So, they must be read and transcoded if the compressed format of the replacement product is different. Introduction of the QIC standards was meant to simplify the interchange of compressed tape cartridges between systems and tape drives conforming to those standards. However, there are now three QIC standards and each uses a different lossless compression technique. Therefore, the interchange and management issues, including the need for transcoding between different formats, really have not disappeared—even for ¼-inch cartridge tape.

6.4   Magnetic Disk Storage

With the introduction of the IBM PC-XT™ in 1983, personal computers began using magnetic (hard) disks for storing computer programs and data. Disk storage capacity grew to 10, 20, and then 40 MB, but programs and data grew even faster. By 1990, personal computer users hungered for more disk storage, but not for long. The manufacturers of data compression technology for computer tapes recognized that their algorithms could be adapted for disk, that data compression could double the apparent disk capacity, and that the Intel and Motorola™ microprocessors used in personal computers were powerful enough to run data compression—in software. Disk data compression programs, including Stacker from Stac Electronics and products from several other manufacturers, quickly followed. By the mid-1990s, disk capacity increased sharply (one gigabyte or more was typical for desktop personal computers in 1996), which provided some relief. But more powerful, larger operating systems and application programs that use more and more multimedia features continue to push the demand for storage, and, thus, disk data compression is still a popular option[2].

The story of disk data compression, like tape, begins in the early 1970s. If tape could be compressed, why not compress disk, too, as it is an expensive resource. For many years, compressing disks was considered too complex because disks allow data to be randomly accessed. When a block of compressed data is accessed, decompressed, updated, and recompressed, the number of bytes can

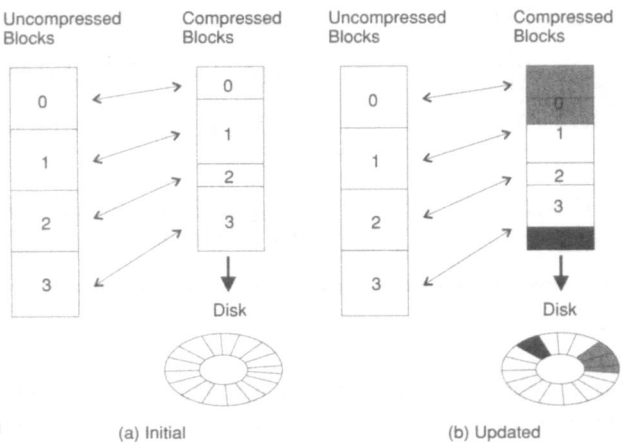

Figure 6.5   Compressed disk.

grow or shrink. As shown in Figure 6.5, block 0 has grown after being updated, and it will not fit back into its assigned disk location. Conversely, block 3 has shrunk, leaving unused space (a "hole"). Early disk compression products could not deal with these situations. They were limited to compressing read-only or infrequently updated data collections. For instance, one product provided online access to compressed, read-only, full-text database files via indexes [Snyd70]. Other products used batch programs to compress entire files, which allowed them to be archived online (or on tape) and restored as needed [Rait87]. Modern archiving utilities such as ARC, PKZIP, and many others provide similar functions [Nels92].

File management systems

For the online environment, what is needed is on-the-fly compression that can handle random updates; older designs for handling disk compression dynamics are not adequate. We will consider two on-the-fly compression schemes used by

---

[2] With disk compression now a standard feature of Microsoft operating systems and with larger disk drives, the demand for Stacker and other stand-alone disk compression utilities has fallen off [Leac96]. Stacker development has been discontinued, perhaps an ironic outcome of the 1994 Stac-Microsoft settlement (described in Section 3.5).

the file management components of modern operating systems. The first, file-by-file compression, is an extension of batch compression archiving programs. In file-by-file compression, user calls to open and close files are intercepted by the computer operating system software. When the user opens the file, the entire file is decompressed; when the user closes the file, it is recompressed. File-by-file compression provides transparent, random access and it is simple to do, but it has limitations. When a file grows large, the opening and closing times can be long [Mons91]. Also, if a file is shared by many users, storage savings are questionable because an uncompressed copy must be available whenever the file is in use. Thus, file-by-file compression may be more appropriate for single-user desktop systems than for large, multiuser systems. File-by-file compression packages are available for Apple Macintosh™ desktop computers [Greh93, Brya94].

A second technique, which we will call block-structured disk compression, works by intercepting disk reads and writes. Whenever the file management system requests data from disk, a small block of data is read from disk, decompressed, and placed in main storage. ("Small" will be defined shortly.) After data within the block is modified, the entire block is recompressed before being written back to disk. This provides for a complete, general-purpose solution that allows random updates and that operates unobtrusively, performing compression and decompression on-the-fly in real time for single-user and multiuser systems. However, it requires new disk storage structures and new disk storage management techniques.

A simplified block-structured disk compression scheme is shown in Figure 6.6. Disk storage is viewed as a logical single-level storage containing fixed-size GOBs (group of blocks); each GOB contains several data blocks.[3] Typically, each block is 512 bytes to 4 KB in size. Each block is stored in one or more disk sectors. A GOB may be 4–32 KB or larger. The GOB size is chosen to balance two constraints: Because all blocks within a GOB are compressed and decompressed as a group, a GOB must be large enough so that the compression algorithm—usually an adaptive Lempel-Ziv algorithm—can be most effective; but the GOB must not so large as to incur obtrusive running times for compression and other disk storage management operations. When compressed, each GOB is stored on disk in one or more physical sectors. Storage management tables (not shown) control the mapping from logical to physical storage.

There are many choices for how to manage disk storage to accommodate the varying number of physical disk sectors needed to store a GOB [Deit83, Pete85, Tane92]. At one extreme is the contiguous file storage scheme shown in Figure 6.6(a), where a GOB is always written to a home area and, if the compressed GOB is too large, the excess is placed in an overflow area. Other designs are

---

[3] Various terms are used to describe GOBs and blocks. MS-DOS uses "clusters" and "sectors." Paged virtual memory implementations, such as UNIX, use "blocks" and "pages."

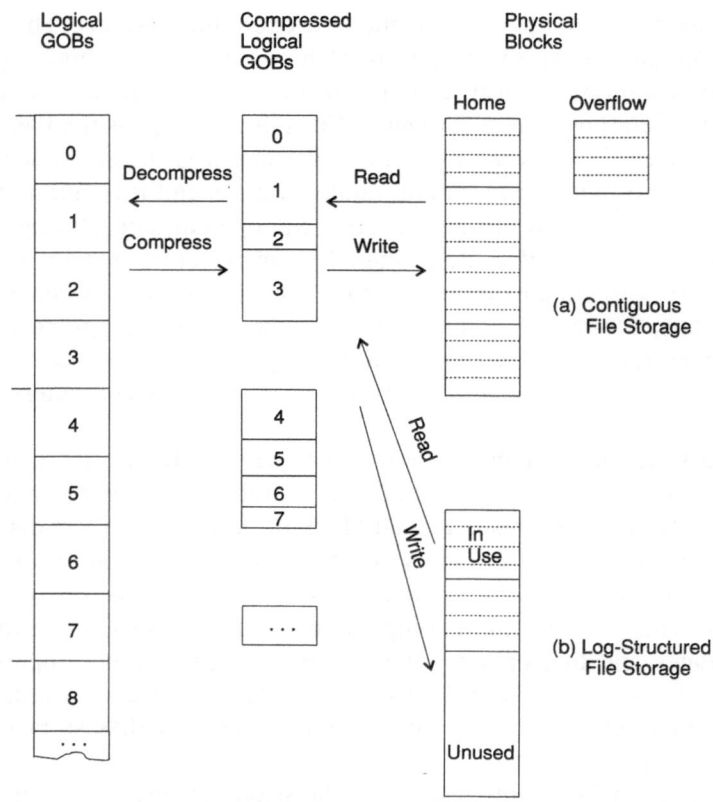

Figure 6.6   Block-based disk compression.

more dynamic, placing a newly compressed GOB into whatever free space is available on disk. The log-structured file system shown in Figure 6.6(b) is the most dynamic of all because it always finds a new location in free space to write a newly compressed GOB [Burr92]. File system design involves many issues beyond the scope of this book. The only point we wish to make here is that compression can be accommodated, no matter which scheme is chosen.

Many on-the-fly, block-based disk data compression products are available for both IBM-compatible PCs and for the Apple Macintosh [Mons91, Trow91, Greh93, Harr93, Stry94]. Although both software and coprocessor hardware products are available, software captured the marketplace in the early 1990s. It is inexpensive, and—by using the idle cycles most desktop and mobile computer systems have available—it is fast enough. Software compression does not require additional hardware, a big advantage for mobile computers where space and power consumption are priorities [Greh93]. Software compression is also used in large systems, including the IBM RISC System/6000, where the IBM AIX™ Version 4.1 operating system offers software for dynamic file system data compression [IBM2], and DEC VAX and Alpha AXP™ systems, where Intersecting Concepts Inc. offers DiskMizer™, a software file compression product [Inte94].

Disk subsystems

Large computer systems have unique disk storage requirements, if for no other reason than they use so much of it. Increasingly, large computers have assumed the role of data servers because they can manage large data collections for a great number of users. Mobile, desktop, and many midrange computer systems may use integrated disks for their storage, but large systems, such as the server shown in Figure 1.5, need disk subsystems. Only by distributing functions—offloading disk data management software and hardware functions from the large-system host CPUs to disk subsystems—can the largest possible storage configurations be managed effectively.

Disk subsystems are logically and physically separate digital systems. They provide the same disk management functions provided by the host CPU and its file system software—but they are expressly designed to manage very large collections of disk storage devices. Data compression is an important new tool allowing disk subsystems to meet the growing demand for more capacity. Data compression is an answer for floor space management because fewer disk devices are needed to contain the data. It also improves the effective data transfer rate of disk devices, causing the data to be delivered faster, which is appealing to both users and disk subsystem manufacturers.

The evolution of disk subsystems has resulted in the outboard migration of caching, processing, and programmability functions once reserved for operating system file management program logic. Modern disk subsystems, particularly those incorporating RAID (redundant arrays of independent disks), already provide many functions that are essential to support data compression. These functions include the following:

- Device space management for relocation and dynamic mapping to manage variations in record, block, or file storage size on update
- Device capacity management of addressable data blocks on the disk drives
- Buffering to manage data rate variations
- Caching of data for read and for update
- Time stamps and other techniques for managing multiple versions of data
- Error handling and recovery

For state-of-the-art disk subsystems, such as the one depicted in Figure 6.7, this allows data compression to be added for a reasonable additional cost. The new functions required for data compression may include file management support such as a log-structured (journaling) file system, garbage collection to keep sequentially accessed data gathered together, and nonvolatile memory for caches and indexes. A significant inhibitor for developing compressed disk subsystems is making compression transparent to the host CPU operating system. For example, the available disk drive capacity—both the real capacity and that consumed by compressed data—is of interest to users of the host CPU and, therefore, to its operating system. One effective solution is to revise the host operating system—to

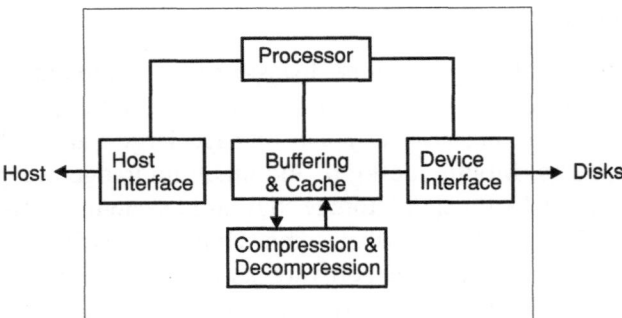

Figure 6.7   Disk subsystem.

make it aware of compression—creating new commands, features, and characteristics at the interface between it and the disk subsystem. Another solution is to achieve compression transparency through device emulation.

The Storage Technology Iceberg™ 9200 Storage System is a disk subsystem that provides transparent data compression through plug-compatible emulation of IBM 3380 and IBM 3390 disk drives [Cost92]. Plug compatibility, a technique widely used by many disk drive makers, means that with minor exceptions all commands and features of the IBM products are emulated, including the disk organization and track format. What is involved here is reformatting data from the host and mapping it to the disk organization and track format of the plug-compatible drives, which Iceberg does, as do products from many other manufacturers. What Iceberg does differently is to compress and compact the data during reformatting. Compression is done by a proprietary variation of the Lempel-Ziv dictionary algorithm, implemented in hardware ASICs (application-specific integrated circuits) designed specifically for this product. Compaction comes about by reformatting records written in count-key-data format[4] to eliminate gaps within records and, ignoring disk track boundaries, by packing records to eliminate unused space at the end of tracks [StoTek2]. In Iceberg, the length changes introduced by compression and compaction are handled by a dynamic disk data management architecture that writes each updated track to a new location and frees the physical storage in the previous location for reuse.

For Iceberg, the combination of compression and compaction typically results in a 3:1 compression ratio, roughly tripling the effective disk capacity [Cost92, StoTek1]. Internally, Iceberg compresses data immediately upon receiving it from the host system, only decompressing data when returning it to the host. This increases the effective data transfer rates on its internal data paths and improves utilization of its internal cache storage. Externally, the host system

---

[4] Count-key-data is the format that IBM disks use for variable-length records. Gaps are inserted between the count, key, and data fields on the disk. A variable number of records are recorded on a disk track, which may leave unused space at the end of each track.

views Iceberg as an IBM 3990-3 storage controller that manages up to 256, 3380 or 3390 disk volumes with a maximum addressable functional capacity of 726 GB. In practice, given the expected compression ratio, the physical storage capacity need be only about one-third the functional capacity. Iceberg can be installed and operated with no host software changes and no proprietary software. However, to optimize Iceberg's functional and performance characteristics, such as using physical storage to its maximum capacity, Storage Technology provides users with a host-based software package that provides reports and tools which allow them to fine-tune operations.

Disk compression issues

All of the disk compression products mentioned above use some variant of the Lempel-Ziv compression algorithm described in [Ziv77]. This algorithm is well suited to the task because it is adaptive, allowing it to effectively compress all kinds of data, and because it can efficiently compress data blocks as small as a few thousand bytes, the size of the data blocks written to disk. There are no standards, nor need there be, as disk data compression is a closed process.

Compression ratio and performance are two issues that affect the application of disk compression to computer systems. For the most part, compression ratio is a concern only when disk storage is running at or near its rated physical capacity. Extensive observations of computer systems, both large and small, show that users should expect a disk compression ratio of 2:1 or 3:1—typically. The problem is that for a specific application it may be lower or higher and it may change; there are no guarantees. The most disastrous consequence occurs when the physical storage is nearly full, for then even what may seem like a minor change to the data can unexpectedly trigger an out of disk space condition. Fortunately, commercial disk compression products anticipate this situation and provide their users with warnings and tools to avoid it.

What about performance: Will disk compression make the computer system slower or faster? The answer is, "it depends." Extensive studies of disk compression in the desktop environment show that compressed systems, even those using software data compression, perform about as well as uncompressed systems [Trow91, Burr92]. Factors that determine how well a compressed system performs include the following:

- Processor speed (if software compression is used)
- Hardware speed (if hardware compression is used)
- Disk speed
- Type and intensity of disk access

Observed results suggest applications that do little other than read and write disk data, in particular, file copy operations that access large blocks of data may run slower with a compressed disk. Applications that randomly access small blocks of data, particularly those that do many reads and few writes, may run faster with a compressed disk. In general, when the data blocks are small, performance depends mostly on the disk seek and rotational delays; compression processing time is minimal. As the block size grows, compression processing time also grows but is offset by a higher effective data rate for transfers from the disk device (because more data is stored per disk revolution). The compression processing overhead in either case can be reduced by making an investment in additional CPU performance (if software compression is used) or in compression hardware. In any event, if, because of deploying data compression, the number of disks in an installation is reduced—for example, to shrink the floor space occupied by a disk subsystem—performance may degrade because there will be fewer disk arms. The only sure way to know how disk data compression will affect system performance is to rely on performance modeling (or measurement).

The disk data compression technology we have described is appropriate for traditional computer data processing applications where information is represented by symbolic data stored in small, randomly accessed blocks. What is appropriate when computers and their disks are used as servers for speech, audio, image, and video data? Do lossless Lempel-Ziv compression and the storage structures described above still apply? They do, but with these limitations:

- Speech, audio, image, and video may already have been compressed before being presented for storage by using algorithms specialized for the particular data type. If so, Lempel-Ziv or any other lossless algorithm is unlikely to further compress the data—they may expand it. In this situation an effective solution is to switch off disk compression when it cannot be effective. This can be accomplished manually if the data type is known, or automatically by testing the effectiveness of disk compression when the data type is unknown. A more sophisticated but costly strategy is to always try several compression algorithms and select the one which affords maximum compression.

- Speech, audio, image, and video data typically occupies much more storage than symbolic data. However, often it is accessed sequentially in large blocks. Furthermore, in many server applications, this data is updated infrequently. Given these conditions, the data storage structures described above can be used, but other less dynamic storage structures, optimized for larger data blocks, may be even more effective.

6.5   Optical Disc Storage

Optical disc storage provides a level in the computer storage hierarchy intermediate between magnetic disks and tapes. Optical discs are used individually or loaded into optical jukebox subsystems that contain several hundred discs, any of which can be accessed within a few seconds. They provide storage of documents and images for medical, legal, government, and many other archival applications. There are many types of optical media that fall into two broad classes, those that are writable and those that are not. In this section we will consider data compression for writable optical discs used for computer storage. In Chapter 9, we will describe both writable and nonwritable optical discs for consumer-electronics products and other applications.

For computer storage, WORM (write once read many), MO (magneto-optical), and the still emerging PD (phase-change dual) discs store information in sectors and concentric track formats that are similar to magnetic disks. They also access data in the same way—randomly, but not as quickly as magnetic disks. Two emerging media, CD-R (CD-recordable) and CD-E (CD-erasable), store data in the spiral track format common to CD-ROM. Like WORM, CD-R is a write-once media. Somewhat tape like, CD-R and CD-E provide semiserial access to large blocks of data that can only be read or written beginning with the file information recorded at the front of each file.

Data compression can be effectively applied to all these optical media. The methods used are essentially the same as those described in Sections 6.3 and 6.4 for tape and disk. Tape like methods apply to CD-R and CD-E; disk like methods apply to WORM, MO, and PD optical discs. Implementations include both CPU software and optical storage subsystem hardware (and software) [Stee91]. Software solutions are appropriate for CD-R and CD-E which require a premastering process to format the data into sectors, add headers, and compute error-correction information [Kals95]. Software has also been used for WORM compression, where, traditionally, software in the host CPU is intimately involved with managing the unique write-once characteristic of this media. Optical storage subsystems are available that handle a mix of WORM and MO writable media and compress both using hardware-implemented, tape like Lempel-Ziv lossless compression [VARB93].

Various compression algorithms are used; there are no standards. This, perhaps, reflects the diversity of today's optical discs—different drives, media, computer system interfaces, and software for running the drives—making interchange of data on optical discs impractical. The optical storage industry, through its trade association, OSTA (Optical Storage Technology Association), is moving to change this situation. They are defining guidelines for implementing the ISO/IEC 13346 standard for media and file interchange of data on removable write-once and rewritable optical discs [OSTA95, Zoll95]. However, whereas the standard does address data compression, the first implementation of ISO/IEC 13346 does not.

6.6 Solid-State Files

Solid-state files are data storage devices that use electronic memory to provide a high-performance alternative to electromechanical storage devices. In computers, solid-state files are primarily used for mobile applications where nonvolatility, small size, low power consumption, and ruggedness are paramount. Among the technologies used are flash memory and RAM with battery backup, both providing permanent, writable storage, and ROM that provides permanent, read-only storage. The same technology is also useful for a variety of consumer-electronics products, including digital cameras, cellular telephones, set-top boxes, and hand-held data collection devices. It is also useful in other portable applications such as heart monitors where these same factors are important. Solid-state files are available in several configurations on PCMCIA cards, a computer industry standard plug-in card for portable computing environments [Ande94]. Solid-state files using flash memory are available on several even-smaller card formats intended for both computer and consumer-electronics applications [Webe96].

Data compression is useful for reducing the cost or increasing the apparent capacity of solid-state files. Even with compression, applications for solid-state files are restricted to a few megabytes of storage as the per-bit cost of electronic memory is many times higher than for magnetic or optical media. Today, cards with up to 16 MB of solid-state storage are available and prototypes containing even more megabytes have been demonstrated. But the cost for many speech, audio, image, video, and other high-capacity applications remains prohibitive, making economical computer applications (and many consumer-electronics applications) years away [Norm95].

Solid-state files are organized so that they appear to the computer system as if they were disk storage devices. Disk like compression techniques such as those described in Section 6.4 are applicable.

6.7   Main Storage

Certainly all levels in the computer storage hierarchy are important, but none is more important than main storage. It is the working storage from which a processor replenishes its cache memory, and it is the storage from which information is moved to I/O devices, including those for lower levels of the storage hierarchy. The major program and data components found in the main storage of modern, full-function digital computers are shown in Figure 6.8. As we learned in Sections 6.3–6.6, there are effective techniques for compressing data stored in online, nearline, and offline storage—the backing storage for main storage. So, too, there are compression techniques for compressing the active contents of main storage. In the immediately following sections of this chapter, we will examine how data compression is used to improve the efficiency of main storage for system programs, databases, user programs, and other data.

6.8   System Software

System software manages the operation of a computer and provides the environment for writing and executing user programs. System software—and here we include operating systems, language compilers, interpreters, editors, communications managers, database managers, and other licensed program products—allows

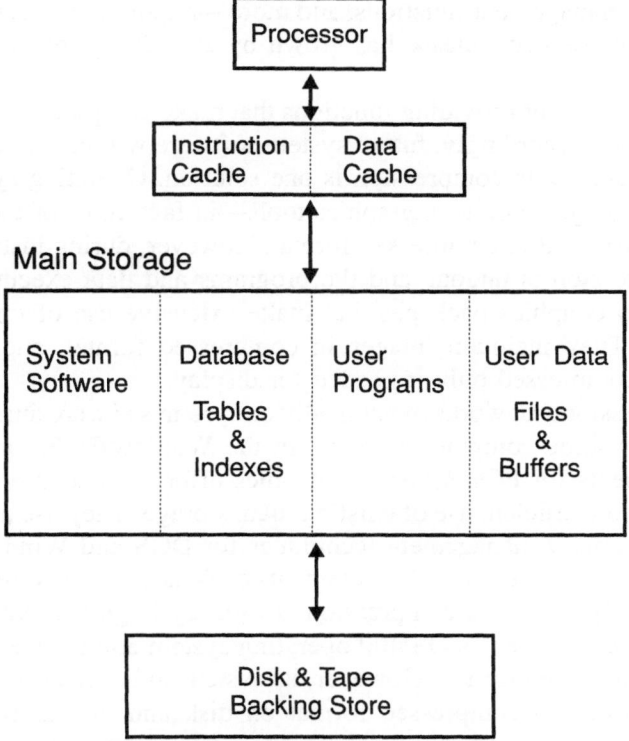

Figure 6.8 Main storage contents.

users to create and execute programs and to access and manage data. System software has grown ever more complex as computers have moved from stand-alone, single-user batch processing to multiuser online processing, and now to networked and distributed processing with complex interactions between computers.

The size of system software has grown too. Whereas the first personal computers required only a few kilobytes of storage for the DOS operating system and a rudimentary text editor, system software for today's desktop computers has grown to occupy huge amounts of storage. However, most would agree that the rewards outweigh the costs, for in the process, personal computer operating systems have become more user-friendly and text editors have been replaced by more powerful word processors. Also, many new productivity aids such as graphics tools and communications packages are now available. This new system software offers sophisticated, customer-pleasing functions but requires hundreds of megabytes of disk storage and 4–8 MB (or more) of main storage to execute it. The system software for large computers also has experienced astounding growth. One example is the IBM AS/400. The 1990 version of its OS/400™ operating system—a fully-integrated operating system containing communications, database management functions, and more—required over 300 MB of disk storage. Each subsequent release has grown by 20–30% as functions continue to be added.

No end is in sight for providing functions that make computers more powerful and easier to use. Accordingly, future system software will continue to consume ever more storage. Data compression is one solution. Operating systems, word processors, language compilers, graphics tools—in fact, most of today's system software is distributed in compressed format. However, during installation, usually the compression is undone and the programs and data execute in uncompressed format. Graphics packages that make extensive use of image data are an exception: They maintain images in compressed format, and, at runtime, images are decompressed only if needed for display.

Data compression that works dynamically on system software during execution is available for some computer systems. In the Windows™ 3.1 and Windows 95™ environments for PCs, several companies offer RAM compression utility programs for more efficient use of existing main storage. They use a combination of improved memory management techniques for DOS and Windows, and dynamic compression for less-essential elements of Windows software applications [IBD95, Conn95]. Dynamic compression is used by large computers too. Like others, AS/400 distributes its OS/400 operating system and its licensed program products in compressed format. However, its system software programs and data modules are stored in compressed format on disk and, in addition, most are maintained in compressed format when loaded in main memory [IBM3]. Only when a particular program or data module is needed for execution is it dynamically decompressed. For example, when error-handling routines and error messages are needed, they are decompressed just before use. Important savings in main storage are realized because only about 15% of the program modules are used so frequently as to warrant keeping them in uncompressed format [IBM4].

There are no standards for system software compression, nor need there be, as both compressed software distribution and compressed software execution are closed processes. Different products use different algorithms. AS/400 uses the Lempel-Ziv compression algorithm described in [Ziv77] for compressing system software. This algorithm is well suited to the task because it is adaptive, allowing it to effectively compress all kinds of data, and it can efficiently compress data blocks as small as a few thousand bytes, a size appropriate for system programs and data. It is lossless, which is a requirement for system software compression. Other techniques may be appropriate, too, particularly for image compression where loss can sometimes be tolerated.

6.9 Database Systems

Database systems are used to store and access data in commercial computers. Although database systems may have begun as mainframe computer tools for managing corporate enterprise information, they have grown to be available on all sizes of computer systems and now manage whatever digital information there may be. Database management system (DBMS) software and hardware allow users to define, manage, and access data in their database while shielding them from details of how the data is stored and managed.

Database organization

A DBMS provides the user a logical view of the database that is a collection of tables similar to the ones shown Figure 6.9(a).[5] Within a table, each row contains the data items that represent information about an entity (i.e., a person, place, thing, or event). Each column contains the data items that describe one attribute of an entity. The table in Figure 6.9 contains character text and numbers, but it could just as well contain digitized speech, audio, image, video, or whatever type of data is needed to manage a business.

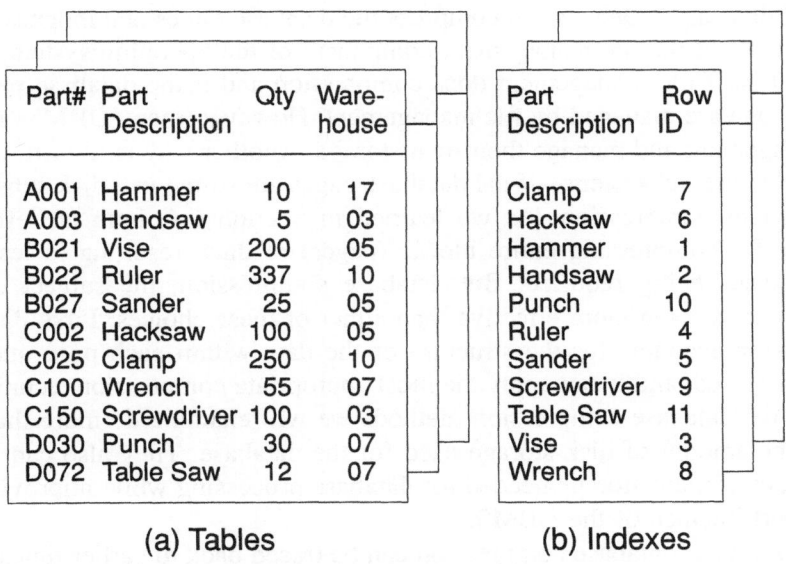

Part#	Part Description	Qty	Ware-house
A001	Hammer	10	17
A003	Handsaw	5	03
B021	Vise	200	05
B022	Ruler	337	10
B027	Sander	25	05
C002	Hacksaw	100	05
C025	Clamp	250	10
C100	Wrench	55	07
C150	Screwdriver	100	03
D030	Punch	30	07
D072	Table Saw	12	07

Part Description	Row ID
Clamp	7
Hacksaw	6
Hammer	1
Handsaw	2
Punch	10
Ruler	4
Sander	5
Screwdriver	9
Table Saw	11
Vise	3
Wrench	8

(a) Tables   (b) Indexes

Figure 6.9 Database objects.

To provide access to the data stored in tables, DBMSs use physical data structures that include several types of objects. One is the index, which is an important object, for it allows users to access data without being dependent on its storage structure. Indexes, shown (conceptually) in Figure 6.9(b), are searchable data structures that contain an ordered sequence of index entries. These

---

[5] We will use the terminology of IBM DB2™, which is a relational database management system. In the more formal terminology of the relational database model, a table is called a *relation*, a column an *attribute*, and a row a *tuple*.

index entries are arranged to place table data in logical sequence, whatever its physical sequence. Each index entry, a data-item and pointer tuple, identifies a row of a table that contains an entity having that data-item value for the indexed attribute. For a particular table, the number of indexes used can be none, one, or many, depending on how many ways that users choose to access the table.

DBMS usage has grown dramatically and so, too, has the storage needed for tables and indexes. Businesses store vast amounts of data online to track their activities and provide service to their customers. They also use many indexes, and indexes use storage. The storage overhead for indexes ranges from a few percent for OLTP (online transaction processing, a particular style of computing), to more for decision support, and perhaps as much as 300% for fully inverted (indexed) text files where every attribute can be searched [Linh93].

Database compression

Data compression is an obvious and effective solution addressing the storage needs of databases. One way to compress the database tables and indexes stored on disk is to let the file management component of the operating system do the job—that is, if file management does compression and if the database pages in main storage are managed by file management. However, many DBMSs bypass file management and manage their own storage. Another way is to turn the task over to the disk subsystem—if the database pages are stored in a disk subsystem that provides compression. As we learned in Section 6.4, both are effective solutions for compressing entire blocks (pages) of data, resulting in less disk storage space being required. But database compression, the subject of this section, can be even more effective than either of these choices: First, database compression accounts for the structure of the data within each page and how that data is used, and it can apply the most appropriate compression techniques.[6] Second, the database compression methods we will examine do more than just reduce the amount of disk storage used for the database. They also can shrink the amount of main storage needed for database processing while improving the access performance of the DBMS.

The origins of database compression can be traced back to earlier times when not only were general data compression techniques such as Huffman coding applied to entire data files on large mainframe computers [Lync85], but row-by-row, data-item-dependent "compaction" methods were also applied to efficiently store data and indexes [Mart77, Regh81]. A sampling of these compaction methods is shown in Table 6.2. Although effective, they do require intimate knowledge of the data content and its structure, which translates to greater user involvement.

In contrast, modern database compression techniques, which we will consider

---

[6] Note that when database compression is enabled, neither file management system nor disk subsystem compression are likely to further compress the database pages and most likely should be disabled.

Table 6.2 Data compaction methods.

Method	Examples
Suppress repeated characters	Truncate leading zeros or trailing blanks Replace runs of characters—run-length coding
Not storing null fields	Store only an indicator that a field is missing
Dictionary substitution	Store a code and look up the data-item in a dictionary; e.g., Code 6 = 'PRINTER IS OUT OF PAPER'
Exploit data order	Store only row-by-row differences
Data format/type conversion	Convert unpacked decimal digits to packed format Convert decimal digits to binary format Convert decimal time-and-date to binary format

next, combine the row-by-row approach of data-dependent compaction techniques with the adaptive data compression algorithms described in Chapter 4. In this way, effective data compression is made available for large collections of data, without requiring users to become data compression experts. The highlights of these schemes are that they

- Store compressed data and indexes on disk
- Transfer compressed data and indexes to main storage
- Store and process compressed data and indexes in main storage

Studies of commercial (business) customer databases show that modern database compression techniques can reduce disk storage space by 30–80% [Iyer94][7]. Furthermore, if the data and indexes remain compressed when loaded into main storage, not only will main storage will be used more efficiently but fewer disk I/O operations will be required—and both contribute to improved performance. As a result, OLTP applications will find more of the data they need cached in main storage. Also, decision support applications, which scan vast amounts of data, can scan more data in fewer I/O operations with less main storage buffer thrashing.

Of course, for these savings in disk storage, main storage, and I/O operations, there is a price to be paid, as additional CPU cycles are needed for handling compressed data. For OLTP applications, where few rows are accessed for each

---

[7] These databases are dominated by symbolic character text and numeric data. Lossless compression such as Huffman coding, arithmetic coding, or Lempel-Ziv techniques are highly effective.

database query, the overhead of software compression may not be intrusive. Several data compression software products that cut the total system cost for OLTP applications are available for mainframe computers [Lync85, Held91]. For decision support applications, where more data is scanned for each database query, the overhead for software compression often is too great [Iyer94]. The solution provided by IBM ES/9000 processors is a hardware assist for compression. It allows DB2 (and other DBMS products that choose to use the hardware assist) to execute both OLTP and decision support queries on compressed databases [IBM5].

Operations on compressed databases

Database pages in main storage that contain compressed tables and compressed indexes are shown (conceptually) in Figure 6.10, where an indexed table reference operation is in progress. Compressed table access proceeds as follows: In this example, the table row containing information on the part described as a "clamp" in Figure 6.9 is accessed via the index. The index is searched with the data-item value "clamp" and the Row ID value "7" is returned. Row 7 of the table, which contains information about the clamp, is extracted from the table and decompressed. When the application has finished processing data in that row, if the row has changed, it is recompressed and returned to the table. As we know, the newly compressed row may have expanded or contracted from its previous size. However, this poses few new challenges for any DBMS optimized for variable-length rows. In DB2 for ES/9000, for example, update-in-place of vari-

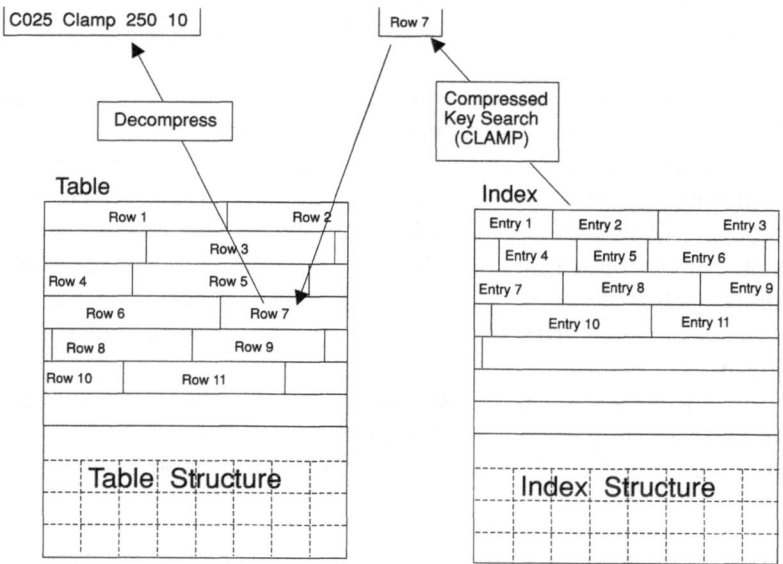

Figure 6.10 Operations on database physical storage structures.

able-length rows is built in, and DB2 uses its standard space management processing functions to handle the expansions and contractions that occur with compression. For those DBMSs that do not have strong variable-length row support, new solutions must be found.

Now, let us consider compressed indexes. Compressed indexes represent only a slight departure from standard DBMS indexes. Balanced-tree (B-tree) indexes [Kroe88] are used in most DBMS products [Iyer94]. For a compressed index, the standard index structure is used, except the keys (i.e., the data-items) are compressed. Index key compression is not new; the techniques described in Table 6.2 for redundancy removal and exploiting data order also have been applied to index key compression [Mart77, Lync85]. What is new is that a data compression algorithm such as the Lempel-Ziv algorithm is used to compress the keys, and—so that the index can be traversed without decompressing the keys—the data compression algorithm must be modified in a way that preserves the sort order [Zand93, Iyer94].

Algorithms for compressing databases

Compressing individual rows in a database table places some unique requirements on data compression algorithms. The typical row of a database table contains only 40–120 bytes[8] [Iyer94]. Studies have shown that adaptive dictionary algorithms provide little compression at start-up until hundreds or thousands of bytes have been processed [Bell90]. Thus, adaptive Lempel-Ziv dictionary algorithms (or other adaptive algorithms such as arithmetic coders) that work well for applications like tape or disk, where data blocks are much bigger, are not going to be effective. A database table row containing 40–120 bytes of nonhomogeneous data (the mixture of character text and numbers shown in Figure 6.9, for example) is not sufficient to initialize these algorithms.

The solution for database compression is to use a priori knowledge about the data to construct either a static or a semiadaptive compression algorithm. Consider how dictionary algorithms might be applied to database compression: One choice would be to use a static algorithm and an existing dictionary that represents the kind of data in the table. For instance, all tables containing payroll information might be effectively compressed by a "payroll dictionary" created from a table containing "standard" payroll data. However, we know this approach will not work well for situations where the data is diverse and there are no standards. Here a semiadaptive algorithm is a better choice. This is the approach offered by DB2 for ES/9000 [IBM5, Iyer94]. DB2 uses a two-pass, semiadaptive Lempel-Ziv [Ziv78] dictionary algorithm, where, during the first pass, the dictionary is created using adaptive techniques. The dictionary is created by scanning the

---

[8] This information was obtained by surveying DB2 customers whose databases contain traditional business data.

entire table if it is small, or by sampling the table if it is very large. During the second pass, adaption is disabled and the dictionary is applied row by row to compress or decompress data.

Modern data compression folklore says that adaptive algorithms are "good" because they extract the highest possible compression—they continually adapt to the changing characteristics of the data. Therefore, are semiadaptive (or static) algorithms always "bad" because they do not? In this case, no. Experiments on real databases show very little difference in compression between semiadaptive and adaptive Lempel-Ziv methods if the dictionary is regenerated whenever the database has changed significantly [Iyer94]. The key is to generate a dictionary that represents the whole table and regenerate it at appropriate times—say, when the data is reorganized. In the intervals between reorganizations the data values within a row may change, but the dictionary, if it represents the whole table, will likely be prepared for those changes. Most important, the data structure of the table does not change between reorganizations.

As we learned in Chapter 4, Lempel-Ziv compression, the technique used by DB2, is most effective on character text, numbers, and some image data. It usually is not as effective on speech, audio, and video. However, databases containing these diffuse data types can be effectively compressed by extending techniques already in place for DB2 and most DBMSs. One method that DBMSs use for handling diffuse data is to include in the table a "tag"—really a pointer—identifying the diffuse data item. The tag is used to access the diffuse data item, which may be stored elsewhere and can be compressed using whatever compression algorithm is most appropriate. All that is needed is to inform the user of how the data has been compressed.

There are no standards for database compression, nor are there likely to be standards. When data is interchanged between database systems, it is extracted from the internal storage structures of the DBMS. Only the data is interchanged, not the internal storage structures. This makes database compression a closed process.

6.10   User Programs

A user program (or any computer program) is a sequence of instructions that describe how the computer will solve a problem. The size of programs has grown, thanks to the ever more complex functions being performed by computers. Another reason for increased program size is RISC (reduced instruction-set computer) architecture. The typical RISC program can consume up to twice as much storage as an equivalent CISC (complex instruction-set computer) program. Increased program size—because of the amount of main storage consumed and the amount of data to be transferred from disk storage—is a concern for all computers. Nowhere is program size more critical than in mobile computers and the embedded processors found in mass-marketed products such as automobiles and appliances. In these computer applications, main storage cost, power consumption, and size are critical issues.

Can data compression be a solution for reducing program size? The answer is in two parts: First, we know programs can be compressed, for when they are archived typical compression ratios range from 1.4:1 to 2:1 [Harr93, Stry94]. Second, as we will learn in this section, it is possible to *execute* compressed programs. We will consider the trade-offs to be made between cost savings for reduced main storage, increased cache management complexity, and decreased processor performance when compressed programs are executed.

We begin by considering how an uncompressed program executes in a computer with a cache. As shown in Figure 6.11, several instructions are packed into fixed-size, blocks of storage—cache blocks. To simplify cache management hardware, the number of bytes of storage in each cache block is a power of 2. In this example, assuming instructions are 4 bytes in length, each cache block shown in Figure 6.11 contains 32 bytes. Instructions normally execute one after the other (i0, then i1, and so on), unless a jump or branch is encountered (i3 to i12, for example). When the processor has executed the instructions in a cache block, control is transferred to the next sequential cache block or to the cache block identified by the jump or branch instruction.

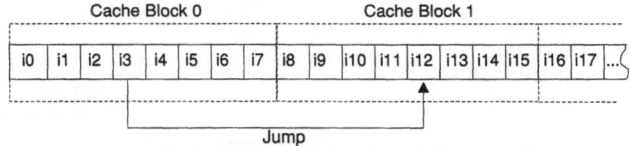

Figure 6.11   Instruction stream.

As shown in Figure 6.12(a), pages containing the active portion of a program are loaded into main storage, and from there the processor dynamically fetches and loads its instruction cache with the blocks of instructions to be executed. Let us focus on the cache management function: To simplify address computation when loading the instruction cache, the cache blocks are not only of fixed size but they also are aligned on powers of 2 main storage address boundaries. When a new portion of the program is needed, the instruction-cache manager selects a block in the instruction cache to be replaced. It performs address computation to locate the new block and transfers that block to the instruction cache. Then control is transferred to the processor which begins executing instructions from the new block.

Now consider how this process works when the program is compressed: Figure 6.12(b) shows the same program stored compressed in main storage. Cache blocks are no longer of fixed size nor are they aligned on powers of 2 main storage address boundaries. This means that while the replacement operation is unchanged, the address computation for locating the new block in main storage becomes more complicated. The solution shown in Figure 6.12(b) is to use an auxiliary map

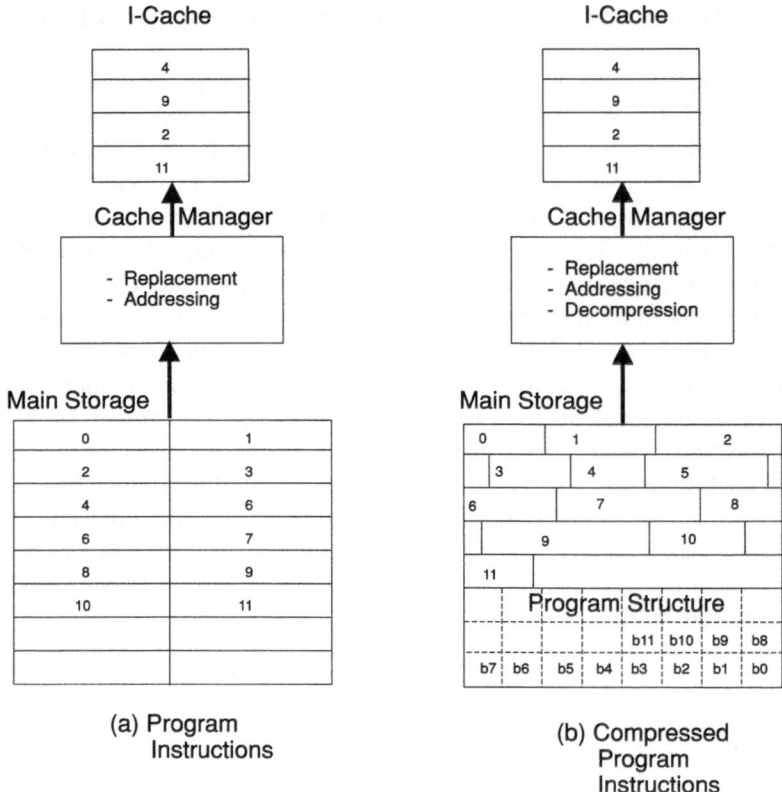

Figure 6.12   Cache memory system.

of main storage, the program structure, which the instruction-cache manager must access to locate the desired cache block. Accessing the program structure to locate the cache block requires an additional main store access for each cache block. This unacceptably degrades performance. The solution is to provide the instruction-cache manager with a lookaside buffer that contains cache block addresses extracted from the program structure. Thus, the need for an additional main storage accesses can be mostly avoided.

Having found a solution for efficiently addressing compressed cache blocks, let us examine what the instruction-cache manager must do to decompress the cache blocks. The critical factor is how quickly the cache blocks can be decompressed, because decompression adds latency to cache block replacement. There is no way to escape additional latency for decompression, but by selecting the correct compression algorithm, decompression can be done in hardware logic to reduce the latency. The issues are which compression algorithm to use and, once implemented, will it decompress data fast enough. State-of-the-art hardware for compression/decompression, as exemplified by VLSI chips that implement Lempel-Ziv compression, operates at speeds up to 40 MBS (megabytes per second) [Wils94B]. However, data rates must be several times faster to sustain cache block replacement for a modern RISC processor [Patt90]. Thus, for now, alternatives to commercially available Lempel-Ziv compression hardware must be considered.

One such alternative is Huffman coding, a generally less effective but simpler coding technique (there is no dictionary to be accessed as with Lempel-Ziv), whose decode tree can be directly hardwired in VLSI logic. Experimental hardware for a modified Huffman decoder was developed by the Compressed Code RISC Processor project at Princeton University [Wolf92]. The Huffman algorithm was modified to generate a bounded-Huffman code with no codes longer than 16 bits. A single, fixed decode tree was generated from average statistics gathered by analyzing a sampling of representative programs. When the compressed programs were generated, compression was disabled for those cache blocks where Huffman code would expand the block. At runtime, the instruction-cache manager detected whether a cache block needed to be decompressed. Typically, program compression was about 1.4:1. Execution time, thanks to the effects of lookaside buffering in the instruction-cache manager, was found to increase by less than 10%.

6.11 User Data

In Section 6.10, we found that by increasing the complexity of the instruction-cache manager and, perhaps, accepting decreased processor performance, data compression can reduce the amount of main storage needed for user programs. It is natural to ask if the compressed program techniques described in Section 6.10 can be extended to the data-cache manager. This would allow the processor to directly operate on compressed data in main storage for even greater savings. As we will learn, processing compressed user data is considerably more complex than executing compressed user programs. Many key issues require further research and development. In this section, we will examine where new solutions are needed—for writing compressed user data from the data cache back to main storage, finding effective compression algorithms, writing compressed user data back to disk, and dealing with data that is already compressed when loaded into main storage.

A key design constraint for the data-cache manager is to define main storage management techniques that are simple, so they can be implemented in VLSI logic, and are fast, so that data-cache write-back operations do not noticeably degrade processor performance. For most computer systems, it is accepted practice to forbid program modification. Therefore, in Section 6.10 the instruction-cache manager for executing compressed programs provides no facility for compressing instruction-cache blocks or writing then back to main storage. In contrast, a data-cache manager must compress and write back to main storage the updated data-cache blocks. Because those blocks may have expanded or contracted with compression, the data-cache manager must also manage, not merely access, the contents of main storage. This requires space management processing for the update-in-place of variable-length data-cache blocks, analogous to that for the database management systems described in Section 6.9.

A second design constraint for the data-cache manager is to define and implement high-performance, effective compression in VLSI logic. The decompression algorithm for the experimental instruction-cache manager described in Section 6.10 was fixed (i.e., not adaptive); there was only one Huffman decode tree, and it was designed to be effective only on program data. Experience with archiving compressed data teaches that adaptive algorithms are more effective in situations where the data statistics are changing—as they will change for the many kinds of data found in main storage. Even semiadaptive data compression algorithms for database management systems (described in Section 6.9) must be customized for each table in the database. So, too, it is reasonable to expect that for compressing user data in main storage—although a fixed algorithm may provide some compression for all data—adaptive compression will make the data-cache manager most effective. This application for adaptive data compression is challenging: Data-cache block sizes are small, perhaps 32–256 bytes. The data-cache manager writes many different kinds of data blocks back to main storage in an unpredictable sequence. The adaption process must track these events, adjusting to provide effective compression for all blocks.

A third design constraint is that compressed main store pages must be written back to disk—efficiently. A fortunate situation would exist if the compression algorithm of the data-cache manager exactly matched the compression algorithm of the compressed file management or disk subsystems described in Section 6.4. Then main storage pages containing compressed data could be written to disk without change. However, this is an unlikely situation because an effective compression algorithm for data-cache blocks, which are small, is likely to have different characteristics than an effective compression algorithm for disk, where data blocks are orders-of-magnitude larger. Otherwise, efficient transcoding will be required to convert from one compressed format to another when moving data to and from disk.

Finally, we must consider what parts of the main storage contents are not already compressed in a modern computer system—what will the data-cache manager find to compress that is not already compressed by some existing software or hardware process? In Section 6.9, we learned that database compression, file management system compression, and disk subsystem compression all compress data stored on disk, but for any given piece of data, only one is necessary. In main storage, a similar situation will exist if some combination of system software compression (Section 6.8), database compression (Section 6.9), and user data compression is in operation. Only one is needed for any given piece of data.[9]

---

[9] A significant portion of the main storage of computers used for multimedia applications will contain compressed speech, audio, image, and video data. None of the (lossless) compression

6.12   Chip-to-Chip Compression

A new trend in digital system design is beginning to appear. In Sections 6.10 and 6.11, we explored how lossless data compression may someday be applied to user programs and data. Underlying these applications is a design principle that will assuredly influence almost all future computers and digital systems. Here is how: As illustrated in Figure 6.13, usually several VLSI chips are needed to build computers and all complex digital systems. Moving data between those chips, fast enough and in large enough quantities, is a continuing struggle for digital system designers. One approach is to improve the performance of VLSI circuitry, sending more bits flying over each wire every second. Still, interchip bandwidth may be inadequate because physical packaging restricts the number of lines between chips. Another widely used approach is to skirt the interchip bandwidth issue by reducing the amount of data transferred between chips. Smart designs intelligently partition computing functions to reduce the interchip data rate, but often this is not economical or simply not possible.

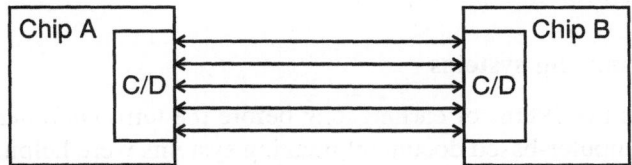

Figure 6.13   VLSI chip interconnection.

Data compression directly attacks interchip limitations by reducing the number of bits transferred. Until recently, this approach was impractical. The hardware needed to compress and decompress data was large and expensive, its throughput was too low, and the latency was too long. However, the VLSI design processes that allow packing more circuits on each chip, the same processes responsible for the interchip bottleneck in the first place, now make it feasible and economical to do on-chip, on-the-fly data compression to more efficiently move data between VLSI chips. On-chip lossless data compression is beginning to pop up at various locations in low-cost computer systems. For example, it is being used by PC graphics controllers to reduce display memory (VRAM) requirements and by RISC microprocessors to reduce instruction bus bandwidth [Wils95F]. One might speculate that data compression will soon be successfully applied to many other VLSI chip interconnections, even to chips that drive the interconnections between computers. The hurdle that system designers must overcome is establishing a favorable trade-off between the latency that compression adds and the additional transmission bandwidth it provides. So far, very simple compression techniques

techniques described in this section are likely to further compress this data. Most likely, all should be disabled.

have been used. Given the affordability of on-chip, dedicated VLSI circuits for data compression, it is conceivable that more complex Huffman coding and Lempel-Ziv algorithms will soon follow.

6.13 Multimedia Computers

In this chapter, we have encountered many instances where traditional computer systems use lossless compression to efficiently store symbolic data and programs. A new type of computer, the multimedia computer, has emerged in the 1990s. In this section, we will begin exploring how these computers use combinations of lossless and lossy compression to deal with diffuse speech, audio, image, and video data. We will look at document imaging systems, perhaps the first true multimedia computers, and multimedia servers, appropriate for image and real-time speech, audio, and video serving applications. Later in the book, we will return to this subject and, in Section 9.11, examine how multimedia PC client computers deal with all types of diffuse data.

Document imaging systems

Beginning in the 1980s, or earlier, long before the term *multimedia computer* was coined, computer-based document imaging systems were helping large businesses and government agencies to effectively automate business processes that handle large volumes of paper or film documents. The information on these documents is captured by scanning them, creating image files that are stored on computer disks. OCR (optical character recognition), bar-code reading, or manual keying allows indexing documents for later retrieval. For some applications, OCR is used to convert the characters on those documents into text. These steps allow the tools that computers provide for managing data and text to also store, organize, retrieve, and process documents. Incidentally, in business computers, until recently *multimedia* simply meant a combination of text and document images.

The original document imaging systems were mostly one-of-a-kind systems created for specific applications. More likely than not, they were stand-alone solutions unintegrated with other data processing activities. By the late-1980s, computer manufacturers began the process of integrating document imaging. This resulted in several thousand, multimillion-dollar document imaging systems being placed in production around the world. Mainframes and minicomputers or, at the least, high-powered UNIX workstations were combined with specialized components such as large-format, high-resolution displays, heavy-duty scanners and printers, and optical disc jukeboxes to build these niche products. Being high end in every way, and obviously expensive, only applications with huge volumes of images could afford them. Then came the PC revolution of the 1990s, totally revitalizing document imaging systems. Now, often document imaging is nothing more than just another application where image and text data coexist in conventional databases on traditional computers. Not only can images be processed and displayed on more-or-less standard PCs, but image scanners and printers are now commonplace and low-cost. Today's document imaging systems are faster, cheaper, better integrated, and more standardized. They now cover the spectrum from the high-end, high-volume systems of old to low-end desktop systems intended for occasional use.

In the strict sense, document imaging involves the scanning of paper or film documents and converting them to digital format. However, in practice, the same system may include electronically received FAX images. It may also include images produced by computer programs such as drawings from computer-aided design programs. Photographs, both scanned and electronically generated, may be included too. Some examples of document imaging applications include check imaging for banks, claims processing for insurance companies, legal documents for law offices, and government records such as arrest records and driver licenses. Also, manuals and drawing for design and service organizations, electronic publishing repositories such as newspaper photo and text morgues (see Chapter 10), and patient records for medical institutions, including medical images (see Chapter 12).

To understand the role that data compression plays in document imaging systems, consider the simplified document imaging system shown in Figure 6.14. Documents are loaded into the system by scanning them into electronic format at an image scanning station. Data compression is applied (for reasons soon to be apparent), and OCR, bar-code reading, or manual keying may take place to capture text information and index the document. The image loading process also includes manual operations to assure the quality of the scanned image and the accuracy of the OCR information (although, software spell checkers and grammatical aids have greatly improved OCR operation). Index information must be created so that, later, the document can be retrieved. When image data leaves the scanning station, it is sent to the image server where it is stored. Later, as needed, image data is retrieved from the server and sent to an image display station for viewing or to a printer for hardcopy. Other types of images that may

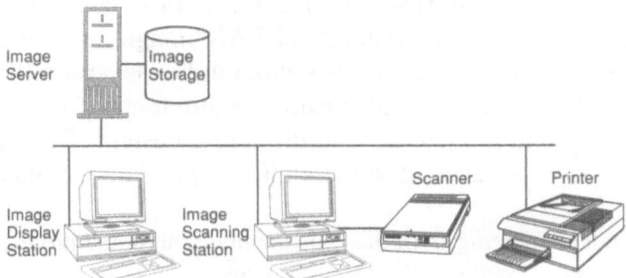

Figure 6.14   Document imaging system.

be included in the system come from sources (not shown) such as FAX servers, computer-aided design workstations, or medical imaging modalities. All these system elements are connected by local-area or wide-area communications networks.

Although conceptually simple, real-world document imaging systems require careful design to enhance the productivity of the people using them while dealing with the realities of processing large blocks of data. For example, it is often acceptable to allow several seconds for retrieving an electronic folder of document images before presenting them to a customer service agent. However, when the folder is presented at the workstation, the agent will expect subsecond display of pages in order to perform the electronic equivalent of riffling through a manila folder in search of a particular document. Almost without exception, to make the system usable, sophisticated system management techniques must be applied to assure that user performance requirements are met. Here, the important role data compression plays in these systems becomes apparent. Even when compressed, an image may be 30–90 KB, many times larger than the database records needed for typical business transactions. Many applications contain millions of documents, requiring enormous amounts of storage, and a multilevel storage hierarchy consisting of at least main storage, online magnetic disk, and nearline optical disc is needed. Image files must be arranged within the storage hierarchy so that the most active are stored in the fastest storage. To assure users at display stations can retrieve and view images with acceptable response times, data staging and prefetching techniques must be used. Transmission times and network bandwidth are critical factors too. To reduce the traffic on the network, data compression is applied at the scanning station so that compressed images can be sent to the image server for storage. To further reduce network traffic and improve response time, compressed images are sent to the image display stations and to image printers where they are decompressed. As to implementing image compression and decompression, it can be accomplished entirely with PC software, whether for scanning, display, or printing. More commonly, image scanners contain compression function and image printers contain decompression function, either built into those products by their manufacturers or added as after-market plug-in cards [Durr94, Guen96].

A broad range of data compression and format options are used in document management systems. The storage required for a JPEG-compressed image of a driver on a driver's license, a compressed FAX image, and an uncompressed image of a work of art ranges from a few thousand to several million bytes. Not only are these different images with distinct requirements for compression, but they are typically found in systems with dissimilar designs. To understand what kinds of compression are used, designers must appreciate factors such as these:

- Diverse standards ranging from those that apply in high-end production systems to those in low-end, casual-use PC-based systems
- Many image types ranging from FAXes to photographs

- Many image representations including bi-level, gray-scale, and color photographic quality; For color images, RGB and many other color-space models; also, various pixel depths with both 8-bit and 24-bit color being common
- Various image resolutions ranging from 100 or 200 pixels/inch for FAX to 300, 600, 1200, or more pixels/inch for more complex images

This all comes together when the image is scanned and an electronic representation of the image is created. Each scanned image is stored in a bitmap data file. Every pixel in the image is represented by a bit or groups of bits in this file. Not only does the number of bits per pixel depend on the above factors, so too do the file structure and the compression technique. The simplest way to illustrate the diversity of compression techniques found in document imaging systems is to examine one widely used file format, TIFF (Tagged Image File Format).[10] TIFF supports various image resolutions and color-space representations. It supports uncompressed images and *six* compression methods, five lossless and one lossy [Andl96]. The lossless algorithms include packbit compression (a byte-oriented run-length coding scheme); also, MH, MR, and MMR from the ITU-T T.4 and T.6 recommendations for Group 3 and Group 4 bi-level FAX image compression (see Section 5.4) and a version of LWZ for color images (see Section 4.6). The lossy algorithm is JPEG (see Section 5.4). So, simply knowing that an image is stored as a TIFF file tells little; extensive decoding of the file header is required to learn what the image is and how it is compressed.

The diversity of file formats and compression schemes makes data interchange between today's document imaging systems difficult, requiring significant investments in software and skill. For organizations seeking to unify image handling, one solution is to convert all images to a common file format. However, today this may not assure seamless interoperation. Continuing with TIFF as an example, many imaging products support this file format; but the TIFF file specification is complex, with many variations and options, leaving room for errors and omissions in its interpretation. The result is that subtle differences have crept into vendor implementations of TIFF [Must94]. Perhaps with time, the strengthening or simplification of image file standards, and the migration to fewer, carefully crafted image compression standards such as JPEG, the interoperation of document imaging systems will be solved. Today, that goal has not been reached. The emergence of electronic document management architectures, the emergence of image data types as actual integral parts of relational databases, and standards for image objects—these are elements of general schemes for open interoperability now being worked on, but much remains to be done [Lidd96].

---

[10] A sampling of other commonly used image file formats includes BMP (a Microsoft bitmapped graphics file format), GIF (a bitmapped color graphics file format defined by CompuServe, as described in Sections 3.5 and 10.3), JPG (a color graphics file format using JPEG image compression, as described in Section 5.4), and PCX (a graphics file format originally developed by Softkey International Inc. for their PC Paintbrush™ program).

Multimedia server computers

Multimedia servers must store and manipulate huge quantities of speech, audio, image, and video diffuse data, making lossy compression an indispensable element needed to control the cost for storage capacity. They are distinguished from traditional computers in that when dealing with speech, audio, and video they must operate in real time. Multimedia servers target market segments beyond the reach of traditional computers. To be sure, multimedia servers are found on client-server computer networks where they are used for more-or-less traditional *business* applications. But they also are, or soon will be, used for not-so-traditional *entertainment* applications such as storing the digital data that communications networks and broadcast channels deliver to television set-top boxes and a variety of consumer-oriented devices. Indeed, entertainment applications are largely responsible for the development of multimedia servers. Table 6.3 lists some existing and potential applications for multimedia servers.

Table 6.3   Multimedia server applications.

Business Applications	Entertainment Applications
Employee training	Video on demand
Desktop multimedia databases	Interactive television
Videoconferencing switching	Home shopping
Security monitoring databases	Multiplayer video games
Interactive kiosk servers	Media production servers
Internet World Wide Web multimedia servers	Broadcast industry audio and video servers

Because multimedia servers primarily handle diffuse data, their operation differs from traditional computers to an extent that requires significant changes in design. The key difference is that they must store and retrieve speech, audio, and video data streams in real time, continuously, and without interruption. This entails transferring large quantities of data at high rates. Multimedia servers must connect to high-speed networks. They must manage storage hierarchies whose capacity, even for modest-sized multimedia servers, can easily rival or exceed that of all but the largest conventional computers. Building a true multimedia server requires new hardware and software. Some of the hardware changes include I/O subsystems than can handle high-speed networks, magnetic disk storage devices that can provide, not just high data transfer rates, but can sustain those rates over long periods of time, and high-bandwidth internal buses to tie it all together. Software changes include file systems that provide real-time scheduling and performance optimization for large blocks of data, often for large numbers of users. Other software changes include bandwidth reservation techniques to assure consistent response times, techniques to synchronize delivery of speech, audio, image, and video data, and storage hierarchy management and buffering techniques that anticipate the demand for continuous delivery of speech, audio, and video with acceptable latency.

The aspects of multimedia server design reach far beyond the scope of this book; more thorough treatments can be found in several sources including [Crut94, Gemm95]. However, we must note that the computer industry is still struggling with the definition and design of multimedia servers, and the capabilities of current systems vary greatly. Multimedia servers come in sizes ranging from PCs to supercomputers, and not all products calling themselves multimedia servers have been totally redesigned to include all of the above changes. The primary criterion that determines how radically their design departs from conventional computers is how many simultaneous, independent multimedia data streams they can support and how efficiently they do this. With few changes, a low-end PC server may support single-stream playback, whereas highly modified designs are needed for high-end systems that can playback thousands of independent data streams.

Our interest in multimedia server design is limited to how data compression enters into the design. We will look at two classes of multimedia servers: store-and-forward servers and full-function servers. Store-and-forward servers essentially act as intelligent storage controllers and database servers for speech, audio, image, and video. They are used in applications where data intended for playback by clients arrives at the server already in compressed format. This data is loaded onto the server and delivered to clients who decompress it during playback. As an illustration of store-and-forward serving, which we will refer to throughout this section, a typical video server application is depicted in Figure 6.15.

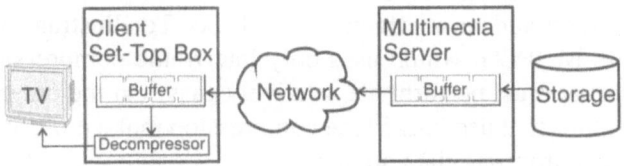

Figure 6.15 Store-and-forward video server application.

In store-and-forward applications, the server is challenged to supply each client's data stream buffers with enough data to ensure the playback process is not starved for data. To do this efficiently, just the right amount of data must be pulled from the server's storage hierarchy and shipped out on the network. The server mainly manages the database and traffic on the networks connecting the clients. It acts as accountant and traffic cop, providing cost-charging services and security, while routing data from its storage to the clients. Given this situation, we might conclude that the server is unaware of data compression, but that is not true. Data compression affects store-and-forward multimedia servers in the following ways:

Assume the client is playing back data at a constant rate, say video at 30 fps (frames per second). When data is compressed with a variable-rate compression algorithm (MPEG for example), the number of data blocks that must be retrieved will vary according to how many video frames the compressor has packed into each block. Obviously, this causes a scheduling problem for the server in that it cannot decide how often to send a data block to the client.[11] There are several solutions. For instance, the server might pessimistically assume each block contains the fewest frames, but this may flood the client buffers with too much data. Perhaps the most effective option is for the server to interact with the compression algorithm and learn how many video frames each block contains. It can then tag each block with this information, using it to pace delivery during playback. The same information is also useful for loading data into the server's storage hierarchy, arranging data blocks on the storage devices in ways that facilitate retrieving a constant number of video frames from a varying number of data blocks.

Many store-and-forward multimedia servers also must support client-initiated interactive VCR-like control functions on video data streams. These functions include pause/resume and variable-speed forward/backward playback. This poses significant challenges to the server because the data rate may vary from nothing to several times the normal rate. A simple but often impractical solution is for the server to deliver data at whatever rate the client requests and let client logic select what information is presented to the viewer. Smarter and more practical solutions move the selection logic to the server. By examining the client requests, it can select the video frames that should be presented to the viewer. There are several approaches, none of which are yet fully developed, but all require that the server "get inside" the compressed video data stream, perhaps to select video frames, or even reconstruct the video data stream to support high-speed playback operations. Here, again, the algorithm used to compress data determines how this is accomplished and how effective it will be. To illustrate, when video is compressed with M-JPEG, which uses only interframe compression, the operations that the server must perform are relatively easy. On the other hand, MPEG and other algorithms that use intraframe compression make it much more difficult to assemble the appropriate data stream.

Turning now to full-function servers, they are distinguished by being actively involved in processing multimedia data, doing more than just storing, indexing,

---

[11] We assume a stream-oriented client-server relationship exists in which after the client initiates stream playback, the server periodically sends data to the client at the selected rate without further requests from the client. This relationship exists between multimedia servers and set-top boxes. There also exists a file-oriented relationship between client and server multimedia computers in which the client computer controls pacing by issuing a read request to the server for each block of data [Gemm95].

and routing it. Some examples of the operations these servers may do include the following:

- Switching and routing audio and video to clients participating in multiparty video-conferencing. This may require compression and decompression transcoding functions to manage and deliver audio and video in different formats and resolutions for clients having differing capabilities.
- Delivering entertainment media to clients having equally diverse needs for transcoding.
- Performing the initial compression of diffuse data, as for music and movies, to allow direct capture by the servers used for media production and distribution. However, today this data is usually compressed by workstations that control the data capture devices, or by the workstations which are used to edit the media. This approach will likely continue to be popular because it is economical and it provides media developers with maximum control over the process.
- Doing decompression to allow data processing operations on objects in the database managed by the server. These operations might include semantic interpretation of speech, audio, image, or video message content. This allows for query retrieval and object recognition.
- Performing OCR (optical character recognition) of decompressed image documents, allowing the text portions of those documents to be stored and processed along with other symbolic data.
- Performing recognition on decompressed speech, allowing spoken words to be processed as text.
- Providing compression and decompression for graphics and image data along with the rescaling, resizing, and format conversions needed to drive shared print servers that generate compound documents, time-series arrays, geographic maps, binary halftone images, and so on.

The market for full-function multimedia servers is not yet well established, and neither are their requirements nor specifications. Therefore, how data compression and decompression will be used or implemented remains to be discovered. One might conclude that because diffuse data compression and decompression will be a widely used functions, they must be done in hardware. However, high-performance parallel server computers, such as the IBM SP1 and SP2, running software compression are used by the entertainment industry to prepare digitized motion pictures and video for distribution [PRNe93]. Thanks to the raw computing power of parallel systems, software-implemented data compression algorithms have proven acceptable for this application. One may speculate that high-performance diffuse data compression will be required in full-function servers of various sizes and costs, and hardware assists will be included in these products, but that scenario has not yet been established.

6.14 Summary

In this chapter, we examined applications in digital computers, where, for the most part, lossless data compression is used for efficient storage of data and programs. We learned the following:

- Data compression reduces the cost, size, weight, and power consumption of mobile computers, and it squeezes the most from the limited available communications bandwidth.

- Software is widely used in desktop computers where abundant free CPU cycles are available for tape, disk, and communications compression. Add-on hardware for compressing diffuse data in multimedia computers is giving way to more integrated solutions.

- Hardware and software are prevalent in large computers for compressing symbolic data but not diffuse data.

- Data compression can be the right solution for interconnecting distributed computers when only low-bandwidth or low-cost links are available.

- Data compression allows more information to be contained in each level of the computer storage hierarchy, allowing it to be used more effectively.

- The running time of computer tape operations may be cut in half with data compression. Hardware and software, proprietary and standards-oriented solutions are offered for all computer tapes, large and small.

- The apparent storage capacity of computer disks can be doubled with data compression. High-performance, on-the-fly, unobtrusive solutions are available for file management software and disk subsystems.

- Data compression techniques similar to those used for tape and disk can increase the storage capacity of optical disks and solid-state files.

- The efficiency of main storage can be improved by compressing system programs, databases, user programs, and other data. Special data compression techniques are available for each.

- Compressed system software can be distributed, stored on disk, and stored in main memory; for most program modules; decompression can be done dynamically just before execution.

- Database compression accounts for the structure of the data within each page and how that data is used. Savings in disk and main storage result, and database access performance improves when data and indexes are compressed with semiadaptive algorithms.

- Compressed user programs can be executed by building an instruction-cache manager that decompresses cache blocks on demand.

- Compressed user data execution requires a data-cache manager that both decompresses and compresses cache blocks while managing the contents of main storage.

- On-chip lossless data compression can help eliminate interchip data transfer bottlenecks.

- Document imaging systems use lossless and lossy compression to efficiently store and transmit images ranging from FAX documents to color photographs. Unfortunately, a plethora of file formats and image compression techniques makes interoperability of existing systems problematical.

- Multimedia server computers use lossy data compression to control the cost for storage capacity. Variable-rate compression complicates scheduling and data selection during media playback. The requirements for lossy compression and decompression functions within multimedia servers are not yet fully established.

7

Communications—
Network Applications

Chapters 7 and 8 describe how data compression is used in communications. For many communications applications, bandwidth conservation is an important reason to use data compression. It can increase the effective throughput of existing transmission channels or, alternatively, reduce transmission costs by allowing lower-speed or shared transmission facilities to be used. Equally important in some applications, data compression can reduce transmission time. Various combinations of lossless and lossy compression are used in communications, with most algorithms being specially adapted for the transmission channels and the data being transmitted on those channels. For each application, we will examine the communications system and the compression algorithms that are appropriate. This chapter deals with applications where voice, data, images, and video are transmitted on communications networks. Chapter 8 describes broadcasting applications.

7.1 Industry Overview

Many businesses are involved with providing products and services for communicating information—between people, between businesses, and from industry to consumers. Everyone from booksellers to television broadcasters provides some form of communications. Our view of "the communications industry" will be limited to applications for digital electronic communications systems and the businesses that provide them. These include traditional telecommunications—telephone, telegraph, and other point-to-point communications services. Also, data communications services, the modern-day blend of computers and communications. And broadcasting services such as radio, television, cable, and satellite.

The communications industry provides rich and varied opportunities to apply data compression. Most assuredly, communications applications provide a study in contrasts. Well-established applications, such as FAX, have clearly defined needs for data compression and mature technology is in place. Newer applications, such as HDTV, also have demonstrated needs, but their data compression technology is still evolving to meet changing definitions of the applications themselves. Sometimes, data compression simply solves a channel bandwidth or cost-of-transmission problem. But some applications, such as direct broadcast satellite television, use it to improve and expand existing services. Still others, like cable TV, plan to use data compression as the springboard for expanding the scope of the application, to do something new, to leverage other industries.

Standards are extremely important in the communications industry because of its global nature and so many diverse elements must work together. This is true of data compression standards too. However, only a few official standards for compressing symbolic data originated within the communications industry, and in some applications, there are no standards—when there should be. In contrast, all of the official standards for compressing diffuse data have come from, are closely connected to, or are strongly influenced by the communications industry. Unlike the computer industry, in the communications industry once a standard is set in place, data compression standards included, usage is widespread because standards compliance usually is compulsory, not voluntary.

In this and the following chapter, we will adopt the conventions of the communication industry and describe services for voice, data (computer data, the symbols found on a keyboard), image, and video transmissions. Moving symbolic digital data between computers is a well-established but relatively new business for the communications industry. However, it is only one component of the communications industry. Granted, the largest part of the communications industry is still involved in the traditional business of moving analog voice, image, and video information. But now all segments of the industry are on a fast path to completely replace the infrastructures of their traditional businesses with digital networks and transmission facilities. Digital data is expected to revitalize the industry and increase its profitability by providing new services that only digital technology will allow. The opportunities for digital data in the communications industry—and for data compression—are enormous, but one should be prepared for a slow roll-out. As we have noted, this industry is standards oriented and it is highly regulated. Expansions or new directions of any kind generate complex standards and regulatory issues, the sort of issues that easily take years to resolve. Communications is also an industry with huge investments in its infrastructure. For that reason (and many others), in the past, changes have come slowly.

Electronic communications systems

The communications industry is built on electronic communications systems that transmit signals containing encoded information over a distance using electrical energy to carry data between a transmitter and a receiver. As shown in Figure

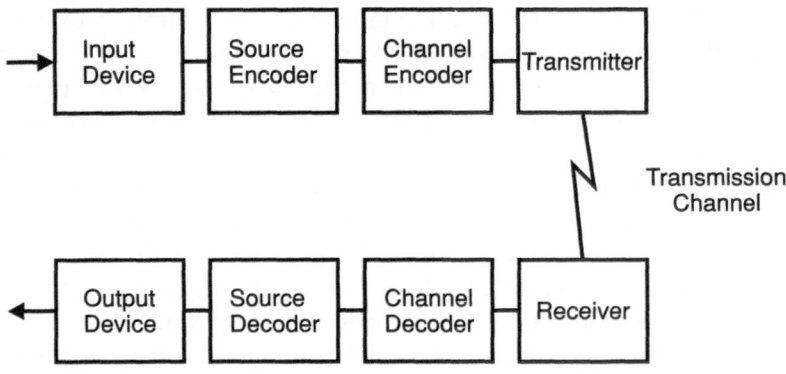

Figure 7.1   An electronic communications system.

7.1, information is conveyed by energy traveling along a transmission channel. That channel may be a wire, a wireless (radio wave) link, or a fiber-optic link.

The first task for any electronic communications system is to convert the information to be transmitted into electrical signals. This is accomplished by input devices such as microphones, computers, scanners, and cameras, where information in the form of voice (speech) or audio, computer data, images, and video are captured. Electrical signals from the input devices are processed in several steps: As previously stated, our interest is limited to *digital* electronic communications systems (for reasons that will soon become apparent). Digital systems transmit information as a sequence of encoded pulses (whereas analog systems transmit continuously varying signals). Therefore, the source encoder must perform analog-to-digital conversion and other transformations—including data compression—to efficiently encode the data. Then the data must be further processed by the channel encoder into a form suitable for transmission. This processing includes adding error-detection or error-correction data to compensate for transmission errors and conversion to an electrical signal that the transmitter can accept. In a wired system, the transmitted signal takes the form of an electrical current that travels along a conductor. In a wireless system, the signal is sent through space as an electromagnetic wave launched by the transmitter. In an optical system, the electrical signal is converted to light that is guided by the glass fiber.

At the receiver, the signal is captured and all the processing steps are undone, allowing the transmitted information to be recovered and reproduced. Output devices include computers, loudspeakers, printers, and image or video display devices. If all goes well, the recovered information will be an exact or acceptably faithful reproduction of the original.

Communications styles and compression

Electronic communications systems are designed to support the communications needs of people who use information in different ways to learn about the world around them. The written word, speech, music, pictures, and even touch and smell are all part of communications. As shown in Table 7.1, there are three styles of communications, each providing differing types and degrees of interactions between people.

Table 7.1 Communications styles.

Communications Style	Interaction Between People	Examples
One way	No direct interaction	Books, magazines, newspapers, radio, CDs, TV, VCR tapes
Bi-directional	Usually not in real time	Letters, FAXes, E-mail, voice messaging, images
Collaborative	Real time	Meetings, telephone calls, audio/video conferences

These different styles of communications call for different types of electronic communications systems and, not surprisingly, different types of compression and decompression algorithms. One-way communications often involve a one-to-many distribution of information—broadcasting and mass distribution—where (in computer terminology) there is one server and many clients. In this situation, getting the highest compression ratio is a good trade-off, for additional compression complexity can reduce transmission time, bandwidth, and implementation costs. Asymmetric compression algorithms (meaning compression can be complex and slow, but decompression is simple and fast) are encouraged. Simple, fast, and inexpensive decompression is highly desirable for all mass-distribution applications because it reduces the complexity and cost of the receivers. Many different situations can occur, but bandwidth and (to some extent) storage capacity—particularly for video information—are usually the major limiting factors. Therefore, compression algorithms may be architected to trade off quality (image resolution and video frame rate, for instance) in exchange for operating within available bandwidth or storage capacity.

Bi-directional communications are two-way and, therefore, each party must compress and decompress information. Here, symmetric compression algorithms are desirable. However, real-time interaction usually is not involved, and processing speed can be traded for higher compression ratios, higher quality, or lower implementation costs. For example, an inexpensive FAX machine that operates at less than the maximum data transmission rate may be perfectly adequate for FAXing orders to the local pizza parlor (but less than adequate if long-distance telephone line charges apply).

Collaborative communications are also two-way, and they demand real-time interaction. This means that compression and decompression algorithms must be symmetric, and they also must provide a low (and controlled) delay time for both encoding and decoding because human interaction is involved. Long delays in processing data for client-server computing increases the response time for transactions, thus negating the advantage of compression. Long delays in processing either audio or video impedes interactions between individuals, and so do erratic processing times that disrupt the smooth flow of information. As with one-way communications, many different situations can occur, but audio and video compression algorithms often must be architected to sacrifice quality (speech intelligibility, audio bandwidth, and image resolution, for example) to operate within available time and bandwidth constraints.

7.2   Voice Telecommunications

For over 100 years, the telephone system has been the most widely used telecommunications service. Voice communications remain a huge revenue producer for the telecommunications industry, an industry whose origins trace back to the transmission of voice and telegraph traffic sent over metal wires and, later, microwave links. Starting in the 1970s, with the integration of computers and communications, the telephone network began carrying computer data traffic. Today, the telephone network has evolved to a network of interconnected networks that carry a mixture of voice, data, images, and video. It uses both analog and digital signals sent over wires and a variety of wireless and fiber-optic links. The major components of telephone networks are shown in Figure 7.2. The subscriber's equipment includes telephones for voice and modems for nonvoice traffic. The local loop connects subscribers to the system. The local exchange switches calls, and the long-distance network routes calls between local exchanges. Traffic within the local exchange and long-distance network complex is handled by a mixture of analog and digital technology. Traffic on the local loop between most subscribers' telephones and the local exchange switching center is still analog. However, with the deployment of ISDN (Integrated Services Digital Network), the local loop traffic is becoming digital too. ISDN provides users with end-to-end digital transmission and increased bandwidth, enabling voice, data, image, and video transmission services.

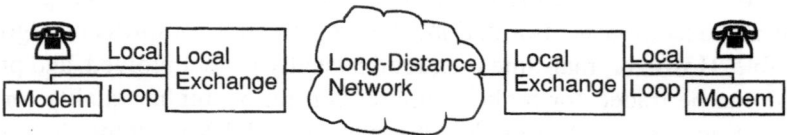

Figure 7.2   Telephone network.

With wireless communications having been added to the mix, wireline telephone networks are no longer the sole providers of telecommunications services. Table 7.2 lists a few of the major services, both operating and proposed [Kobb95].

Table 7.2   Telecommunications services.

Telecommunications Service	Status	Signal Encoding	Capacity Limits
Wired telephony	> 500 M telephones	Analog Digital	Signal encoding Wireline circuits
Cellular telephony	> 20 M Users	Analog Digital	Signal encoding Radio frequencies
PCS - Personal Communications Services	Emerging	Digital	Signal encoding Radio frequencies
LEO - Low-Earth Orbit satellite systems	Future	Digital	Signal encoding Radio frequencies

Although voice traffic continues to dominant all these services, from an economics viewpoint, the ability to efficiently mix voice and data is critical for growth and survival of all telecommunications networks; so, too, is the ability to accommodate the growing demand for image and video transmissions. However, the carrying capacity of all telecommunications systems, be they wired or wireless, is limited. More efficient signaling techniques (to pack more information into existing systems) are not always practical. Expanding the system may not be practical either due to the cost for additional wireline circuits or the lack of additional radio-frequency spectrum allocation. These factors constrain the number of channels and bandwidth each system can provide.

The solution to providing more capacity for all these services is digitally encoded transmission—with data compression. Why digital networks? Technical advantages include noise immunity, the ability to transmit information over great distances without degradation, and computerized network control, to name a few. Economic advantages relate to providing all the communications services that customers need, thanks to the ease with which a mixture of data types may be transmitted. Another advantage of digital transmission is that data compression, which conserves bandwidth and increases information-carrying capacity, can be implemented far more effectively than for analog-encoded transmissions.

Speech coding

Let us focus on how data compression is used for voice transmission: Research on speech coding (voice compression) began in the 1930s, but early accomplishments were limited. The signals were analog, and although simple techniques provided some bandwidth reduction, more powerful methods like vocoders were difficult to implement in the analog domain. Speech coding did not really take hold until the telephone network began going digital in the 1970s. Not only did digitally encoded transmission make voice compression more feasible, but compression soon became a necessity.

Throughout the 1980s and 1990s, voice traffic continued to increase, stressing the capacity of the public-switched telephone network. The standard telephone analog voice circuit provides a 3-KHz frequency bandwidth (200–3200 Hz) and can carry one conversation. DS0, the equivalent digital voice circuit, mimics the analog voice circuit using 64 Kbps PCM coding (8-bit samples at an 8-KHz sampling rate), and it, too, can carry but one conversation. Speech coders, which reduce the bit rate needed for each conversation, thus conserving bandwidth for voice transmissions, are clearly useful for increasing network traffic capacity. With rapid progress in the effectiveness of digital speech coders, and faced with growing voice traffic, the ITU-T released a series of recommendations (standards) aimed at doubling and quadrupling the capacity of public-switched telephone network circuits. Using speech coding, the digital transmission rate was cut from 64 Kbps to 32 Kbps and subsequently to 16 Kbps. (See Section 5.2 and Table 5.2 for more information about the ITU-T G.726 and G.728 standards.) New standards for 8 Kbps have been developed, and 4 Kbps and lower are now actively being researched. By continuing to cut the coding rate, the existing telephone network can be made to carry more voice traffic; alternatively, more bandwidth is made available for nonvoice transmissions.

On another front, the spread of wireless communications systems intensifies the need for very low bit-rate speech coding. Cellular telephones and other wireless systems have a problem—they are just too popular. There are too few radio channels to go around, and allocating more is unlikely in an already overcrowded radio-frequency spectrum. The cellular telephone industry found a solution by going to digital transmission and sharing existing channels. For instance, in North America the standard 30-KHz cellular telephone channel carries one analog voice transmission or, via modem, can transmit data at 14.4 Kbps. Using the same bandwidth, IS54, the North American digital cellular telephony standard, provides three 13-Kbps channels for voice (or data) transmissions [Rapp94]. Obviously, there is too little bandwidth for telephone-line standard PCM speech coding. As a result, the IS54 standard specifies speech coding at 7.95 Kbps with the remaining bandwidth used for error protection. (See Section 5.2 and Table 5.2 for more information on IS54 and several other cellular telephony speech coding standards, all of which use low-bit-rate speech coding equally aggressively.)

7.3   Data Communications Networks

Advances in communications technologies and the merging of computers and communications have created a world in which it is hard to imagine *not* computing at a distance. Not long ago, remote computing, meaning computing from afar, was nearly unknown, and distributed computing, meaning linking several computers together by a network, was confined mostly to short distances over computer channels or buses. Only large organizations could afford private networks for medium or high-speed, long-distance data transmissions. Today, nearly everyone has access to economical remote and distributed computing. The connection may be wired or wireless, over short distances on LANs (local-area networks), or over great distances on WANs (wide-area networks). All LANs and WANs are now enabled for data traffic. These include the public telephone network and private leased communications lines from telecommunications providers, public cellular and other wireless networks, and the ever-growing number of public and private packet-switching, broadband data networks.

   With advances in technology have come changes in how computers and communications are used to meet the needs of individuals, businesses, and society. Personal computers are linked to networks. Larger computers on a network serve smaller client computers. Computers of all sizes are distributed and work together through networks to solve large computing tasks. All these networked computing styles are on the increase, whereas stand-alone computers connected to unintelligent dumb terminals are not.

   Data compression is used in many different networked computing environments. Figure 7.3 provides an overview of those considered in this chapter. Included are low-speed telephone lines and modems for connecting individual users to remote and client-server computing environments; also included are multiplexed, medium-speed links carrying a mixture of voice, data, and FAX traffic between sites within organizations. Other uses for medium-speed links are to provide LAN-to-LAN internetworking connections in distributed computing environments and to connect mainframe computers with remotely located I/O devices. Another element of networked computing to be examined is the high-

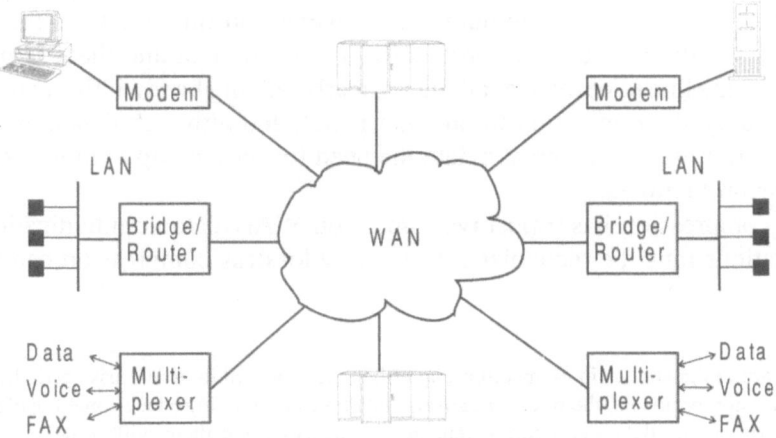

Figure 7.3   Networked computing environments.

speed links that provide the transmission capacity needed for network backbones. We will also look at how compression is used by the communications software that manages the network and allows computers to communicate.

All these networked computing environments share a common element—WAN connections. WANs are essential for long-distance transmission, but they restrict network computing in the following ways: their bandwidth may be less that what is needed, their response time may be too long, and they also can be quite expensive. Fortunately, data compression can attack all these restrictions. It can improve WAN performance by providing higher effective throughput or shorter response times, and it can reduce WAN costs by allowing the use of lower-speed or shared transmission lines. With the introduction of high-speed broadband links that use fiber optics and high-speed transmission protocols—frame relay, ATM (asynchronous transfer mode), SMDS (Switched Multimegabit Data Service), and BISDN (Broadband ISDN) to name a few—WAN bandwidth has grown dramatically. Unfortunately, many individuals still face the "last mile" problem, where the only way to get to this new world of high-speed communications is through old-world, low-speed telephone lines. For them, data compression that squeezes every last bit possible through those lines is a good investment. On the other hand, users connected to modern-day LANs—where not only is the bandwidth high, but the styles of computing that users favor require it—need high-bandwidth links to continue doing high-bandwidth computing across a WAN. True, communications costs have dropped dramatically, but, still, the monthly charges for medium to high-bandwidth WAN links can put a sizable dent in anyone's computing budget. For them, making the most efficient use of the lowest-possible bandwidth lines becomes an economic necessity. For all users, the volume of bits to be transmitted continues to grow, requiring more time for transmission. This makes data compression, which eliminates redundant bits, a wise choice for everyone.

To illustrate the interplaying roles of WAN bandwidth and data compression, consider the time needed to move a 1-MB file from a server computer to a user's PC. Table 7.3 shows the minimum data transmission time required for various line speeds if the data transfer protocol is 100% efficient and there is no delay waiting for the line to become available.[1] Clearly, adding bandwidth can transform an intolerably slow operation to one that is not, and although data compression cannot work miracles, it can alleviate the need for moving up to more expensive transmission facilities.

Data compression has a positive impact on WAN data communications, but its limitations must be recognized. First, only lossless compression can be used

---

[1] Lines are designated as low-, medium-, and high-speed according to discussion in this section. All transmission protocols, the rules that govern data transmission, introduce some hopefully small overhead for routing data and assuring reliable transmission, and there will be delay, unless the line happens to be idle.

Table 7.3   Minimum data transmission time for a 1-MB file.

Line Type	Line Speed	Uncompressed	Compressed (2:1)
Low-speed			
Analog telephone	28.8 Kbps	4.63 min	2.31 min
ISDN telephone	128 Kbps	1.04 min	0.52 min
Medium-speed			
Sub-T-1	0.768 Mbps	10.4 sec	5.2 sec
T-1	1.544 Mbps	5.2 sec	2.6 sec
High-speed			
Cable TV modem	10 Mbps	0.8 sec	0.4 sec
ATM	155 Mbps	0.052 sec	0.026 sec

for data transmissions between computers. Computer application programs expect error-free transmissions, making information loss unacceptable. So, data compression cannot improve transmission efficiency much more than 2–4 times. Second, only uncompressed data can be compressed. This means there will be little reduction for images, video, and other data that is normally precompressed before transmission; only text files, programs, and messages will be transmitted more efficiently—if another program has not already worked compression magic on them. To deal with the mix of compressed and uncompressed data that may be encountered on communications networks, data compressors must test the data (or respond to user directives) and only enable compression when it will actually reduce the number of bits to be transmitted. A third factor is that data may be encrypted for secure transmissions. The encryption process, which randomizes data, making it virtually incompressible, renders compression totally ineffective. As discussed in Chapter 14, the only workable solution for transmitting compressed, encrypted data is to apply compression before encryption and do decryption before decompression.

When data compression operates across a network, limitations are encountered that occur nowhere else. To appreciate why this is true, we need to understand how communications between computers take place. Computers connected to networks are controlled by communications software that runs in each computer and device connected to the network. To facilitate the exchange of data, each computer or device must adhere to a common *architecture* (the hardware and software structure that implements the communications function) and a common *protocol* (the conventions for sending and receiving data). There are many different communications architectures and protocols for computer networking; some are proprietary, some are not. Proprietary examples include DECnet™ (Digital Equipment Corporation networking) and IBM SNA/APPN™ (IBM System Network Architecture/Advanced Peer-to-Peer Networking). Nonproprietary examples include TCP/IP (Transmission Control Protocol/Internet Protocol) and the protocol specified by the OSI (Open-Systems Interconnection) reference model, a communications architecture developed by ISO. Like all communications architectures, the OSI protocol is implemented by a layered stack. Each layer does part of the functions required for communications to take place. It provides these services to the next higher layer and, in so doing, depends on the next lower layer to carry out more primitive functions. The OSI layers, whose functions are typical of those found in all communications protocols, are described in Table 7.4.

Table 7.4 OSI layers.

Layer	Function
7. Application	Provides the interface for user application programs to send and receive data (messages)
6. Presentation	Provides a standardized format for data exchange between applications and may provide data transformations such as compression and encryption
5. Session	Controls communications dialog between applications including establishing and terminating connections, recovery, and other services
4. Transport	Ensures reliable data delivery by providing end-to-end error recovery and optimizes network usage by flow control and other techniques
3. Network	Provides logical addressing and isolates the upper layers from details of the data transmission and switching technologies visible at lower layers
2. Data link	Provides physical addressing, flow control, and (sometimes) the error detection or correction needed to reliably send blocks of data (frames) across the physical links
1. Physical	Deals with the mechanical and electrical interfaces to the hardware and the transmission of an unstructured bit stream over the physical link

As to the limitations encountered when data compression operates across a network, Table 7.4 suggests that data compression, if it is present, operates within layer 6, the session layer, but that is not always true. Many WAN data communications products that use data compression work at layer 2 or 3 of the protocol. They use adaptive LZ77 or LZ78 compression algorithms (described in Section 4.6) that depend on passing information to the decompressor, allowing it to synchronize its history buffer or dictionary with the one in the compressor. The Lempel-Ziv algorithms assume this to be an orderly, error-free process.[2] The problem is that communications networks sometimes scramble the order in which information is transmitted or, worse yet, garble or lose information during transmission. Now, essentially all computer communications network protocols solve these problems; somewhere within the protocol stack, they order the parts of a transmission and apply both error-detection and recovery techniques so that the chances of an end user receiving anything but a bit-identical copy of transmitted data are vanishingly small. However, this may not be true at low levels of the communications protocol where transmission may be neither orderly nor error-free. Therefore, as we will see, manufacturers of WAN data communications products have been forced to develop special (often proprietary) error detection and correction schemes to keep history buffers and dictionaries in synchronization. This solves the compression integrity problem, but there is little that can be done when a network loses information, except retransmit the data and restart the adaptive compression process. The only choice may be to trash the history buffer or dictionary and restart from zero, a situation not good for maintaining high compression ratios and high throughput or short response times.

Data compression involves making trade-offs. For data communications, processing time and resources are invested to shrink and expand data in the hope that the time and expense for doing that will be more than offset by the improved throughput on the WAN link. As we know, some algorithms compress more than others, and the more that data can be compressed, the less there is to send across the link. But obtaining more compression usually means spending more time, or spending more money to make it happen faster, or both. In data communications, obtaining the highest compression ratio to minimize the number of bits sent across the line is not always the best choice. The reason is the effective throughput increases only when the time spent compressing and decompressing data is less than that saved by transmitting compressed data. Figure 7.4 illustrates this point by showing timings for both uncompressed and compressed file transfers. With uncompressed file transfers, the file transfer time is that needed to transmit the uncompressed data across the line. With compressed file transfers, the data transmission time (see Table 7.3) shrinks by a factor of 2 or more. But the actual file transfer time is data transmission time plus the time spent compressing and uncompressing data.

Transfers on low-bandwidth, "slow" lines make the time spent compressing and decompressing data less critical. In fact, as Figure 7.4 suggests, even a serial compression process—something that users at both ends of the line might do in software—could reduce the file transfer time for a low-bandwidth line. How-

---

[2] For that matter, all adaptive algorithms must pass synchronization information and all assume the transmission will be error-free.

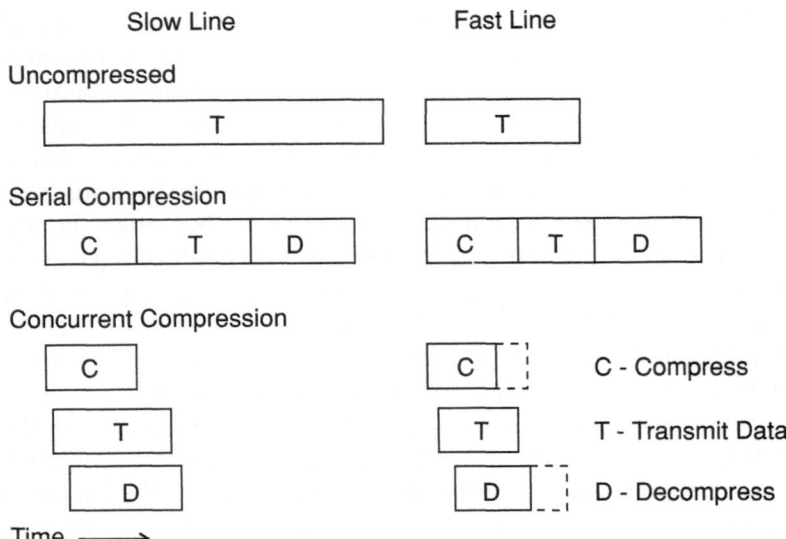

Figure 7.4   WAN file transfer timings.

ever—and there are many variables to consider including processor speed, how much and how fast the data compression algorithm squeezes and unsqueezes data, and more—serial compression is an unlikely choice when line bandwidth is greater than, say, 10 Kbps.

To reduce the file transfer time for higher-bandwidth, "fast" lines, concurrent compression is needed. With concurrent compression, independent processing functions compress and uncompress data while data transmission is in progress. Assuming they operate fast enough, most of the compression and decompression time can be overlapped with the time spent transmitting the compressed data. This must happen for the effective line bandwidth to be increased by an amount equal to the compression ratio. Here, too, line bandwidth is a factor because data transmission time decreases as bandwidth increases but compression and decompression times do not. As Figure 7.4 shows, we must find a way to shrink the compression and decompression times too. Two approaches are found in products now in the marketplace. Microprocessors dedicated to doing compression and decompression provide adequate speed for lines whose bandwidth is less than 128 Kbps (to pick a number, which will change with time and technology), whereas dedicated hardware compressor/decompressor chips are used for higher-bandwidth lines. By using dedicated hardware, the fastest currently available products can handle line speeds in the range of 1–2 Mbps [Heyw95]. This undoubtedly reflects customer demand—not the limitations of compression hardware—because lossless compression chips that operate at speeds up to 40 MBS are available [Wils94B].

Data compression has yet another effect on WAN performance when a line is shared by many users. If several users try to send data at the same time, they will experience queueing delay, the time spent waiting for traffic on the line to clear. Users perceive this as lengthy response times for transmissions that pass through the shared line. Client-server computer users doing interactive computing are highly sensitive to increases in response time, for they often depend on sending many small messages across the network and receiving second or subsecond responses. From the classic queueing theory delay curve shown in Figure

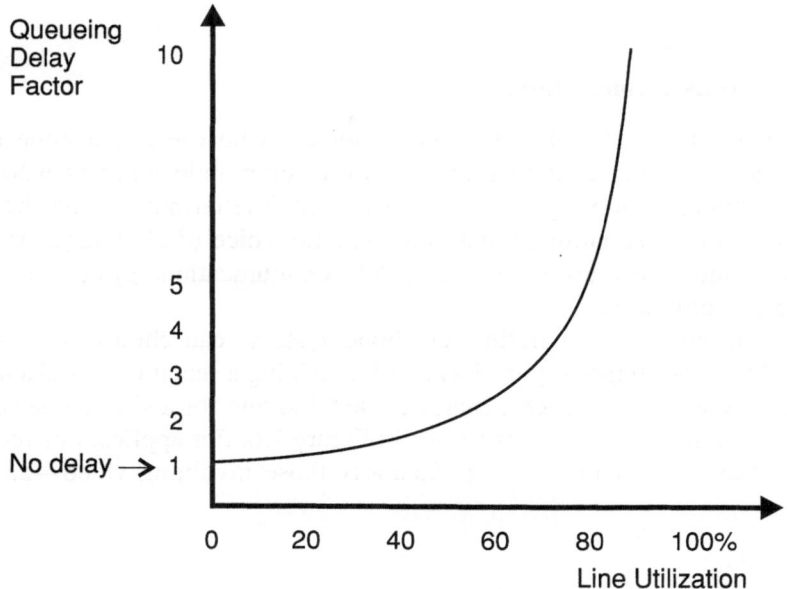

Figure 7.5 Shared-line queueing delay.

7.5, we can see that on a heavily loaded line shared by many users, the response time can grow tenfold or more. Compressed transmissions can dramatically improve response time on a shared line because the line is less busy than when carrying the same volume of uncompressed traffic. In fact, there are three ways that data compression can be used to enhance a shared line:

- Maintain the same throughput and improve the response time (at the same cost)
- Increase the effective throughput and maintain the same response time (at the same cost)
- Maintain the same throughput and response time (but cut the cost by using a lower bandwidth line)

Now let us examine the compression technology used for networked computing. The environments and products considered are as follows:

- Individual users connected via modems to remote and client-server computing environments

- Shared lines where multiplexers allow a mixture of voice, data, and FAX traffic to be carried between sites within businesses and organizations
- LAN-to-LAN internetworking where bridges and routers establish a WAN connection
- Remote I/O devices where computer channel extenders establish a WAN connection
- High-speed links used to form the backbone of WANs
- Computer networks where communications software is used for managing the network

Individual user connections

This environment is typical for telecommuters who use a telephone line to connect their personal computer to a network, or mobile workers who use a wireless communications system to connect a mobile terminal to do the same. The most common situation is that voice and nonvoice (data, image, or video) information must be transmitted over a telecommunications system optimized for voice transmissions.

Users who connect to wireline telephone systems can choose from several options. One solution (see Figure 7.2) involves adding a second line and a modem to connect a computer or FAX machine. Users looking for a single-line solution can choose from the two options shown in Figure 7.6. For applications requiring the highest-available data rates—particularly those involving video—an ISDN

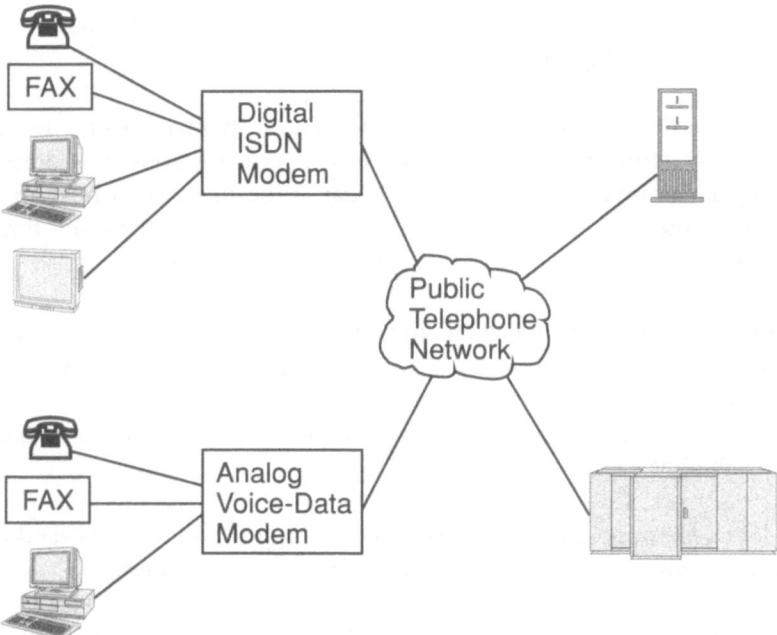

Figure 7.6   Integrated voice-data telecommunications.

digital line is attractive. The basic-rate interface ISDN service provides an aggregate uncompressed data rate of 144 Kbps that can be shared by voice, data, image, and video transmissions. However, ISDN lines are more expensive, and they are not yet available to everyone in the United States or elsewhere.

In contrast, voice-data modems for analog telephone lines are widely available. They allow voice and data (images and video too) to be transmitted during a single call. Some voice-data modems alternately transmit either voice or data. Simultaneous voice-data modems transmit both voice and data concurrently.

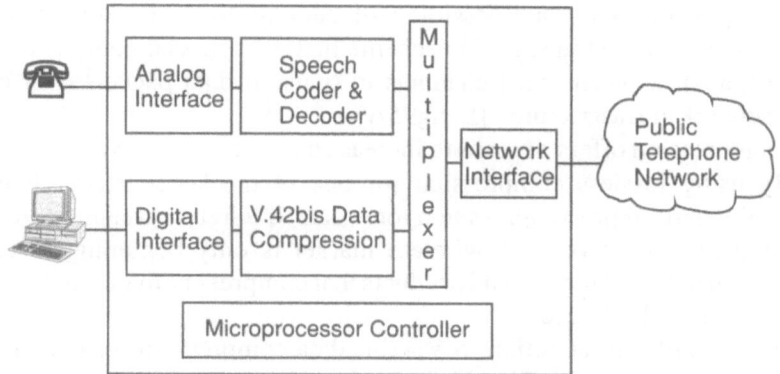

Figure 7.7   Simultaneous voice-data modem.

As shown in Figure 7.7, they incorporate speech coding and data compression functions. State-of-the-art modems provide uncompressed data rates of 28.8 Kbps, and 33.6 Kbps modems are beginning to appear.[3] Currently available voice-data modems use speech coding to reduce voice transmissions to 8 Kbps, leaving 20 Kbps (uncompressed) for data or FAX transmissions [Klei95, Mann95]. V.42bis data compression, a modem option to be discussed shortly, can multiply the data transmission rate by a factor of 2:1 or more.

Users who connect to wireless communications networks will find their options for mixing voice and nonvoice transmissions are restricted. First, let us consider how wireless systems transmit voice: As learned in Section 7.2, digital cellular telephone systems depend heavily on speech coding to increase their carrying capacity. Earlier (in Section 5.2) we learned that some speech coders can handle a mixture of voice and nonvoice; some cannot. Unfortunately, the speech coders that provide the most compression, the ones that cellular telephones use, work only for voice. They must be disabled during nonvoice transmissions, reverting the wireless channel to PCM format. The channel bandwidth for digital cellular

---

[3] Technology for modems operating at 56 Kbps exists [Wall96]. Actually, most users may not see much benefit if faster modems come to market. Today's 28.8-Kbps modems often are forced to operate at far less than their rated speed because of the noise on analog telephone lines. Modems that attempt to push to higher data rates will face increasing noise limitations.

transmissions in the United States is about 13 Kbps, but not all of that channel bandwidth is available for voice (or nonvoice) transmissions. Channel error rates are high, and extensive error correction or retransmission is required, especially for nonvoice transmissions, where data loss cannot be tolerated. As a result, today's digital cellular telephone channels provide minuscule PCM bit rates for nonvoice data transmission. For data transmissions over digital cellular systems, expect less than 9.6 Kbps after error correction is applied. The situation for analog cellular transmissions is not much better. When connected to cellular telephones, currently available analog cellular modems provide up to 14.4 Kbps. Data rates up to 19.2 Kbps are possible with cellular digital packet data (CDPD) services, an alternative transmission scheme that uses special equipment and the air space (gaps) between voice channels to transmit data packets over existing cellular network infrastructures [Lang95A].

Data compression offers a means to increase data rates for all wireless transmissions. By using lossless compression (or one of the specialized schemes for images and video) to precompress nonvoice data, a wireless channel can be used more efficiently. However, the wireless market is only beginning to consider how voice and data will merge, and products that compress nonvoice transmissions lie somewhere in the future.

Let us now shift our attention to V.42bis data compression for telephone-line modems. V.42bis is an ITU-T standard for data compression in V-series modems (9.6 Kbps V.32, 14.4 Kbps V.32bis, 28.8 Kbps V.34, and more to come). V.42bis uses LZ78 dictionary compression. (See Section 4.6 for a description of LZ78 type algorithms.) Beginning with the LZW version of LZ78, a series of modifications was made to produce an algorithm adapted for communications and cost-limited modem implementations. Here are the highlights of those changes:

- Each modem uses a pair of dictionaries—one for the compressor and another for the decompressor. Two dictionaries are required—one for each direction of transmission—because only one function, either the compressor or the decompressor, can be responsible for updating a dictionary. Then, too, the characteristics of transmitted and received data can be quite different.

- Maximum dictionary size is negotiated between the calling modem and the answering modem during call setup. The key parameters are the maximum number of tokens that each dictionary can contain and the maximum number of symbols allowed in each token. The V.42bis standard specifies each dictionary must contain a minimum of 512 tokens, each containing at most 6 symbols. Larger dictionaries are allowed, which will provide more effective compression, but this increases the modem cost because storage must be provided for the dictionaries. A well-configured V.42bis-enabled modem might provide 2048-token dictionaries, giving it somewhat better compression characteristics, but it must still work with a fully compliant but less capable V.42bis modem that provides only the minimum values. The number of symbols each token may contain is restricted both to limit the size of the dictionary and to limit the time spent searching for long string matches. Here, time considerations won out over compression efficiency.

- A procedure is defined for deleting infrequently used tokens from a dictionary. This frees space in the dictionary for reuse, allowing the fixed-size dictionaries to better track changes throughout lengthy data transmissions.
- A two-character escape sequence is provided to allow a transparent mode for sending uncompressed data whenever this provides greater compression. A V.42bis modem can shift back into compressed mode at any time by sending another two-character sequence.
- An escape-code sequence is also provided that causes the current dictionary to be discarded. This sequence can be transmitted by the compressor whenever it chooses; for example, an old dictionary may no longer be useful when a new transmission begins.

The V.42bis standard allows for a range of cost-performance trade-offs to be made in designing a compressing modem. Sometimes it is not necessary to obtain the highest compression (or to use compression at all) for data transmission. There are many other performance bottlenecks in data transmission, beginning with the data source itself. For instance, V.42bis compression will have little effect on transmissions involving short messages created by a person at a keyboard or by some client-server programs. Only when the telephone line is the bottleneck—as it will likely be when large, uncompressed data files are transferred between computers—can a V.42bis-enabled modem increase end-to-end bandwidth and have a positive influence on performance. To learn more about how data compression applies to real-world data transmissions over telephone lines, and about implementation trade-offs for V.42bis modems, see a fascinating account provided in [Thom92].

Shared line connections

This environment is typical for connecting a branch office to the corporate network, particularly in countries having limited telecommunications infrastructures. Line sharing is also important for international networks where transmission costs are much higher than within the United States. In these situations, by consolidating voice and data (images and video too) on a single transmission line and, thus, averting the need to install separate lines for each type of traffic, communications costs can be dramatically reduced.

As shown in Figure 7.8, multiplexers allow voice traffic, FAX transmissions, and data communications between computers, or between terminals and computers, to share a single line. Multiplexing and data compression are two techniques for maximizing the amount of information that a shared line can carry. Multiplexing subdivides the line's capacity, whereas data compression reduces the number of bits each source must transmit. Together, these techniques allow multiple sources to share a communications line whose bandwidth capacity is less than the sum of the capacity requirements of the individual sources.

There are several multiplexing techniques for subdividing communication line bandwidth [Stal94A, Stal94B, Tayl95A]. Voice-data multiplexers may use any

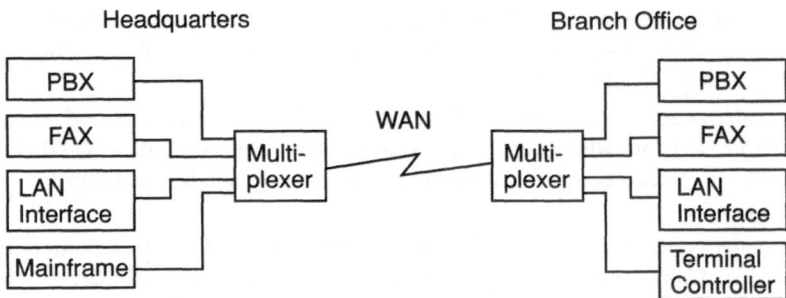

Figure 7.8 Shared-line connection.

or all of the following: Time-division multiplexing (TDM) assigns time slots to each data source. Data from many sources can be carried simultaneously by time-interleaving bursts of data from each source. This form of multiplexing is suitable for carrying voice and other delay-sensitive traffic because each source is guaranteed some fraction of the line bandwidth. The disadvantage of TDM is that if any data source does not fully utilize its time slots, the line will not used to its full capacity. Statistical time-division multiplexing (STDM) allows any time slot to be used by any source, which allows the line capacity to be used more effectively. However, as no one source is guaranteed a specific amount of bandwidth, the basic STDM technique must be enhanced for this application.

Fast-packet multiplexing, a generic term applied to many different high-speed transmission technologies, sends data across the line in packets (small blocks) that may contain data from any of the sources.[4] Essentially an extension of STDM, this multiplexing technique makes the entire line bandwidth available for all types of traffic. To assure that time-sensitive sources receive the bandwidth they need, all traffic on the line is prioritized. Packets from time-sensitive sources receive the highest priorities and are transmitted first. Packets from other sources such as LANs are given lower priorities; these packets are held in a buffer memory until packets with higher priority clear the line. Should the buffer overflow, packets will be dropped, forcing retransmission of packets from lower-priority sources.

Data compression techniques are important to multiplexers for sending both voice and data. Today's multiplexers allow voice and data to be sent over medium-speed lines as data rates as low as 56 Kbps. In many countries, 56 Kbps may be the fastest WAN link available, and throughout the world, if faster lines are available, they (usually) cost more. As learned in Section 7.2, a single uncompressed voice line requires a bandwidth of 64 Kbps, making the transmission of

---

[4] High-speed transmission protocols that use fast-packet multiplexing include frame relay where variable-size packets are transmitted and cell relay protocols such as SMDS and ATM, where small, fixed-size packets are transmitted.

even one voice channel impossible at 56 Kbps. With ITU-T standardized speech coding (compression), each voice line can be reduced to 32, 16, 8, or even 5.3 Kbps. For users who have a PBX (private branch exchange) with many voice lines to connect and have a lot of voice traffic, a multiplexer that provides efficient voice compression can mean real savings. Many multiplexer vendors go beyond the standards to provide proprietary speech coding algorithms operating at rates as low as 2.4 Kbps [Tayl95A]. Some use silence suppression, a technique that transmits no voice packets during lulls in the conversation, which can be quite effective because rarely are people at each end of the line speaking at the same time.[5] However, as with all low-bit-rate speech coding techniques, speech quality is a concern and users should be prepared to accept less than telephone-system speech quality.

Multiplexers also employ a full range of compression techniques for data transmission. The data packet compression techniques used by bridges and routers (discussed below) apply here too. Indeed, it becomes difficult to distinguish products sold as voice-data multiplexers from bridges and routers because many multiplexers provide optional bridge and router hardware modules that eliminate the need for additional equipment. It must be noted that, except for voice, multiplexers do not conform to any standards for data compression. This means that products from different manufacturers that do provide data compression usually cannot interoperate.

LAN-to-LAN internetworking

This environment is typical for large and not so large organizations whose workers are geographically dispersed. Within a site, PCs, workstations, printers, and other I/O devices, servers, minicomputers, and even mainframes and super-computers are connected to a LAN. This allows computer users within a site to access data and resources beyond those available on their own system. When their collaborative efforts are spread across sites, these same users will need access to data and resources on LANs that serve other sites. The solution is to interconnect various LANs so that any two devices on the interconnected networks can communicate. Interconnecting LANs may be as simple as snaking a cable to the next floor or building and tying the networks together with appropriate interface devices. However, as shown in Figure 7.9, when LANs are separated by greater distances, their interconnection often requires sending data through an intermediate WAN. Today's LANs operate at 10–100 Mbps, whereas afford-able WAN links may operate at no more than 56 Kbps to 1.5 Mbps. The problem, which even a moderate-sized organization is likely to encounter, is that LAN-to-LAN traffic tends to be occasional and bursty and can easily saturate a WAN link, causing intolerable queuing delays. A higher-bandwidth WAN link is the

---

[5] See the discussion of variable bit-rate coding in Section 5.2.

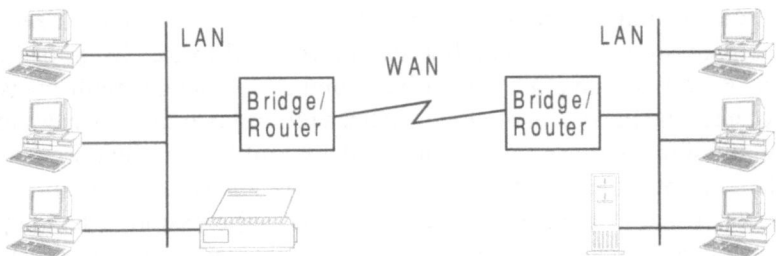

Figure 7.9   LAN-to-LAN internetworking.

answer, but faster WAN links are not always available, and if they are, they will definitely be more expensive. Data compression often is a much cheaper solution.

Several types of devices are available for internetworking LANs. Our interest is in bridges and routers, devices that establish remote connections through a WAN link, and in so doing, compress data. Bridges and routers that use compression increase the effective bandwidth of the WAN link, thus, more closely matching its bandwidth to that of the LANs, or they lower the cost of transmission by allowing a lower-bandwidth WAN connection to be used. Briefly, bridges are appropriate when interconnecting two similar LANs that use the same signaling and message transmission protocols, whereas routers connect two networks that may be similar, or different, but use the same message transmission protocol.[6] As the name implies, routers deal with selecting and sending data over multiple WAN links, but so do bridges. The real difference is that bridges are faster because they operate at layer 2 of the transmission protocol, whereas routers operate at layer 3 [Davi94].

To appreciate how data compression works in bridges and routers, we must understand that high-speed WANs use some form of packet switching. To efficiently handle the data traffic that computers generate, they transmit data in short bursts. As shown in Figure 7.10, a user message is broken into a series of packets. The entire message might contain (to pick a number) 1500 bytes, but, depending on the WAN protocol, the packets can be much smaller. Each packet contains a header and part of the user message—the payload. The header contains control information including source and destination addresses that allow each packet to be routed through the network from its source to the destination. When all the packets arrive at the destination, the headers are stripped off and a copy of the message is assembled.

From this brief introduction of packet switching, it is clear there are many

---

[6] There are also gateways for connecting two computer networks that use entirely different communications architectures. Depending on whether incoming and departing messages are compressed or not, gateways may use data compression as they transfer information from one network to the other.

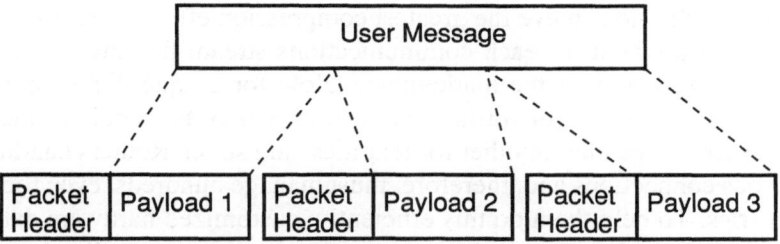

Figure 7.10 Message packets.

opportunities for data compression to reduce the volume of bits flowing across the network. Let us begin our discussion of the ways data compression can be applied with two operating modes—packet-by-packet mode and continuous mode. As mentioned earlier, most network-compression products use some variation of Lempel-Ziv, the algorithms that use a history buffer or dictionary. Packet-by-packet mode starts a new history buffer or dictionary for each packet and discards it when packet transmission is finished. Continuous mode creates a history buffer or dictionary and refines it over many packets in a communications stream, discarding it only when the connection is closed down.

Packet-by-packet mode cannot achieve much compression unless the packets are very large, which they often are not. Its advantage is that the compressor and decompressor dictionaries need only be synchronized within a packet. Continuous mode can achieve higher compression ratios because there is more data to which to adapt. But this requires the dictionaries at both ends of the link be kept in synchronization across many packets, using some type of error correction that can compensate for lost or corrupted packets. Without this, dictionaries can diverge, and it becomes impossible to correctly decompress subsequent packets. If this happens, both dictionaries must be flushed, outstanding packets must be discarded, and the entire transmission must be restarted. Because not all network protocols provide the necessary error detection (much less correction) in the network protocol layers where bridges and routers operate, manufacturers of networking products that use continuous-mode compression must provide their own.[7] Lacking standards for keeping dictionaries in synchronization, as one might expect, different proprietary error-handling schemes have been developed [Heyw95].

Another difference between packet-by-packet and continuous-mode compression is the number of dictionaries. Packet-by-packet mode uses only one set of dictionaries at each end of the link (one for the compressor, another for the decompressor); all packets moving across the link share the same dictionaries.

---

[7] To take advantage of the high data rates and low error rates of modern transmission facilities, broadband technologies such as frame relay eliminate error checking and correction at low levels, moving the function closer to the end users [Davi94, Stal94B].

Continuous mode—to achieve the greatest compression effect—requires the dictionaries be customized for each communications stream flowing on the WAN link. Many routers now in the marketplace allow for unique dictionaries to be associated with each type of traffic that each user may be sending; one set of dictionaries for image files, another for text files, and so on. Routers handle many simultaneous connections and, therefore, must manage hundreds, even thousands of dictionaries. To help them do this efficiently, customized hardware data compression chips have been created for network compression applications, chips that allow rapidly switching between many different dictionaries [Chil95].

Now, let us discuss what part of a packet should be compressed. There are three options: header compression, payload compression, and frame compression (that compresses the entire packet). Header compression makes sense when the packets are very small. The header for TCP/IP, a popular network protocol, contains 40 bytes of data; the headers for other protocols may be larger (or smaller). For typical interactive computing sessions, each message contains only a few bytes of data, which makes most of the bits on the WAN line overhead—there just to escort packets from their source to their destination. To address this situation, a standardized header compression scheme has been defined for TCP/IP that reduced the 40-byte header to just 5 bytes [Jaco90]. It recognizes that much of the per-packet header information remains unchanged from packet to packet for a sequence of packets traveling between specific addresses during the life of a connection. By keeping track of active connections, the sender can transmit only what has changed from the previous packet and the receiver, who maintains an identical history, can reconstruct the packet header. Header compression is protocol-specific; a different algorithm must be developed for each network protocol. Unfortunately, not all network protocols have standards for header compression, leaving manufacturers of networking products that use it to develop their own implementations.

In payload compression, only the data payload portion of the data packet is compressed, leaving the header intact. Besides the obvious, that payload compression makes sense for the large data packets used when data files and images are being transmitted, it has the advantage that network latency is not increased. With the header information left unchanged, packets can be routed through a multihop network without decompressing and recompressing any part of the packet, just as they would be if uncompressed. In addition, it is the only option for virtual-packet switching network services such as X.25, frame relay, and ATM, where the unchanged header information must be available to switch the packets through the network.

Frame compression, which compresses the entire packet, provides the best compression ratio, and is insensitive to network protocols, might seem the best choice, but that is not always true. Because the entire packet is compressed, information in the header is not available for switching the packet through a WAN switching network. For routing packets through multihop networks, the intermediate routers must decompress and recompress the packet at each step to recover routing information from the header, which can only delay packet transmission through the network. This makes frame compression a good solution for point-to-point connections, such as leased lines and ISDN, where switching and routing are not issues. Here, compressing the entire data stream to be transported across the link, as if it were one application, will maximize the compression ratio.

Our discussion of LAN-to-LAN internetworking would not be complete without mentioning other effective "compression" (i.e., data reduction) techniques that many routers use to increase the effective WAN bandwidth. All LAN protocols create packet traffic whose sole purpose is to aid in managing the LAN [Darl95]. Some of this traffic can be eliminated from WAN links by filtering information that is of no interest to distant LANs. Other traffic can be eliminated by protocol spoofing whereby the router responds to "are you still alive" requests as if it were the distant LAN, rather than passing the request through the WAN link.

In the marketplace, today, there is a wide range of WAN-link bridges and routers that provide compression, and there are stand-alone compression products for use with routers that do not have integrated compression. Routers use various combinations of all the techniques we have described. Bridges and stand-alone compressors, which work at the lowest level of the network protocol, are limited to frame compression. The performance of these products—both how fast they operate and how much compression they deliver—and their cost varies. The key factors are whether special-purpose hardware is dedicated to data compression and the effectiveness of the compression techniques. However, WAN line speeds up to 2 Mbps and, depending on the network traffic mix, compression ratios of 2:1–4:1 or more are not unusual [Quia94, Toll94A, Toll94B, Darl95]. Finally, we must note there are no standards for data compression in LAN-to-LAN internetworking. This means that bridges and routers from different manufacturers which do provide data compression usually cannot interoperate.

Mainframe Computer I/O
Channel Extension

Large mainframe computer systems, as shown in Figure 7.11(a), use I/O channels to connect their I/O (input/output) devices. Independent of the main processor(s), an I/O channel provides special-purpose processing for I/O data and device control; it also defines a protocol and physical interface for connecting I/O devices to the computer. Originally, the physical I/O channel connection for IBM mainframe computers was a parallel copper-wire interface, limited to not more than 3 MBS (24 Mbps) and limited to distances of about 400 feet (120 meters). More recently, a dedicated fiber connection, ESCON™ (IBM's Enterprise System Connection Architecture), has been developed that allows data to be sent at speeds up to 133 Mbps over distances up to about 10 kilometers. This allows greater flexibility for locating I/O devices within a site, but many organizations have need for locating printers and tape libraries, for instance, off-site at even

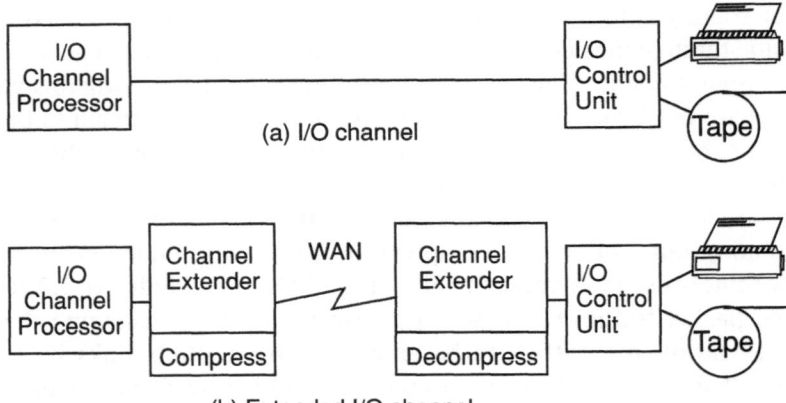

(b) Extended I/O channel

Figure 7.11   Mainframe computer input/output.

greater distances. For them, various manufacturers offer channel extender products that greatly increase the maximum distance.

As shown in Figure 7.11(b), some channel extenders use medium-speed WAN links to transport I/O data and device control information over great distances. Clearly, the WAN bandwidth determines how well the extended I/O channel performs, and data compression can provide the same type of benefit that we have seen in other WAN-link applications. By reducing the number bits to be transmitted, it reduces the WAN bandwidth required, reduces the communications costs, and maximizes the throughput and capacity of the extended I/O channel. There are several ways in which I/O channel data compression can be accomplished. However, precompressing the I/O data in the mainframe processor is not one of them because I/O control units have no decompression facilities. Instead, as shown in Figure 7.11(b), compression and decompression can be integral functions within the channel extender, or (not shown) external compressors and decompressors can be connected between the channel extender and the communications link. Somewhat akin to the differences that separate bridges and routers, integral compression will likely provide the most data reduction: An external compressor is limited to using a single history buffer or dictionary for compressing the entire WAN-link bit stream, no matter what mix of I/O devices is active. Because the channel extender recognizes I/O channel commands and it knows which I/O device that data is intended for, an integral compressor can maintain a unique history buffer or dictionary for each I/O device. (Recall that similar techniques are used in routers.) This allows the data stream for a tape unit, for instance, to be treated differently than printer data that may have quite different compression characteristics. Experimental results show data compression is highly effective for extended I/O channels. Whereas external compression techniques may provide a 2:1 reduction, compression ratios of 5:1 or higher have been observed for integral compressors [Levi95]. However, results do vary. For example, data compression will work quite differently on an I/O channel carrying precompressed image traffic when compared to that same I/O channel carrying highly compressible printer data. As with bridges and routers, there are no standards for I/O channel data compression, and different manufactures channel extenders that provide data compression usually cannot interoperate.

High-speed links

So far we have discussed data compression for WAN links whose bandwidth ranges up to 1–2 Mbps. As shown in Figure 7.12(a), the approach taken is to

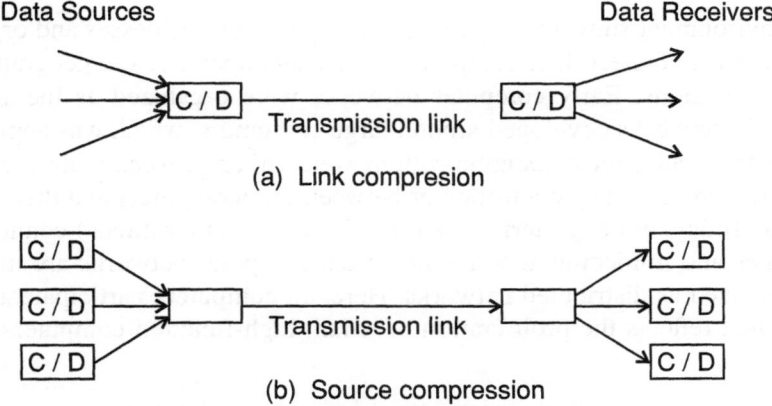

Figure 7.12 Communications compression.

position a compressor/decompressor at each end of the link and compress traffic on the link. One might also consider doing data compression in the same way for high-speed broadband LANs and WANs. However, the need for data compression on high-speed links is not as clear in that new protocols for copper links and the adoption of optical technology have roughly kept pace with user demands for bandwidth. Also, there is the issue of data rate. Broadband LANs and WANs are pushing ever closer to gigabit-per-second data rates—far faster that what any existing single piece of data compression hardware or software can handle.[8] This combination of factors makes direct application of compression to broadband LANs or WANs questionable, at least until faster data compression technology becomes available.[9] Today, if data compression is to be used for broadband LAN and WAN transmissions, a more workable approach is the indirect one shown

---

[8] Wireless LANs are a different story. Their bandwidths are much lower, making data compression more feasible, and their usage is spreading, making it more desirable. As a result, one might speculate that data compression technology could someday be adapted to wireless LANs.

[9] However, there are situations where broadband transmissions must be sent over lower-bandwidth links. One manufacturer has introduced a product that compresses ATM traffic for transmission over an intermediate satellite link. It operates at speeds up to 45 Mbps [Gree96].

in Figure 7.12(b). Here, each source of traffic precompresses data before sending it to the network and, after transmission, postdecompresses it. Given the data compression technology currently available, this is the most practical approach for amassing enough computation compression power to match the transmission bandwidth of broadband LANs and WANs. Indeed, it currently is the approach used to handle video transmissions where the transmission of uncompressed video overtaxes the capacity of broadband WANs and LANs, making precompression and postdecompression a necessity.

Computer networks

The environment shown in Figure 7.13 is typical for businesses and organizations who must connect their computers to manage operations at geographically dispersed locations. Early computer networks were organized as hierarchical, host-centric networks developed around large computers, which was appropriate for the time because most communications were either between mainframes and the remote terminals they controlled or between minicomputers and their remote terminals. Today, although terminals (or PCs emulating terminals) connected to mainframes and minicomputers are still used, computer networks are more apt to be organized as distributed networks. Here, all computers participate as equal peers, which reflects the proliferation of small, high-function computers.

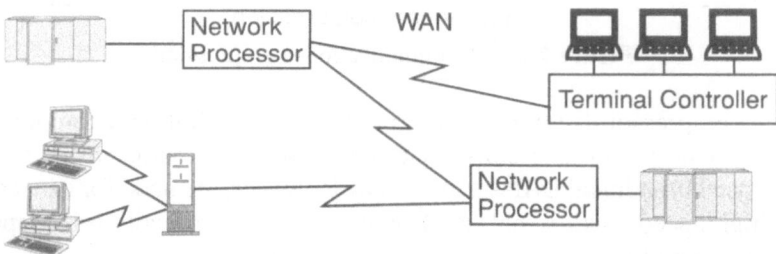

Figure 7.13   A computer network.

Efficiently managing networked computer and communications resources is critical for organizations having sophisticated distributed systems interconnected over LANs and WANs. When faced with designing and managing a complex, multilink computer network, managers must decide where to place network processors, select the types of links to use, and determine the capacity of both the nodes and links within the network. One aspect of this task is deciding how data compression should be applied to the network to maximize its performance and, of course, minimize the cost for communications. This task is complicated by factors such as the diversity of tariffs for domestic and international communications, the differences in line speeds throughout the network, the processing power at each node that can be devoted to data compression, and the diversity of traffic flowing on each link within the network. Fortunately, there are network design tools to assist in this effort, such as the one described in [Cahn91]. These tools can help to understand how data compression will affect the total cost and/ or the average performance of the network. They also can help decide how the existing design should be modified if data compression is added to a network, including selecting the links, routings, and locations for compression and decompression. As seen in the environments described earlier in this section, data compression may be, and often is, introduced to meet the performance and/or cost problems associated with a specific link or set of users. However, by taking a more global view, network design tools often allow managers to discover that the best network configuration for compressed traffic is not a scaled-down version of a network designed for uncompressed traffic [Cahn92].

As discussed earlier in this section, computer networks are controlled by communications software that runs in each computer and device connected to the network and provides a common architecture and protocol to facilitate the exchange of data. Although a full discussion of computer communications architectures and protocols is beyond the scope of this book, we are interested in one aspect—how this software uses data compression to reduce storage and transmission costs for computer communications.[10] There are several approaches for using data compression in computer communications: One is for user-application programs to compress data before handing it off to the communications software. However, many communications architectures provide for data compression as a function within one of their layers. When setting up the communications network, users must decide which links in the network will carry compressed traffic, which conversations on a link will be compressed, and, naturally, which data compression method to use. Some communications architectures do not specify the data compression method, allowing the user to make an application-specific selection. Others provide support for data compression as a general facility within the communications software itself. For instance, SNA (IBM System Network Architecture) provides two (proprietary) data compression techniques, a run-length coding algorithm similar to the HDC algorithm described in Section 4.3 and an LZ78 dictionary algorithm of the type described in Section 4.6 [Guru84, IBM6]. These algorithms may be used individually or in combination.

Another type of data compression has been used in computer network software for a very long while. In an era when communications lines operated at 1.2–9.6 Kbps, and much of the traffic on those lines consisted of text-based data being sent between terminals and mainframes or minicomputers, the introduction of terminal controllers (see Figure 7.13) was a significant step forward. Not only could the transmissions from several terminals be concentrated onto a single line but, because the terminal controller was programmable, there was opportunity

---

[10] Descriptions of computer communications protocols and architectures can be found in many references, including [Stal94A, Stal94B].

to apply data compression to reduce the number of transmitted bits. Here is what was done[11]: Figure 7.14 shows a screen that might be presented to a terminal user as part of an order-entry program. To add an item to the order, the terminal user keys data into the (shaded) product code and quantity fields. If standard programming techniques are used, when the enter key is struck, the entire screen is transmitted back to the host computer where a program updates the order, fills in the description, unit price, amount, and total fields (designated by boxes), and sends an updated screen back to the terminal. Smart programming recognizes that the user has changed only two fields, extracts those fields, and sends them to the host. Similarly, the host program returns only the fields it changes. Of course, even further reduction will occur if each field is compressed before transmission.

```
┌─────────────────────────────────────────────────────┐
│              ACME Tools Incorporated                  │
│  Customer:                                            │
│  Smith Company                                        │
│  Anywhere, USA                                        │
│                                                       │
│  Product   Description  Quantity   Unit      Amount   │
│  Code                               Price             │
│                                                       │
│  A001      Hammer          2       $5.17     $10.34   │
│  C025      Clamp          10        0.39      3.90    │
│  C100      Wrench          1        9.87      9.87    │
│  [D072]    [        ]     [2]      [    ]    [     ]   │
│                                                       │
│                                    Total [ $24.11 ]   │
└─────────────────────────────────────────────────────┘
```

Figure 7.14   Order-entry screen.

Looking back, we might dismiss what was done as just smart programming or data reduction—not data compression. However, in reality, two sound principles for applying data compression to digital systems were exploited—differential coding and dictionary substitution. Differential coding allows that when both the sender and receiver retain the last message transmitted, only the differences between messages in a sequence of messages need be coded and transmitted. In this application, most of the screen remains unchanged, and differential coding greatly reduces traffic on the communications line. Dictionary substitution allows for a token or code to be transmitted, and when received, it is replaced by an entry from the local dictionary. In this application, dictionary substitution operates in the following way: At any given time, there are a finite number of screens that can be sent to a particular terminal connected to a particular application. Most of the data on a screen is "boilerplate" that remains unchanged no matter how often the screen is used. There is no need to transmit this information but

---

[11] For examples of products which use these techniques, see [Held91].

once if the receiver (in this case, the terminal controller) can store the screen panels. Later, when a particular screen is needed, only a byte or two of data must be sent to allow the receiver to extract a copy from its "dictionary." Then, data for the variable fields on the screen is sent (compressed, of course), and the screen panel is reconstructed. Smart programming or data compression? Either way, both techniques are effective and remain in widespread use.

7.4   FAX

Business applications for facsimile began to appear in the 1960s, but the only available FAX machines used analog technology and they were expensive. They were also hard to use and their copy quality was not good. Most distressingly, they were slow. There was just too much data to send over ordinary telephone lines. Transmitting an 8½-inch × 11-inch page required 6 minutes. Improvements in the 1970s cut the time nearly in half, but transmission was still far too slow and far too expensive over long-distance telephone lines. A more reasonable goal was to send at least two pages each minute. Thanks to the development of effective compression algorithms, that goal was met in 1980 when the ITU-T adopted the Group 3 standard for coding, compressing, and transmitting digital facsimile [Mcco92, Arps94]. However, at that time, digital technology was still expensive, but costs were dropping rapidly. By the mid-1980s, FAX machines went from being rare and expensive to becoming everyday equipment for business and home use.

Standards for transmission and data compression are important in the FAX marketplace. The early ITU-T Group 1 and Group 2 standards for facsimile applied to analog facsimile equipment, which no longer is widely used. Today's Group 3 standard applies to all equipment intended for digital facsimile transmission of bi-level (black-and-white) images over PSTN (Public-Switched Telephone Network) analog transmission facilities. It specifies scanning, coding (compression), transmission, and printing for equipment intended for person-to-person communications. Group 3 equipment, including stand-alone FAX machines and FAX modem attachments for computers, is widely available. Also, computer-generated documents can be converted to the format specified by the standard and, using a computer with a FAX adapter card installed, transmitted either to another similarly equipped computer or to a stand-alone FAX machine. There also is a Group 4 standard that applies to all equipment intended for digital facsimile transmission of bi-level images over the digital transmission facilities of the ISDN (Integrated Services Digital Network). It is intended for computer-controlled, business applications such as electronic mail, electronic document storage and retrieval, integrated text and graphics document handling, and so on. Group 4 facsimile equipment is not yet widely deployed, because ISDN is not widely deployed and because the function and speed of Group 3 equipment continue to improve. Also, Group 3 equipment is now allowed to work on ISDN digital lines, transmitting at 64 Kbps, several times faster than today's typical PSTN-connected FAX machine [Coop93].

Our discussion will focus on the workings of Group 3 facsimile, which consists of scanning, transmission, and printing—the three operations shown in Figure

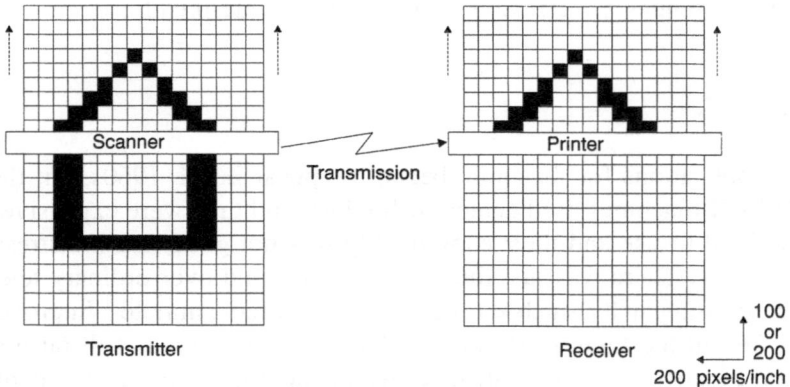

Figure 7.15   Group 3 bi-level facsimile.

7.15. Each page is treated as an image represented by a two-dimensional array of pixels. The page being sent is scanned one line at a time starting at the top of the page. The scan line, which is oriented across the width of an 8½-inch page, corresponds to a row of pixels. Within the scanner, the scan line is focused on a CCD (charge-coupled device) chip that contains a line array of 1728 photosensors; each photosensor reads the brightness of one pixel and produces an electrical signal. For bi-level images, the signal is interpreted as either a binary 1 or 0, corresponding to a black or a white pixel. After the signals for an entire scan line have been read out, buffered, encoded, and transmitted, the page is stepped forward one scan line. The resolution of this scanning process is (approximately) 200 pixels/inch horizontally and 100 or 200 pixels/inch vertically, depending on whether standard or fine resolution is selected. At the receiving end, the signals are decoded and converted into a format suitable for a thermal or laser printer. Synchronization signals are transmitted along with the page image data to keep the printer and scanner locked in step.

From Figure 7.15, we can see why transmitting an uncompressed FAX page requires so many bits. Not only does each object on the page produce bits to be transmitted, but so do the white spaces between objects. Within objects, large features are represented by many bits and adjacent horizontal scan lines can be nearly identical. Early digital facsimile pioneers recognized these conditions as opportunities for data compression. Specialized algorithms were developed that not only compressed the long strings of 0's representing white space and the shorter strings of 1's representing black features, but the algorithms also vertically correlated the horizontal scan lines for further compression.

So far, we have described facsimile methods suitable for transmitting bi-level, black-and-white images. Facsimile transmission of more complex images is also possible. JBIG is a joint ITU-T and ISO/IEC standard for both bi-level and multilevel (several bits per pixel) images. For bi-level, black-and-white images, when compared to the algorithms specified in the ITU-T T.4 and T.6 recommendations for Group 3 FAX, JBIG offers more compression. JBIG is also effective when halftone black-and-white images, gray-scale, or color images are directed to image printers. Another advantage of JBIG is that it allows progressive encoding. This allows, for example, a low-resolution image to be quickly sent to an image display for browsing. Then, if requested, more detail can be sent.

JPEG, a joint ITU-T and ISO/IEC standard for photographic-quality color (gray-scale and black-white too) images, is the standard specified for color facsimile. Although JPEG is usually thought of as a lossy algorithm, it also provides lossless coding for facsimile images. However, there has been little interest in stand-alone color FAX equipment because costs are higher than black-and-white facsimile and business needs have not yet developed. Long term, the prospects for color facsimile may hinge on the growing number of low-cost color printers and color photocopiers, which can easily double as color FAX devices.

Characteristics of the algorithms applicable to facsimile compression are summarized in Table 7.5. Detailed descriptions can be found in Chapter 5. All of

Table 7.5 Compression algorithms for facsimile.

Algorithm	ITU-T Recommendation	Lossless Coding Techniques Employed
MH (modified Huffman coding)	T.4 (Group 3)	Sequences of black or white pixels in one scan line are run-length encoded followed by static Huffman coding.
MR (modified READ coding)	T.4 (Group 3)	The differences in two adjacent scan lines are coded using the vertical correlation of black and white pixels. Periodically, an MH-coded line is inserted to limit error propagation.
MMR (modified-modified READ coding)	T.6 (Group 4)	MRR adapts MR for error-free transmission. The differences in two adjacent scan lines are coded using the vertical correlation of black and white pixels. MH-coded lines are not needed.
JBIG	T.82	Bi-level images are coded with an adaptive two-dimensional model that uses either two or three lines of the image followed by adaptive arithmetic coding. Multilevel grey or color images are similarly coded with a three-dimensional model.
JPEG	T.81	Continuous-tone, grey-scale images and color pictures are coded, employing transforms, Huffman, and arithmetic coding.

these algorithms provide lossless compression of facsimile images. The JPEG algorithm also provides for lossy compression of color facsimile images.

7.5   Teleconferencing

Teleconferencing means "meeting at a distance," using telecommunications links to bridge the distance and bring people together. Teleconferencing allows physically separated groups or individuals to meet, to collaborate, and to share information without traveling. Teleconferencing is nothing new; the telephone is the most basic of all teleconferencing systems. What is new are affordable teleconferencing systems that allow sharing voice, data, images, and video. Moreover, the public-switched telephone network has become more robust, providing the digital bandwidth needed to support these systems. The result is, among other things, telecommuting, a new life-style that allows working electronically from a distance without commuting.

As shown in Table 7.6, there are a variety of teleconferencing solutions. Some are low-cost, some are more integrated, and some are more functional. The simplest of all is plain old telephone conferencing (via speakerphone) in conjunction with FAX. It provides adequate function for many applications without any

Table 7.6   Teleconferencing solutions.

Teleconferencing Solutions	Voice	Still Images (B/W and Color)	Specialized Input/Output Devices	Document Sharing and Annotation	Computer Data File Sharing and Annotation	Video
Telephone and FAX	✓	✓ (B/W)	No	No	No	No
Audiographics systems	✓	✓ (Optional)	✓ (Optional)	✓ (Optional)	No	No
Videophone	✓	✓ (Optional)	No	No	No	✓
Videoconferencing	✓	✓ (Optional)	✓ (Optional)	✓ (Optional)	✓ (Optional)	✓
Desktop computer conferencing	✓[1]	✓[1]	✓ (Optional)	✓ (Optional)	✓	✓[1]

Notes:
[1] With desktop videoconferencing.

additional expense to users who already have telephones and FAX machines. Audiographics systems are more sophisticated. They offer a mix of voice and graphics information of all types, and some allow document sharing. Video solutions now lead the teleconferencing marketplace. The cost of video transmission has declined, as have costs for videophones and videoconferencing systems, making video far more affordable. Then, too, many users already have networked desktop computers; when equipped with computer conferencing software and videoconferencing hardware, desktop computers provide an integrated, cost-effective solution offering all teleconferencing services. In the immediately following sections of this chapter, we will examine how data compression applies to graphics-based and video-based teleconferencing systems.

7.6 Audiographics

Audiographics systems combine two types of data—audio and graphics—and transmit them over telephone lines. These systems are useful in applications where visual illustrations are needed to complement telephone conferencing. Examples include collaborative efforts in business, education, government, and personal communications, where images, drawings, copies of documents, sketches, computer graphics, and other visual information must be exchanged. Applications where audiographics systems have proven useful include planning, project management, problem-solving sessions, and training, among others. The primary advantage of an audiographics system is the low-cost means for interconnecting to any site in the world via public telephone lines.

Audiographics systems use a variety of technology including the following [Park94]:

- Telewriting equipment, including pens, tablets, and boards for capturing freehand messages and graphics
- Freeze-frame video systems for transmitting images, documents, graphics, or still pictures of conference participants
- Computer systems for transmitting text, graphics, and annotation of documents or images

Other equipment may be used to complement an audiographics system. FAX machines, scanners, and any device whose output can be sent over telephone lines may be used together with an audiographics system.

The function (and cost) of audiographics systems ranges widely. The simplest may provide one device such as an electronic tablet for sending handwritten drawings or messages. Moving up the scale, one finds products such as the AT&T Picasso™ Still-Image Phone. It allows users to send full-color, compressed still images and, optionally, do freehand annotations with a user-supplied mouse and a standard television display [Viza93]. More functional systems offer a variety of specialized input/output devices—video cameras for capturing drawings, documents, slides, and microscope images, scanners for capturing high-resolution documents and images, video monitors for displaying images, and high-resolution printers. Also, it is not uncommon to find audiographics systems that use a computer to control the system and have storage devices for digitized graphics data. From a hardware viewpoint, a well-configured audiographics system may not be all that different than a computer conferencing system or a videoconferencing system, and therein lies a problem—the high cost of audiographics systems in relation to their competition.

Telephones and FAX machines are everywhere and they are inexpensive. Small videoconferencing systems sell in the same price range as audiographics systems and can connect the same specialized input/output devices. Users of networked desktop computers, who choose to equip them with computer conferencing software and videoconferencing hardware, can enjoy all the conferencing services of an audiographics system—plus video—often at far less cost. Thus, with the availability of affordable, more integrated, more functional teleconferencing solutions, the appeal of specialized audiographics systems has declined.

Standards for interconnection and interoperation are important for all teleconferencing solutions. However, standards, including those for data compression, have not played a big role in developing audiographics systems, other than voice transmission standards. For graphics information, audiographics system manufacturers have chosen to use various compressed file formats including JPEG and many de facto standards such as GIF. But the marketplace focus is shifting to computer conferencing (and videoconferencing) and there has been new interest in standards that cover all aspects of teleconferencing. In Chapter 5, standards for voice (speech) and videoconferencing were described. Only recently has a standard emerged that augments these standards, covering graphics and the other forms of information used for conferencing. The ITU-T T.120 suite of recommendations for data sharing allows exchanging (computer) data and images and provides protocols for linking whiteboards, scanners, projectors, and other conferencing equipment [Sull95, Mess95A]. It remains to be determined whether these recommendations will be adopted by all who provide teleconferencing solutions, including suppliers of audiographics systems.

7.7   Videophone

They're (almost) here! That statement summaries the status of the videophone (video telephone), long a staple item on futurists' "look what's coming next" lists. After many years of tantalizing promises, conditions appear right for bring the videophone to market. Whether people want or need video to accompany their telephone conversations is another story, but the technology issues holding videophones off the market have been ironed out.[12] Of course, data compression played a major role.

Videophones are desktop, telephone like devices that combine voice and video for transmission over telephone lines. These products are aimed at personal one-on-one communications. Their video screens are generally not much larger than 4 or 5 inches, and as video systems go, current videophones are definitely low end. Video resolution typically is not more than 128 × 112 pixels. Color depth is limited. So, too, is motion handling, as frame rates are much less than 30 fps television standards.

The first videophone, the AT&T Picturephone™, was showcased at the 1964 World's Fair. It was truly an innovative product, but it proved to be unmarketable. Users may have been ready for video-enabled telephones, but the telephone network certainly was not. When Picturephone service was introduced in 1970, the black-and-white video signal was transmitted a rate of 6.3 Mbps, the equivalent of 100 telephone lines [Trow94]. That much bandwidth was not widely available, and where it was, the service was not affordable for customers to use on a regular basis.

Now, move forward in time to 1992-1993 when a new generation of video-phones was introduced by AT&T and British Telecom [NewS93]. These products offered all the features of Picturephone and color images too. The advances made in data compression during the intervening years were clearly apparent, for these products could transmit video and voice signals over a single (analog) telephone line. One product, the AT&T VideoPhone 2500™, transmitted audio (at 6.8 Kbps) and video at a nominal 10 fps using a total of 19.2 Kbps [Earl93]. Other products operated at similar or lower rates. The only problem was that these videophones were not compatible!

That brings us to the next generation of videophones. From all indications, they will be compatible—with each other, with group videoconferencing systems, and with desktop and (in the future) portable videoconferencing computers—and they may be constructed quite differently than previous videophones. The keys to compatibility are standards for video and audio compression and for data transmission. There are two choices: Videophones that connect to analog telephone lines will conform to the ITU-T H.324 suite of standards [Mess95B]. H.324 specifies a data rate of 28.8 Kbps—8 Kbps for voice, using G.723 speech coding, and 20 Kbps for video, using H.263, a video coding scheme capable of interoperating with H.261. The other choice, videophones that connect to digital ISDN lines, will conform to the H.320 suite of standards [Crou93]. H.320 specifies

---

[12] There are those who argue video is unnecessary because through choice of words and inflections, the speaker's voice conveys most of the information. But the increasing use of video for business communication seems to prove them wrong. Also, there are those who argue video will be a nuisance in personal communications—who wants to bother with combing your hair and checking your wardrobe before answering the phone? That issue you, the reader, must decide.

a data rate of p × 64 Kbps. p = 2 (128 Kbps) is sufficient for videophone service—16 Kbps for voice, using G.728 speech coding, and 112 Kbps for video, using H.261 video coding. (See Chapter 5 for further discussion of the ITU-T standards mentioned in this paragraph.) As for how future videophones will be constructed, there are indications that the desktop paradigm may give way to a modular system based on a television set-top box that connects to a standard telephone and to a television receiver [Wirb95]. (Set-top boxes are discussed in Sections 9.4 and 9.10.) This approach not only reduces videophone cost by eliminating the need for special video displays, but it allows users the freedom to choose screen size and use their VCRs to record conversations. Essentially, it provides a low-cost videoconferencing system, the subject we will discuss next.

7.8   Videoconferencing

The story of videoconferencing begins in the 1960s when, realizing the power of television, educational institutions began televising classes to remotely located sites. Analog television technology was used and video transmission, often just one way from the instructor to the classroom, was expensive. The 1970s were a time of great promise: educational uses for video expanded, two-way video was in vogue, commercial businesses became interested, and videoconferencing equipment manufacturing companies were chartered. But, alas, video was still too expensive. Only those educational institutions and top Fortune 500 companies with the deepest pockets could afford videoconferencing equipment and the bandwidth to connect it. The technology went digital in the mid-1970s, and data compression was introduced, but hard-to-obtain and expensive T-1 (1.544 Mbps) lines were needed to carry the compressed video. Compression technology improved rapidly in the 1980s. First 384 Kbps, then 224 Kbps, and late in the decade affordable videoconferencing systems that could transmit acceptable quality video at 112 Kbps became available. In the same time frame, digital network connections grew easier to obtain and connect-time charges dropped rapidly. The videoconferencing industry was launched.

It is said that to be successful, videoconferencing must overcome three obstacles [Trow94]:

- Transmission costs must be reasonable.
- Integrated videoconferencing systems must be available (and they must be affordable and interoperate).
- Business people must be willing to replace face-to-face meetings with electronic tools.

The first two obstacles have been overcome. The introduction of ISDN and switched-56 Kbps telecommunications service has cut the cost for a video call within the United States to about twice that for a voice-only long-distance call.

Furthermore, the near-term deployment of compression algorithms that allow video to be transmitted over an ordinary analog telephone line will drive the cost even lower. Easy-to-use videoconferencing equipment is widely available and costs are falling—at double-digit rates—thanks to VLSI technology, volume production, and PC-based designs. In addition, thanks to standards for compression and transmission, interoperability is becoming the norm. As for any reluctance to use videoconferencing, this obstacle has been overcome too—judging from its popularity among educational institutions, government agencies, and especially among businesses where projects are spread over far-flung locations. Another indicator is the growing number of public rooms, making videoconferencing available to anyone for an hourly fee [Schm94]. The most obvious appeal of videoconferencing is that it reduces travel expenses. However, the features businesses find most attractive are how it accelerates decision making, improves communications, and enhances business processes, including contract development, product development, and customer service, to name a few [Port94, Trow94].

Videoconferencing systems provide for real-time transmission of moving images (video) and sound between two or more sites. These transmissions are often augmented with still-image graphics and computer data. Most videoconferences involve two-way, interactive exchanges, although one-way broadcasts are still important tools for distance learning in educational institutions and for business television (information dissemination and training) in corporate communications. Typical specifications for various kinds of videoconferencing systems, intended for different audiences, are provided in Table 7.7. High-end boardroom systems provide the highest-quality presentations to large groups, in a fixed-room setting, using the best available data capture and display devices, and lots of bandwidth. Initial cost and operating costs are high, limiting the market for these systems. Portable rollabout systems offer technical capabilities appropriate for smaller groups and are far more affordable. As a result, the market for rollabout systems is much larger, with an estimated 50,000 systems installed by 1995 [Trow94]. Desktop videoconferencing systems are aimed at meeting the needs of individual users. Although market estimates for this emerging technology vary widely, considering the number of PCs installed, forecasts of several million units per year in the late 1990s seem believable [Leav95].

The codec

The heart of a videoconferencing system is the codec (coder-decoder). The dataflow of a typical videoconferencing system is shown in Figure 7.16.[13] A codec

---

[13] Figure 7.16 shows a two-site configuration. Multisite videoconferences require that the various locations be bridged together into a single conference. Users have the option to purchase a multipoint conferencing unit that performs this function or purchase the service from long-distance carries including AT&T, Sprint, and others [Trow94].

Table 7.7 Videoconferencing systems specifications.

Typical System[1]	Boardroom Systems	Large-Group Rollabout	Small-Group Rollabout	Desktop Videoconferencing
Price (1995)	$50,000 - $1 M	$30,000 - $70,000	$20,000 upward	$1,000 - $6,000
Number of users	Many	10 - 15	6 - 8	1
Monitor - Size - Number	Large screen 2 or more	≥ 27 in. 2	≥ 20 in. 1	≥14 in. 1
Transmission speed	384 Kbps - 2 Mbps	≤ 384 Kbps	≥ 112 Kbps	28.8 - 128 Kbps
Resolution - pixels[2]	100 - 200K	≤100K	25 - 100K	≤25K
Frame rate[3]	30 fps	15 - 30 fps	15 - 30 fps	6 - 30 fps
Hi-resolution graphics[4]	Optional	Optional	Optional (Low resolution)	No
Document/computer conferencing	Optional	Optional	Not typically	Personal computer software

Notes:
[1] Sources for detailed videoconferencing system specifications include boardroom and group systems [Trow94] and desktop systems [Heck94, Kobi95A, Labr95, Leav95, Pere95, Tayl95B].
[2] Resolution: 25K pixels = H.261 QCIF, 100K pixels = H.261 CIF, 200K pixels ≈ broadcast-quality television.
[3] Frame rate depends on resolution and available bandwidth.
[4] H.261 Annex D allows attaching graphics systems which double CIF vertical and horizontal resolutions.

must be installed at each videoconferncing site, along with cameras, monitors, microphones, and loudspeakers. The codec's main task is digitizing and compressing video and audio signals, multiplexing those signals, and delivering the combined signal to a network for transmission. The codec also must accept a similarly encoded signal from the network, demultiplex the signal, decompress the video

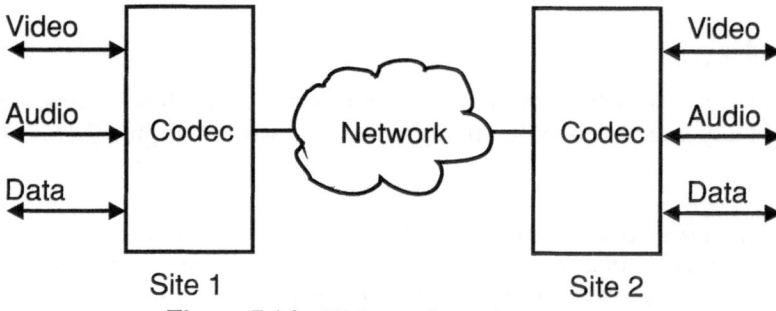

Figure 7.16 Videoconferencing system.

and audio, and provide analog video and audio outputs. When videoconferencing is done on the desktop, these codec functions can be reduced to a single board installed in a PC. For group and boardroom videoconferencing systems, the codec contains more function and is larger. In addition to video, audio, and network functions, boardroom and group system codecs accept and multiplex data from graphics devices and computers. These codecs also accept inputs from control panels and hand-held remote units, allowing users to operate devices in the conference room. Users may select cameras, control tilt, pan, and zoom for local and remote-site cameras, adjust audio volume and muting, and more.

Let us now take a closer look at how a codec digitizes and compresses video and audio. Codecs use the following techniques for video:

- Picture resolution is reduced to less than broadcast television standards.
- Color information is transformed and subsampled.
- Frame rates are reduced (if necessary).
- Intraframe coding is applied.
- Interframe coding is applied.
- Entropy coding is applied.

Picture resolution and frame rate are important in the following way: The typical videoconferencing scene to be televised contains a group of people seated at a table or, with desktop videoconferencing, the face of a person seated at a desk. The televised objects are large and they do not move much. All that is necessary is to provide enough resolution to show the expressions on people's faces in close-up shots and provide a frame rate that is high enough to avoid jerky hand motions. This means video transmissions can be reduced to less than broadcast television standards, cutting the amount of information to be digitized, compressed, and transmitted. As to resolution, the ITU-T H.261 standard for videoconferencing specifies CIF and QCIF, two reduced resolutions that require transmitting approximately one-half and one-eighth the pixels, respectively, needed for broadcast-quality television programs. (Details of the ITU-T H.261 standard and the techniques described in this paragraph are found in Section 5.5.) This standard also reduces the number of bits for each pixel by half, without apparent loss of color fidelity, because the human eye is more sensitive to luminance and less sensitive to color. As to frame rate, 30 fps is always desirable, and well-designed codecs resort to frame-rate reduction only when all other methods fail to meet transmission bandwidth objectives. Often 15 fps (or less) has proven acceptable for videoconferencing. Therefore, the ITU-T H.261 standard allows for 30, 15, 10, and even 7.5 fps transmissions; proprietary methods also allow (or require) reduced frame rates. The remaining steps (intraframe, interframe, and entropy coding—what some might call the genuine compression steps) reduce the information within and between pictures and efficiently encode what remains for transmission. Typical reductions (after entropy coding) are 25:1

for intraframe coding and an additional 3:1 for interframe coding. When all the digitization and compression techniques used by codecs are combined, the video data rate is reduced by 300:1 to 1200:1, or more, as shown in Figure 7.17.

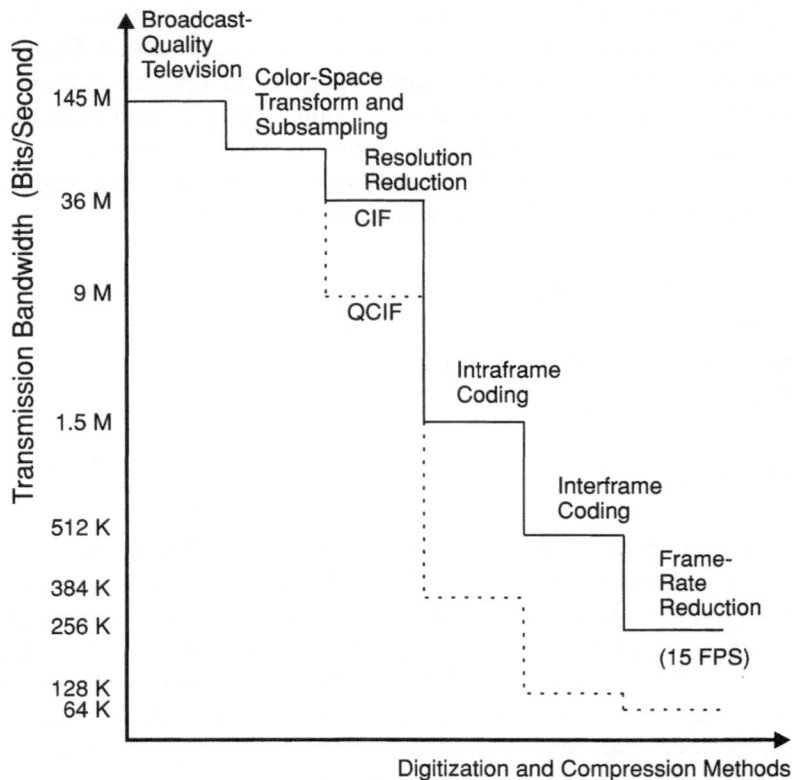

Figure 7.17   Codec video processing.

Consider now the audio portion of the videoconference. The audio content of videoconferences nearly always is people speaking. What is most important is that their speech be clearly intelligible. There are many factors that contribute to speech intelligibility including room reverberation and noise control, microphone placement, audio feedback control, and echo control during transmission [Port94]. A codec deals with audio transmission much in the same way the telephone system deals with voice transmission, and codecs use the same coding (compression) and transmission techniques. Four standards are used for coding the audio portion of teleconferencing transmissions: High-end products use ITU-T G.722 to provide wideband-quality speech at 64 Kbps. Other choices are ITU-T G.711 and G.728, which respectively provide telephone-quality speech at 64 and 16 Kbps, and for desktop video systems connected to the PSTN, G.723 which provides telephone-quality speech at 6.3 Kbps. (See Section 5.2 for a discussion of these speech coding standards.) Why are so many different speech coding standards needed?

Obviously, there is the speech-quality issue, but more important is how much bandwidth is used for audio in relation to the total available transmission bandwidth. Audio and video are multiplexed, and as Figure 7.18 shows, audio robs bandwidth-starved video of a significant part of the transmission bandwidth. Each advance in videoconferencing equipment has squeezed audio and video into less and less bandwidth. Thus, to assure adequate bandwidth be available for video, new reduced-bandwidth speech coding standards have been and will continue to be needed.

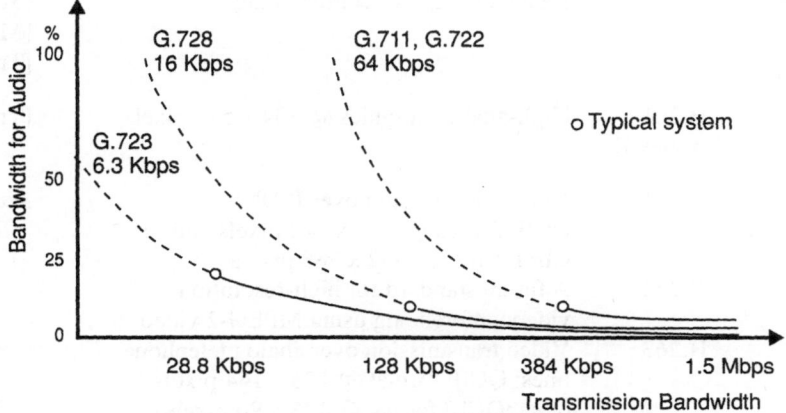

Figure 7.18   Videoconferencing audio bandwidth.

There are ITU-T standards that address all aspects of videoconferencing.[14] The videoconferencing standards, discussed in this section and elsewhere in the book, which relate to data compression are summarized in Table 7.8.

Videoconferencing issues—video compression and transmission

Our description of videoconferencing, which has been based on the ITU-T standards, would not be complete without mentioning the many nonstandard techniques for video compression and transmission used by boardroom and group systems and by desktop videoconferencing products. The ITU-T standards now in place do not provide the highest-resolution video, nor are they always the most efficient for transmitting pictures at the lowest possible bit rates. Some high-end boardroom videoconferencing systems continue to transmit NTSC (or PAL) analog video or use high-bandwidth digital video transmitted at T-1 (1.544 Mbps) rates or greater for the clearest pictures in large-group settings. High-definition picture transmission techniques also are used by specialized telemedi-

---

[14] For a complete list of videoconferencing standards see pages 118-119 in [Port94], and page 97 in [Trow94].

Table 7.8   ITU-T Videoconferencing compression standards.

Function	ITU-T Standard	Description	References
Audio	G.711	Telephone-quality (3-KHz) speech @ 64 Kbps	Section 5.2
	G.722	Wideband (7-KHz) speech @ 64 Kbps	[Port94]
	G.723	Telephone-quality (3-KHz) speech @ 6.3 Kbps	[Trow94]
	G.728	Telephone-quality (3-KHz) speech @ 16 Kbps	
Audiographics	T.120	Data and graphics conferencing	[Sull95] [Mess95A] [Trow94]
Graphics	H.261 Annex D	High-quality graphics @ 704 x 576 pixels	[Trow94]
Video	H.261	Video transmission over ISDN: QCIF format @ 176 x 144 pixels and CIF format @ 352 x 288 pixels	Section 5.5
	H.262	A future standard for high-resolution videoconferencing using MPEG-2 video	
	H.263	Video transmission over analog telephone lines: QCIF format @ 176 x 144 pixels or subQCIF format @ 128 x 96 pixels	

cine consulting systems. Then, too, most manufacturers of group videoconferencing systems offer proprietary digital video solutions that offer improved resolution. There are many examples [Trow94]. Included is the CLI (Compression Labs Inc.) CTX Plus™ compression algorithm that transmits 368 × 480 pixels in NTSC-compliant systems and 368 × 576 pixels in PAL-compliant systems, doubling the resolution of ITU-T CIF. Also, the PictureTel's SG3™ compression algorithm that efficiently encodes video for low-bandwidth transmissions and allows it to be transmitted along with a wideband (7-KHz) audio over 112 Kbps (two switched 56-Kbps) links. Another approach adopted by some group system manufacturers is to improve picture quality by enhancing the ITU-T standards, as does the PictureTel 320*plus*™ product. It takes advantage of a feature in the ITU-T H.261 standard (see Section 5.5) which allows for proprietary compression algorithms.

At the time of this writing, the desktop videoconferencing picture remains clouded (pun intended!) with proprietary solutions for video compression and transmission. Whereas a variety of approaches are not unusual for *any* emerging technology, the desktop videoconferencing marketplace offerings are uncommonly diverse. Forging a single solution for desktop videoconferencing with universal, agreed-to video compression standards, networking protocols, and communications standards is complicated by the following factors:

- Cost must be very low, causing many desktop videoconferencing product manufacturers to seek software solutions for video compression and transmission.

- Few early to mid-1990s vintage PC microprocessors are sufficiently powerful to run their normal work load and run H.261, MPEG, or any other standard video compression algorithm. As a result, many desktop videoconferencing products rely on nonstandard but computationally-simpler video compression algorithms that deliver low-resolution images at reduced frame rates. Typical values are 160×120 pixels at 10 fps or less.

- Within an enterprise, usually networked PCs are connected to a LAN (where there are no agreed-to standards for video or audio transmissions), and if connected to a WAN, often the connection is not ISDN (where H.261 applies). Outside this environment, for individuals with PCs connected to analog phone lines, only recently has a standard (H.263) for video communication emerged.

Another complicating factor is that videoconferencing is but one of many video applications moving to the desktop. This means video compression algorithms for multimedia and entertainment data also play an important role. Given the nature of the PC marketplace to seek out low-cost, one-size-fits-all solutions, it is not surprising that videoconferencing solutions have appeared which are based on MPEG, M-JPEG, and totally proprietary algorithms.

With desktop videoconferencing still a technology in transition, what the common solution for desktop videoconferencing will be, or if there will be one, remains to be discovered. However, there are indications of what the direction may be: One factor is, with the growing importance of video, PCs will quickly become video-enabled platforms, delivering high-quality video for all applications. As a result, interest in compromise video solutions is likely to wane, favoring standardized, high-quality video compression algorithms. Another factor is that many businesses and organizations already have group or boardroom videoconferencing systems; they may seek out interoperable desktop videoconferencing products that comply with ISDN-based ITU-T H.320 videoconferencing standards, and they undoubtedly will want to use the same solution for desktop-to-desktop videoconferences. However, for now and some years to come, analog phone lines are the only connection affordable to many PC users and, for them, the answer may be ITU-T H.324-compliant videoconferencing. A third factor is the millions of PCs connected to the Internet, where video transmissions of all kinds are on the increase. Recently, the ITU-T approved H.323, a new standard for data, audio and videoconferencing over packet-switched data networks such as Internet [Mess96, Yosh96]. H.323, which controls functions such as call setup and packet exchange, uses the same audio and video codecs developed for H.324-compliant videoconferencing over analog phone lines. The Internet may prove to be the consummate environment for desktop-to-desktop videoconferencing—although predicting future developments for the Information Superhighway is beyond the scope of this book and definitely beyond this author's knowledge!

7.9   Telemetry Systems

Telemetry systems use sensors to make measurements on people, places, or things at remote, inaccessible, or hazardous locations, and they transmit data to receiving equipment where monitoring, display, and recording takes place.[15] All of this may conjure up visions of orbiting spacecraft and scientists hovering over exotic equipment, as well it should, but telemetry systems have everyday uses too. Consider automobiles: All one needs to do to start the engine is turn the ignition key; it is that simple. While turning the key, most drivers are not thinking about what goes on under the hood where a telemetry system is hard at work. There the engine management computer busily checks sensors for the coolant temperature, air temperature, manifold air pressure, and more. If it decides that a cold-start condition exists, for instance, it then initiates a program that sets up the fuel injectors to deliver just the right amount of gasoline for starting the cold engine. When the engine starts, before driving off, the driver unwittingly makes more use of telemetry by checking the warning lights and the gas gauge—displays that are activated by even more sensors to tell the driver that everything is (or is not) OK.

There are many kinds of telemetry systems. The first systems formally described as telemetry systems were developed for aerospace applications, including monitoring rockets and satellites, collecting data from unmanned deep-space probes, and doing the same for manned spaceflights. Earth-bound telemetry systems are widely used in biomedicine, nuclear reactors, and mechanical equipment of all kinds, including pipelines and railroad diesel engines.[16] Remote sensing is an application for telemetry that involves not only collecting and transmitting data but also analyzing and interpreting the data. Although long used for seismic exploration and oceanography, recent advances in remote-sensing technology relate to orbiting satellites and the information they collect about the earth and its oceans and atmosphere. Through the development of satellite-borne digital imaging, data can be collected that provides information on weather, pollution, global warming, plant-growth patterns, and much more. The difficulty with digital imaging telemetry is it generates tremendous amounts of data. For

---

[15] Telemetry systems, although not a traditional communications industry application, are included here for completeness.

[16] The author was once engaged in developing telemetry and pattern recognition techniques for diagnosing the "health" of mechanisms in computer punch-card equipment [Hoff70]. Unfortunately, thanks to the limited signal processing methods of the day and implementation expense, automated mechanical diagnostics for computer equipment was an idea far ahead of its time.

example, each image captured by the thematic mapper on board one of NASA's LANDSAT satellites contains 200–300 MB of data [Rabb91, Bell95]. Collecting a terabyte a day from a remote-sensing satellite is not considered unusual [Gers93]. Needless to say, transmission and storage problems abound.

The difficulty with *all* telemetry systems is that they generate too much data. As a result, scientists have developed a diversity of specialized techniques for efficiently coding data, particularly for aerospace telemetry where transmission bandwidth is low. Before transmission, it is standard practice to process the data collected by sensors. This may mean simply eliminating noise in the electrical signals produced by the sensors or providing error control, but it can also involve transforming the signals for efficient transmission, including data reduction and data compression. According to one source, the earliest application for modern digital data compression was in space digital telemetry and military communications, where limited power aboard rockets and spacecraft and limited bandwidth for transmission makes on board data reduction and compression mandatory [Capp85]. When applied to telemetry, data compression is a tool that accomplishes three objectives: It allows telemetry bandwidth to be used more efficiently, it decreases the time and cost for transmitting data, and it decreases the volume

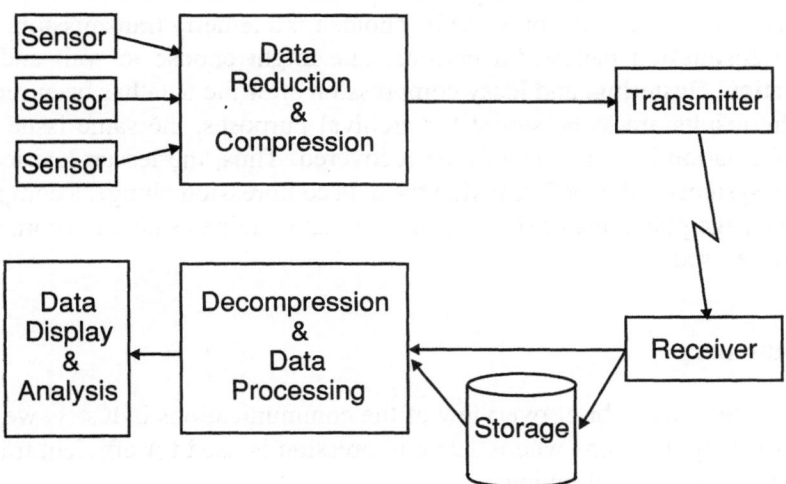

Figure 7.19   Telemetry system data compression.

of data that must be archived. Figure 7.19 shows how data compression is incorporated in modern telemetry systems.

What kinds of data compression *techniques* are used in telemetry? They *all* are! What is not used are standardized data compression *algorithms*.[17] Telemetry

---

[17] We note that large volumes of the data collected by satellite-borne telemetry systems are archived and available to the public for processing. If the use of this data becomes more widespread, the need for compression standards will become more important too.

systems are specialized. They transmit a diversity of information ranging from an indication of whether an electrical switch is open or closed to video. Electrical waveforms, sequences of floating-point numbers, highly structured data such as multispectral images—anything is possible. For example, special differential coding methods have been developed for compressing sequences of integer and floating-point numbers [Hune89, Lell92, Webe93]. Sifting through the literature on telemetry, one finds all the compression techniques described in Chapters 4 and 5 and many others. Rather than attempting to enumerate them, let us consider how three categories of compression techniques apply. These are classification and clustering, lossless compression, and lossy compression [Sayo92]. Classification and clustering attempt to extract particular features from data. Vocoders are an example of this approach. Classification and clustering methods sometimes are described as data reduction, but they, too, along with lossless and lossy compression, allow information to be transmitted with far fewer bits.

The key issue that telemetry system designers face when using data reduction and compression is loss of information. When a particular technique is incorporated on board a satellite or deep-space probe, it is difficult to change. This may make it impossible to extract additional information from the sensors and it limits what new data processing techniques can do with the received data in the future. Lossless compression is the only "safe" choice for telemetry transmission. Therefore, if transmission bandwidth permits, one might choose to wait and apply classification, clustering, and lossy compression after the data has been received. But if the results are to be stored for archival purposes, the same issue exists. Once information is lost, it cannot be recovered. Thus, the lesson learned from telemetry systems is that before taking the data compression plunge, a comprehensive long-range plan must be developed, one that anticipates how the compressed data will be used.

7.10   Summary

In this chapter, after a brief overview of the communications industry, we examined network applications where data compression is used for efficient transmission. We learned the following:

- Data compression improves the effective throughput of transmission channels or reduces transmission costs by allowing lower-speed or shared transmission facilities to be used.
- Data compression is used with all styles of communication—one-way, bi-directional, and collaborative—but each style places different demands on compression and decompression algorithms.
- Data compression is used by all segments of the communications industry, telecommunications services for point-to-point and broadcast communications, and data communications services for connecting computers, to address bandwidth and transmission issues.

- Speech coding, data compression specialized for voice, increases the traffic capacity and conserves bandwidth for both wired and wireless telephone networks.

- Data communications networks use data compression to increase throughput of slow lines, to allow faster lines to be shared for lower transmission costs, and to reduce the queueing delay for transmitting messages.

- Data communications networks require lossless data compression algorithms that can operate in error-prone environments and that can operate within time constraints.

- Hardware is required to perform data compression for all but the slowest data communications lines and, as yet, no hardware is fast enough for high-speed broadband networks.

- V.42bis, a standardized scheme for data compression on telephone lines, allows modem designers to make cost-performance trade-offs.

- Multiplexers that allow voice and data to share a single line require efficient data compression for both types of traffic.

- Bridges and routers, for LAN-to-LAN internetworking across WANs, use data compression to reduce WAN traffic saturation and to reduce data transmission costs.

- Specialized data compression algorithms are required to deal with packet-based data transmissions.

- Channel extenders for mainframe computers use data compression to reduce WAN transmission costs and to increase extended I/O channel capacity and performance.

- Tools are available to set up and define how data compression can most effectively be applied to complex computer networks.

- Computer network communications protocols now allow generalized data compression to be used for all types of traffic, whereas special-purpose data compression has been used for many years to reduce terminal-to-computer traffic and improve application program performance.

- FAX machines, once rare and expensive, quickly became commonplace products for office and home following the development of digital transmission and data compression standards.

- All forms of teleconferencing depend on data compression for efficient transmission of voice, graphics, images, and video.

- Videoconferencing, an industry segment that owes its existence to data compression, expanded greatly with the availability of low-cost products that comply with H.320 videoconferencing standards, including the H.261 data compression standard. Further expansion is expected as PC-based desktop videoconferencing products become available that comply with H.324 videoconferencing standards, including the H.263 data compression standard.

- Telemetry systems that use data reduction and lossy compression must be designed to anticipate future uses for the collected data because lost information cannot be recovered.

8

Communications—
Broadcasting Applications

In this chapter, we continue our examination of communications and consider television and radio broadcasting applications where data compression is used to reduce the bandwidth needed for delivering digitized data. Various combinations of lossless and lossy compression are used, with most algorithms being specially adapted for the transmission channels and the data being transmitted on those channels.

8.1 Broadcasting Overview

Profound changes are taking place in television and radio broadcasting. Today, broadcasters are largely focused on new digital products and services. As pointed out in Chapter 3, no fewer than four approaches now compete to deliver analog video (and audio) to our homes. All of them—terrestrial broadcasting, cable, satellite, and in-home boxes, including VCRs and video disc players—are moving to digital. Telephone and computer networks also have plans for home delivery of digital audio and video, and, in so doing, they hope to capture some portion of the consumer dollars now going to broadcasters. In the past broadcasters engaged strictly in mass distribution of home entertainment and information services using one-way communications. Today, reflecting the changing needs of consumers, they are moving toward providing a more personal, more customized delivery of enhanced home entertainment and information services and to using two-way, interactive communications. Make no mistake—much remains un-known about what consumers really want and how the broadcasting industry will reshape itself to meet their needs. Major questions remain unanswered, particularly in television broadcasting where the demand for high-definition television and the requirement for interactivity is unknown. But, clearly, consumers do want—and will pay for—more freedom of choice and more quality. Examples include multichannel cable and satellite television versus a few terrestrial broadcast television channels; also, FM radio (and, soon, digital audio broadcasting offering CD-quality audio) versus AM radio. Without question, to move forward, the broadcasting industry needs digital technology—first for delivering more choice and more quality and later, perhaps, for providing computer-controlled interactivity. Existing analog broadcasting facilities provide neither the bandwidth nor the interactivity and, essentially, are incapable of providing the desired functions. Digital broadcasting—with data compression—does provide the needed capacity and function.

In this book, our exploration of the heady events taking place in broadcasting centers around data compression and how it is used to expand the effective bandwidth (carrying capacity) for broadcast channels. The immediately following sections of this chapter examine several different broadcasting methods, each of which must deal with the limited carrying capacity of the media. As in all communications, bandwidth is a limiting constraint for broadcasters, whether the transmission channels are wireless, wired, or optical fibers. For wireless and wired broadcast methods, there simply is no more bandwidth available; for optical-fiber-based methods more bandwidth means investing more dollars. In both situations, data compression is the enabling technology.

8.2   Terrestrial Broadcast Television

In the United States, for nearly 50 years commercial television has provided home entertainment and information using over-the-air terrestrial broadcasts in analog NTSC standard format. Elsewhere in the world, the PAL and SECAM analog standards have been used for nearly as long. Over the years, analog broadcast standards have been upgraded to include color, stereo audio, and a few specialized data services. Although few technology-based standards have lasted so long or served so well, the convergence of computers and communications—in the home—foretells their giving way to new digital-based broadcasting standards. Digitized television, when integrated with computers, telecommunications networks, and consumer products, holds promise for providing a new array of products and services never before available.

In 1987, the FCC formed ACATS [the Advisory Committee on Advanced Television (ATV) Service], a committee to assist in establishing a new television standard for the United States. Their mission was to develop a new standard for high-definition television that could deliver wide-screen, movie-theater-quality pictures and CD-quality sound to home television receivers. Various systems were considered including an analog HDTV system on the air in Japan since

1991 and four proposed digital HDTV systems[1] [Yosh93A, Hopk94]. In 1992, the FCC committee decided the future U.S. standard would be digital, and it would be broadcast on 6-MHz terrestrial channels, using the same bandwidth and the same channels as for regular-definition (NTSC) broadcast television. The problem was how could HDTV fit into a 6-MHz channel, as it displays more than twice the resolution of the existing NTSC standard, both vertically and horizontally. Also, it has a wide-screen format (16:9 rather than 4:3), and its high-quality video signal uses a component format that requires more bandwidth than the composite-format NTSC signal. It also provides 5.1-channel CD-quality audio. In total, HDTV would need as much as 60 times the data rate provided by the 6-MHz channel [Zou92]. Obviously, as any reader of this book knows by now, the solution is data compression. The MPEG-2 compression algorithm, which evolved along with the definition of HDTV, is now an integral part of the HDTV standard. The HDTV standard is now in the final stages of formalization.

While the HDTV standardization effort was in progress, broadcasters began to recognize the power of digital television could be used in ways other than for supporting HDTV. Although HDTV is technically intriguing, the downside is, initially at least, that it will be very expensive for both broadcasters and consumers. New production and distribution facilities are required, and HDTV receivers will cost several times more than standard NTSC (PAL or SECAM) receivers. According to many industry observers, this translates into a long period of waiting for HDTV to become widespread and profitable.[2] Meanwhile, terrestrial broadcasters petitioned the FCC—and received permission—to use the channels allocated for HDTV to broadcast lower-resolution SDTV (standard-definition television). The advantages of SDTV are that it provides studio-quality (NTSC CCIR-601 standard) video, which never before could be broadcast to home receivers. It is digital, which means it can be compressed and transmitted over standard broadcast channels, and it can be received and displayed by NTSC-standard receivers when equipped with set-top converter boxes. Also, SDTV, which uses MPEG-2 compression and conforms to the HDTV standard, requires not more than 5–6 Mbps of bandwidth, a fraction of that needed for HDTV. As shown in Figure 8.1, this allows some combination of several SDTV channels and other digital data services to be packed into one 6-MHz terrestrial broadcast channel. It is argued this will allow terrestrial broadcasters to compete with other home entertainment and information providers to deliver the variety and type of services consumers desire [Leop95D].

---

[1] A significant detail is that the Japanese HDTV system was transmitted via satellite because it required several times more bandwidth that standard television.

[2] The plan for phasing in HDTV in the United States allows each of the more than 1400 terrestrial broadcasters who choose to air HDTV programming to apply for a second (UHF) channel [Hopk94]. Conventional analog NTSC programming will air on the channel they now have been granted, simulcast along with digital HDTV programming on the second channel. At some point in time, analog broadcasts will be phased out.

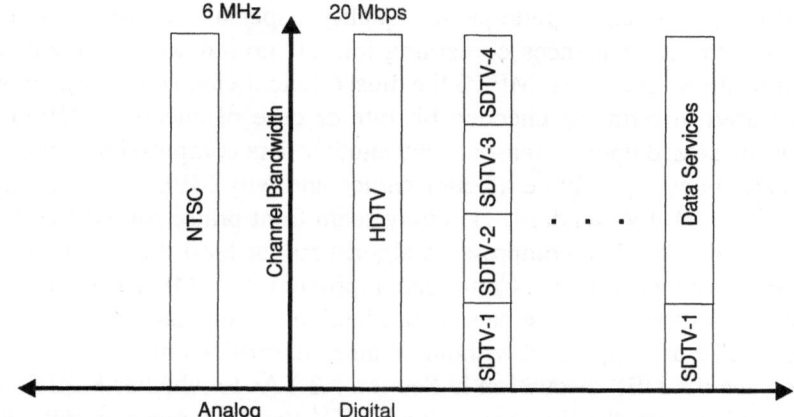

Figure 8.1 Terrestrial television channel bandwidth assignment options.

Plans for digital terrestrial broadcast television in the United States continue to move forward, with FCC approval on an ATV standard for HDTV and SDTV expected in 1997. In Europe and Asia, efforts leading toward digital television are moving forward too [Yosh95C, Yosh95D, Yosh95E]. In Europe, the Digital Video Broadcast (DVB) project is defining standards for terrestrial, cable, and satellite digital television broadcasts. The move from analog to digital television in Europe was delayed by a since-abandoned effort to create an analog HDTV standard [Fox95]. In Asia, the move to digital television lags behind both North America and Europe, in part because analog HDTV has been available in Japan for several years. Thanks to differing existing transmission standards and a host of other factors, a single worldwide standard for digital television is doubtful. However, all digital television proposals do share one common element: They all specify MPEG-2 compression. (See Section 5.5 and Table 5.8 for further discussion of MPEG-2 and HDTV formats.)

We will close our discussion of terrestrial television broadcasting, as we begun, with some thoughts on the durability of the new HDTV standard. The question is, Will it serve well for years and years, as the NTSC standard has done, or will advances in information handling technology cause the HDTV standard to self-destruct at a tender age? Throughout the process leading to its creation, lots of people, supporters and foes alike, have offered up strong opinions, and reasons to back up their position, on whether the HDTV standard will (or will not) endure. Reams have been written to explain, justify, or debate almost every conceivable subject relating to the HDTV standard, and several comprehensive overviews and introductions have been published, including [Hopk94, Basi95, Chal95]. Here, just one aspect of the HDTV standard will be addressed—the inclusion of MPEG-2 data compression and its effect on the durability of the standard.

Section 5.5 (Video Compression, State-of-the-art video coding and beyond) described some technical limitations of MPEG. Most notably, it does introduce coding artifacts that can degrade picture quality, especially at low bit rates and in fast-action image sequences containing lots of motion with frequent scene-to-scene transitions. Neither is MPEG the most efficient video encoding algorithm when measured in terms of encoded bit rate or ease of encoding. Often these limitations are seized upon as reasons why another data compression technique—and there are many—would be a better choice and why MPEG will shorten the life span of the HDTV standard. This may seem faint praise for MPEG, but the truth is that *all* video data compression algorithms (at least those that use lossy compression) produce artifacts. Continued improvement in MPEG encoding techniques, which will assuredly reduce its production of noticeable artifacts during decoding, can be accomplished without changes to millions of HDTV receivers. (For proof, see the DBS discussion in Section 8.3.) As to whether MPEG coding efficiency will shorten the life span of the HDTV standard, one can only observe that the encoded bit rate is sufficiently low for broadcasting HDTV and, because it is a broadcast medium, the complexity (and cost) of encoding affects only the broadcaster, not the receiver.

There is one additional point: Should *any* data compression algorithm that compromises picture quality be part of the HDTV broadcasting (or any) transmission standard? Here, the assumption is that when (not if) some sufficiently better compression technique comes along, and everyone agrees the standard needs to be updated, millions of HDTV receivers will be obsoleted. Given that video compression is hardly a mature science, this could happen sooner than anyone expects. One proposal is to define HDTV without regard to bandwidth (and without compression) and transmit it over those broadband media able to provide sufficient bandwidth [Simo95]. Unfortunately, no existing transmission media reaching U.S. homes, not terrestrial, satellite, or cable broadcasting, nor telephone or computer networks, provides the bandwidth needed for uncompressed HDTV. So, if we want HDTV, it is going to be compressed, and that compression will be MPEG—for better or worse.

8.3   Direct Broadcast Satellite

The era of direct broadcast satellite (DBS) television service arrived in 1994 when Digital Satellite System (DSS™) broadcasts became an "overnight" sensation.[3] Simple in concept—digital signals are transmitted from satellite television broadcasters' ground stations to orbiting satellites, where the signals are then beamed to homes equipped with receiving dishes and decoders—DBS actually proved tremendously difficult to turn into a profitable commercial enterprise. This is

---

[3] Digital Satellite System is a joint effort of DirecTV-GM Hughes Electronics, RCA-Thompson Consumer Electronics, and United States Satellite Broadcasting-Hubbard Broadcasting. DSS began broadcasting in 1994 with 175 channels of video and music.

what the backers of DSS learned after traveling a long and arduous path strewn with technical obstacles, financial roadblocks, and the failure of half a dozen other DBS ventures. Beginning in 1982, when the FCC authorized the orbital satellite slots needed for the service, many companies invested hundreds of millions of dollars to give consumers a low-cost, widely available, small-dish alternative to large-dish satellite, cable, and terrestrial broadcast television and videocassette rentals [Marr95]. To attract viewers, DSS backers knew they must offer consumers more than just low cost and wide availability. They concluded that DSS must provide near laser-videodisc-quality S-VHS video, CD-quality sound, and 100+ channels for video, music, and future broadband data services— all specifications in excess of what viewers could find on competing cable television systems. The backers of DSS, although they may not admit it, probably were surprised along with everyone else at its explosive growth. Within the first year, nearly one million DSS receivers were sold, exceeding by many times the first-year sales for VCRs, CD players, and big-screen televisions, all highly successful consumer products of their time. Among the many features of DSS, surely the enormous array of channels and the high-quality pictures and sound provided the push that consumers needed.

How could DSS afford to provide so many high-quality channels? Compressed digital video and audio provided the answer. Satellites are well known for being notoriously expensive to build and put in orbit, each costing perhaps 50-100 million dollars (or more) [Barr93], and satellite transponder bandwidth is limited. Data compression allows transponder bandwidth to be used far more efficiently. With compression, the 27 Mbps bandwidth of each DSS transponder can provide four to eight or more channels of high-quality, SDTV-resolution digital video. DSS also provides about 30 digital radio channels and, in the future, may offer digital data services. Data compression makes DSS economically feasible, and it provides the picture and sound quality consumers want.

DSS uses MPEG-2 compression, and herein lies an interesting tale. At the time DSS service was launched in 1994, the final MPEG-2 specification was still in process. However, the lack of a final specification had not stopped chip makers who, as soon as drafts of the MPEG-2 standard were available in 1993, rushed to put MPEG-2 decoder chips into production for use in DBS receivers and many other products. The problem DSS faced was that MPEG-2 encoder chips, which were needed for live broadcasts, would not be available for many months in the future.[4] The solution DSS chose was to use MPEG-2 decoder chips in its receivers but to begin operating with MPEG-1 encoded broadcasts. This allowed all DSS receivers, beginning with the very first unit shipped, to receive broadcasts encoded

---

[4] The complexity of MPEG-2 encoding delayed the arrival of encoder chips that could compress live broadcasts in real time. Non-real-time encoders, whether in hardware or in software running on powerful computers, which suffice for compressing programs stored on film or tape, could not handle sports events and other live DSS broadcasts.

in MPEG-2 whenever they became available. Meanwhile, the receivers could decode MPEG-1 encoded broadcasts because MPEG-2 is backward compatible with MPEG-1. Surprisingly, the less-detailed MPEG-1 encoded pictures produced little reaction from consumers who were more concerned with the picture artifacts that appeared in fast-action image sequences containing lots of motion or in sequences containing frequent scene-to-scene transitions [Pohl95B].

Picture artifacts are the bane of all image and video compression algorithms, MPEG included. MPEG-2, however, by providing great latitude for how video is encoded, with the only rigid requirement being that the end result conform to the MPEG-2 bit-stream syntax, reduces the problem.[5] One of the flexibilities of MPEG-2 is that it allows variable bit-rate encoding. For instance, fewer bits per second can be used to encode low-resolution images, or image sequences that contain little motion, or image sequences captured at less than 30 fps (as with 24-fps movies). On the other hand, more bits per second can be used for encoding when these conditions do not prevail, the most important being to reduce visible artifacts for high-motion scenes and during scene-to-scene transitions.

DSS incorporates several innovations for reducing the visibility of picture artifacts. Initially, as shown in Figure 8.2(a), channels were assigned a bit rate

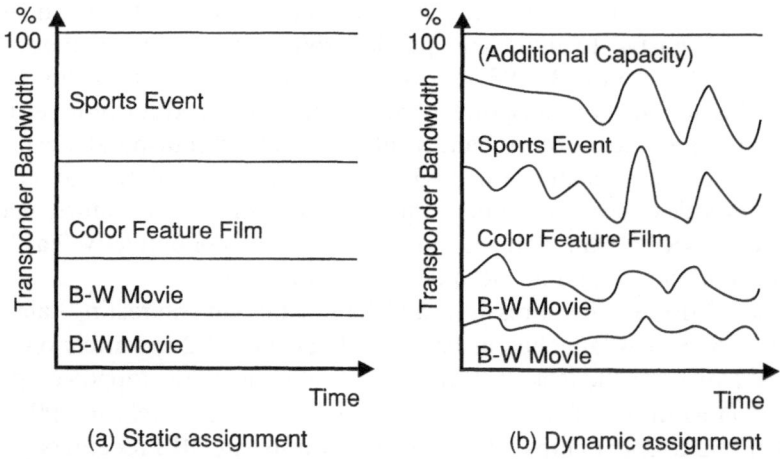

Figure 8.2 DSS transponder bandwidth sharing.

that did not vary with time but did vary according to program content and importance. For example, old black-and-white movies received fewer bits per second than first-run color, action-intensive, pay-per-view features, and all movies (running at 24 fps) received fewer bits per second than full-motion, action-intensive sports events. Over long periods of time the average results of this

---

[5] Although DSS uses MPEG-2 compression, its bit-stream packet protocol is different than that found in the MPEG-2 specification.

approach may be satisfactory, but it cannot address the instantaneous demand for bits, which leads to consumer concerns about visible artifacts. DSS subsequently introduced the dynamic bandwidth sharing method shown in Figure 8.2(b), a statistical multiplexing process that continuously varies the bit rate according to program content. In case you were wondering—yes, its operation is similar to STDM, a method for multiplexing data packets on the shared data communications lines discussed in Section 7.3; only here, the packets contain MPEG encoded pictures. Like STDM, no channel can be absolutely guaranteed all the bandwidth it may need, but the overall effect of dynamic bit assignment has two positive outcomes: First, the total available satellite transponder bandwidth is used far more efficiently, which means each transponder can carry more channels. Second, when compared to static bit assignment, the number of times when not enough bits per second are available is greatly reduced for every channel. The consequence, of course, is that the encoding and multiplexing processes are far more sophisticated.

The unquestionable success of DSS has encouraged companies around the world to begin providing digital DBS television service. In 1996, similar services are in operation or are planned to go into operation for Canada, Latin America, South America, Europe, Japan, and other Asian countries. Also, four DBS television services are available in the United States (see Table 8.1), and others are being planned [Warr95, Arns96]. Two important groundrules for a successful DBS service are to provide a large number of channels and allow viewers to use a small receiving dish. Thus, all DBS providers are on or planning to move to high-power satellites (a requirement for small dish size), where space for DBS transmissions is now at a premium. The prospects for placing additional satellites in orbit are dimmed in that few orbital satellite slots remain available for DBS transmissions. This has increased the price for admission for other potential DBS providers, with MCI Communications Corporation paying nearly $700 million for a satellite slot and license to operate its 300-channel DBS system planned for the late 1990s [Shiv96].

8.4   Cable Television

Cable television is available to most U.S. households; by 1992 more than 60% of U.S. households were connected [Pres93]. Of the remainder, some choose not to be connected, and some 10–20 million of us live in mostly-rural areas not served by cable. Not only has the number of cable television subscribers grown, but so too has the number of cable television channels. With typical cable systems offering, perhaps, 40–60 channels, this still leaves content providers scrambling to find a place on crowded cable systems for at least 100 new special-interest cable channels. Technology exists for cable systems to provide no less than 150 channels, but cable system operators have moved slowly on expanding existing (analog) systems, as adding channels requires new electronics and laying new

Table 8.1   United States DBS television services circa 1996.

	DSS	PrimeStar™	EchoStar™	AlphaStar™
Receiving dish size	18 in.	39 in.[1]	18 in.	30 in.
Channel capacity[2]				
1990	—	10^3	—	—
1994	175	67	—	—
1996	200	95	95	100
1997	200+	140	200	300
Compression algorithm	MPEG-2[4]	MPEG-1[5]	MPEG-2	MPEG-2
References	[Pohl95D, Taki95A, Taki96]	[Edge95B, Taki95A, Nice96]	[ElNe95, Edge96, Nice96]	[Edge95D, Taki96, Nice96]

Notes:
[1] Dish size will decrease with move to high-power satellites.
[2] Total - video and music.
[3] Analog transmission. In 1994, PrimeStar upgraded to digital.
[4] Bit-stream packet protocol differs from the MPEG-2 specification.
[5] May move to MPEG-2 in 1997.

cable, or replacing cable with high-capacity optical-fiber links.[6] This, a hugely expensive undertaking, which could, at most, triple the channel capacity, would leave them with a cable system having more channels but not more function.

Instead, the cable industry sees a future where subscribers will be provided with individualized programming and real-time two-way interactive communications will be supported. To accomplish this, cable systems must remake themselves using digital television and computer technology. With digital television—and data compression—the channel capacity of existing systems can be multiplied tenfold.[7] Most important, the merger of digital television and digital computer technology allows cable systems to move from just providing one-way broadcast

---

[6] Cable systems operate within various bandwidths. Modern urban hybrid coaxial/fiber cable systems provide a forward (headend-to-user) bandwidth range of 54–750 MHz, allowing up to 110 (6 MHz analog) broadcast channels to be carried. All-fiber networks provide 1 GHz bandwidth, allowing 150 channels.

[7] Each 6-MHz cable channel can carry 40 Mbps of digitized video. With MPEG-2 compression, 10 high-quality SDTV video data streams can be carried by each channel.

television to offering two-way interactive television and a host of data transmission services. A potpourri of services is envisioned for digital interactive cable systems including the following:

- On-demand movies and news
- VCR-like function for viewing movies
- User selection of camera angles for sporting events
- Interactive videogames with far-off competitors
- Home shopping and interactive advertising
- Electronic Yellow Pages browsing
- Internet access, E-mail messaging
- Subscriber-to-subscriber services including telephone, video telephone, videoconferencing, and more

In the early 1990s, the cable television industry, along with programming-content providers and a slew of computer and silicon vendors, engaged in what can only be described as frantic efforts to form strategic alliances and launch ambitious plans for full-service interactive networks. (Telephone companies, having the same goals in mind, engaged with these same groups in similar activities.) By the mid-1990s, many of the grand plans had fallen by the wayside and the early morning marathon dash to interactivity took on the characteristics of an evening stroll. Cable system operators point to the substantial costs for rebuilding their networks for two-way interactivity. Then, too, there are regulatory issues to resolve, and the uncertainty about what customers want on their digital interactive cable—and will pay for—remains, as it was in the beginning, a nagging concern.

To appreciate the challenges, consider the two cable systems shown in Figure 8.3. A conventional analog cable system, as shown in Figure 8.3(a), distributes broadcast channels through what is called a tree and branch network [Mill94]. Terrestrial and satellite broadcasts are distributed down through the network to all subscribers, whose set-top converter boxes determine which channels they may view. The first cable networks were built from coaxial cables, amplifiers, and distribution gear. In theory two-way communications are possible on all-coaxial cable systems, but, in practice, amplifier noise makes this impractical. The solution, which is well underway, is to eliminate the amplifiers by replacing coaxial cable with optical fiber. Hybrid fiber/cable networks not only increase the channel capacity, picture quality, and reliability of the cable system, they also make limited forms of two-way communications possible. Nevertheless, this still does not provide for the kind of fully two-way interactive communications that cable television visionaries dream of as a goal. For that, a network similar in concept to the one depicted in Figure 8.3(b) is needed. Here, by means of circuit switching, every subscriber is essentially provided a private path that links them to any one of thousands of video (or data) sources. In computer terms, one

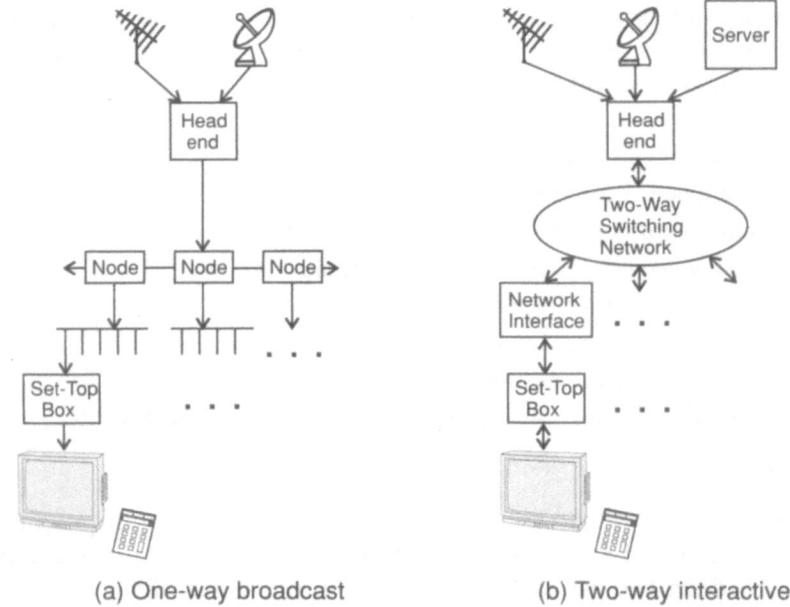

(a) One-way broadcast   (b) Two-way interactive

Figure 8.3 Cable television systems.

might think of this as a gigantic client-server network, where, instead of receiving a huge number of channels, each user has a single channel that carries personalized video or data.

To move from one-way broadcast to two-way, fully interactive cable systems, the subscriber's set-top box must grow more sophisticated, and therein lies one reason that interactive television for the masses may be a long time in coming—cost. Current set-top (analog converter) boxes, which essentially provide little more than channel selection, must be replaced with set-top boxes that contain a high-powered microprocessor and its operating system, peripheral chips for decompression, video and graphics processing, and copious amounts of memory. This is needed just to provide digital one-way television and limited two-way interactive services.[8] Advanced interactive services such as subscriber-to-subscriber videotelephony and videoconferencing require even more processing power and memory, real-time compression chips, camera interfaces, and more—endowing the set-top box with the characteristics (and cost) of a well-configured multimedia computer. Even with silicon integration and high-volume production, for sometime to come the cost of set-top boxes will delay the onset of interactive television services [Cole95]. Additional information about set-top boxes can be found in many sources, including [Cici95].

---

[8] DAVIC (the Digital Audio-Video Council) has set a cost target of $300 for the first standardized digital set-top box [Leop95C].

Details of how cable television systems will be reconstructed to provide interactive television reach far beyond the scope of this book. For those readers who wish to learn more, your attention is directed to several survey papers [Mill94, Blah95, Larg95]. Our interest is limited to the role data compression plays for cable to go digital and provide interactivity. The simplest scenario is one where data compression (and digital television) is used to increase the channel capacity of a conventional cable system. Compressors placed at the headend, or in the video sources themselves, will allow up to tenfold more channels to be squeezed into the space occupied by a single analog channel. The compressed digital video is then transmitted to set-top boxes where, under microprocessor control, a decompressor will reconstruct whatever channel the viewer selects. This might seem to be every channel surfer's dream, having 500 or more channels on tap, but not so.[9] Channel surfing is all but impossible with compressed digital video because (recall the MPEG group of pictures discussion in Section 5.5) when a new channel is selected, it can take several seconds to build up a viewable picture. Rather than offering viewers a bewildering array of channels to pick from, some channels will likely be reserved for program guides, similar to those found on DBS systems, that help viewers navigate through the sea of programming choices. Although new program content will be added, the first use for the increased channel capacity is predicted to be for enhancing pay-per-view offering [Cici93]. Similar to the approach taken by DBS, a movie will be offered on several channels with staggered start times, thus, allowing near-on-demand video.

A far more advanced scenario, one that only the most visionary of visionaries expect to be realized any time soon, will find set-top boxes that contain both compressors and decompressors. This, perhaps the full realization of the Information Superhighway, will allow subscribers to originate information, providing for true subscriber-to-subscriber communications.

Finally, note that throughout all the struggles and debates about what interactive cable television will be, and when it will happen, and everything seemingly up for grabs, there has been unwavering support for MPEG compression by all participants [John95A]. However, MPEG, a highly asymmetric algorithm, is best suited to one-way mass distribution applications. Consequently, as the story of two-way, fully interactive television unfolds, one might expect other algorithms such as H.261 for videoconferencing, H.263 for videotelephony, or advanced forms of MPEG will be needed at the set-top too. Stay tuned!

8.5 Telco Video

Under the 1992 FCC "video dial-tone service" ruling that permitted telcos to transport video services on their telephone networks, the portion of the network

---

[9] Channel surfing is the fine art of using the remote control to quickly scan through channels to determine what to watch.

used for these services is regulated and must be made available to all companies seeking to distribute video programs [UPI92]. The FCC decision was followed by numerous court actions that cleared the way for telcos to someday provide video programming services nationwide [Leop95A]. With AT&T in the lead, long-distance companies and local exchange carriers (LECs) have begun efforts to define and demonstrate the types of video programming services they believe customers want[10] [Zieg93, EET95A]. This places them in direct competition with cable television systems for providing, not just video-on-demand but all the services described in Section 8.4. Telcos definitely have some technology advantages over cable systems, but they also have some liabilities: They have broadband switching networks in place (which must and are being upgraded for video distribution). They have interoperability standards that will allow nationwide operation (whereas cable systems tend to be localized and not conform to widespread standards). The piece of technology that telcos are missing is bandwidth on the local loop (see Figure 7.2), the connection between subscribers and the telephone network. When running standard telephone line protocols, the local loop provides data rates ranging from 28.8 Kbps or less (analog) to not more than 144 Kbps (ISDN)—bandwidth sufficient for videoconferencing, perhaps, but far less than sufficient for high-quality video entertainment. At least 1.5 Mbps are needed for even moderate-quality MPEG-compressed video.

To solve their bandwidth problem, telcos have several choices: One is to replace existing twisted-pair copper wire local-loop connections with coaxial or fiber optic cables. Although this is where telcos see themselves ultimately heading, the large installed base makes it very expensive, and most expert observers both inside and outside the telephone industry agree that the time for completing this transition is far in the future. AT&T has proved another choice in the form of ADSL (Asymmetric Digital Subscriber Loop) technology. ADSL is a new signaling method that allows downstream (network-to-subscriber) video transmissions to proceed at 1.5–6 Mbps rates over twisted-pair copper local loops that are not longer than 18,000 feet.[11] As shown in Figure 8.4, ADSL also provides a low-bit-rate bi-directional (digital) control channel and a conventional bi-directional analog voice channel [Lin95]. Although intended primarily for downstream video transmissions (which explains the asymmetric part of the ADSL acronym), in the future it may be used for two-way applications, such as videoconferencing, where upstream video transmissions proceed at much lower rates [Sant93].

In combination with MPEG compression, ADSL makes it possible to transmit

---

[10] LEC is the name given to the Regional Bell Operating Companies (RBOC) and independent telephone companies that provide subscribers with local-loop connections to the telephone network.

[11] Standard telephone line protocols are designed to allow low-cost, reliable communications over great distances and over lines of widely variable quality. ADSL takes advantage of advances in digital filtering, advances in VLSI that make more powerful coding techniques economical, and the fact that many LECs are using fiber optics to reduce the length of the copper portion of the local loop [Chen94].

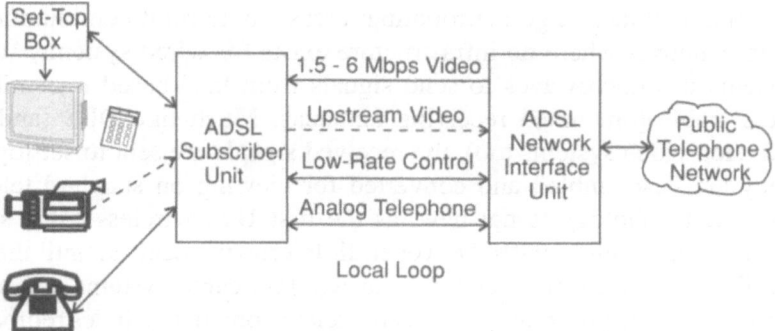

Figure 8.4 ADSL architecture.

a small number of high-quality video channels over existing copper telephone lines. The bandwidth and distance restrictions for ADSL are obvious, but, as it turns out, they are not debilitating. First, video switching is done within the telephone network. Because most subscribers are content to view one channel at a time, a local loop that carries a single video transmission is quite adequate for many video services, including video-on-demand. Second, in the United States, nearly 75% of the 100 million local loops that connect homes to local exchanges are less than 18,000 feet in length. Thus, ADSL, which is positioned as a low-cost gap-filler prior to the arrival of broadband, may be the technology that telcos need to quickly get into video distribution.

There are several versions of ADSL [Chen94]. The first, ADSL-1, operates at 1.5 Mbps for up to 18,000 feet. It allows a single VCR-quality, MPEG-1 compressed video transmission. But the competition (cable and DBS) has moved beyond MPEG-1 to MPEG-2. An updated version of ADSL, which is specified in the ANSI T1.413 ADSL standard, operates at a downstream rate of 6.1 Mbps and an upstream rate of not more than 640 Kbps for distances up to 12,000 feet [Bain95, Lieb96]. This will allow one very high-quality MPEG-2 encoded video transmission or several transmissions at lesser quality.

An important point must not be overlooked: Our discussion and the development of ADSL focuses on video transmission, but ADSL is a transmission technology that can transport any type of digital data over twisted-pair telephone lines at megabit rates. As a result, ADSL-based modems allow high-speed connections to digital data networks such as the Internet [Gree95B]. Also, complementary and competing symmetrical transmission technologies are under development that will increase the data rates in both the upstream and downstream directions [Gree95A, Bell96].

8.6 Wireless Cable

Wireless cable provides yet another means for delivering video, one that has proven popular where, for a variety of reasons, wired cable systems are difficult to install. This includes large metropolitan areas, some rural communities, and developing countries where no infrastructure exists for wired systems. Wireless cable systems use microwaves to send signals from land-based transmitters to subscribers' rooftop-mounted receiving antennas. Much like DBS (and wired cable and telco video systems too), the received signals are sent to set-top boxes where they are descrambled and converted for viewing on standard television receivers. The technology is not new, as the first U.S. wireless cable systems went on the air in the mid-1970s. However, little growth occurred until the 1990s when the FCC allocated more channels to wireless cable systems and allowed them to offer the same programming as cable television; this includes rebroadcasts of local-broadcast television stations, an advantage not currently shared by DBS. Now, in the mid-1990s, U.S. telephone companies are heavily investing in wireless cable systems as a short-term solution for providing video services [Wyli95]. What makes it attractive is that, when compared with the technical and economic problems of upgrading their wired infrastructure to carry broadband traffic and considering that wireless cable systems do not obey the regulations and requirements restricting wired cable franchises, wireless cable offers telephone companies the prospect of lower investment costs and shorter deployment times to enter the video delivery business.

Existing wireless cable systems use a technology known as multipoint multichannel distribution service (MMDS) to broadcast analog video to subscribers. They operate at microwave (2-GHz band) frequencies that lie above the standard broadcast channels. This limits reception to, typically, a radius of 25 to 30 miles because the path between the transmitter and a receiver must be essentially free of any obstructions for what is sometimes called line-of-sight transmission. MMDS operates within a 200-MHz bandwidth and, therefore, existing systems can carry no more than 33 analog 6-MHz television channels, which, in today's marketplace, makes them noncompetitive with DBS and wired cable. The solution is to go digital and use MPEG-2 data compression to boost carrying capacity to more than 125 channels. With FCC authorization and digital technology comparable to that used by DBS and digital wired cable systems, the first digital MMDS system went on the air in 1996 [Piet96].

An emerging technology for wireless cable systems known as local multipoint distribution system (LMDS) has the potential to greatly increase their carrying capacity. Not only is it digital, but LDMS is allocated far more bandwidth than MMDS. There is also the potential for interactivity because LDMS allows two-way transmissions. LMDS uses ultrahigh-frequency (28-GHz band) microwaves. Because these signals are greatly affected by obstructions, they must be sent from lower-powered transmitters over shorter distances. Reception is limited to approximately a 3-mile radius in experimental systems now being tested and, therefore, these systems follow the model of cellular telephony, depending on multiple transmitters to cover a larger area. With more than one GHz of bandwidth allocated to LDMS, hundreds of compressed video channels can be transmitted. With its cellular structure and two-way transmission capability, in the future, it may support data and telephone transmissions, too, although the technology for this does not yet exist. It is too early to tell what services LDMS will offer, how it will compete with other wireless services for digital-bit delivery (such as those listed in Table 7.2), or, more important, who will bring it to market. As of this writing, LMDS technology exists only in prototype one-way wireless cable systems; 200 MPEG-2 compressed video channels were provided by a system tested in Atlanta, Georgia [Anto96].

8.7   Digital Radio

Digital radio is a new technology that will enable broadcasters to transmit CD-quality digital audio without interference or perceptible loss of quality. Digitization not only eliminates the noise that accompanies AM broadcasts and the multipath fading of FM broadcasts, but with error detection and correction, it allows error-free reconstruction of the audio signal just as it was originally broadcast. No one yet believes digital radio will totally replace either AM or FM, but its backers expect digital will quickly become the premier radio broadcasting method. It is not just the superior sound quality that makes digital radio attractive, for digital radio also can transmit text-based information. This will allow broadcasters to offer a host of ancillary services such as audio-visual programs, value-added services, and other new program features. Receivers equipped with text displays will provide listeners with station call letters, song titles, information about the artist, and about the recording being aired. Other possibilities include program guides describing upcoming broadcasts, traffic reports for motorists, weather reports including maps, and (yes!) advertising.

Digital radio goes by several names: The FCC calls it digital audio radio services (DARS) which is sometimes shortened to DAR. In Europe and most of the world, it is known as digital audio broadcasting (DAB), the term we will use. Part of the confusion is that many different systems have been proposed for both satellite and terrestrial transmission. There are a variety of schemes for allocating broadcast spectrum to DAB, with little agreement on how to use it [Jurg92]. Satellite broadcasting proposals abound in the United States and in Europe and elsewhere in the world [Jurg93, Leop95B]. Terrestrial DAB systems are equally diverse. In Europe, the EUREKA 147 DAB system has been demonstrated by commandeering portions of the television broadcast spectrum [Pros94]. In Canada, EUREKA 147 DAB is being tested using newly allocated spectrum; it is planned to be a replacement service for existing AM and FM stations. In the United States, the favored terrestrial broadcasting scheme is IBOC (in-band, on-channel), which uses existing AM and FM radio broadcast and transmission facilities. With IBOC, DAB signals are placed within the broadcaster's existing frequency assignments, making it a somewhat compatible scheme. FM broadcasters, for instance, could simultaneously broadcast an analog and a digital signal within the 200 KHz frequency spectrum they are currently allocated.

Broadcasters recognize that CD-quality digital audio sounds great, but, due to spectrum scarcity, the data rate is far too high to transmit in any economical or feasible way—unless data compression is used. This most assuredly is true for terrestrial broadcasting, where radio channels are allocated only a fraction of the needed bandwidth; and satellite broadcasting, where more bandwidth is potentially available but is mostly given over to higher-paying video services. As observed in Section 8.3, DSS airs about 30 MPEG-compressed audio channels. All current and proposed DAB systems include audio compression, some variant of, or proposed extension to MPEG-2 audio coding [Jurg96]. ITU-R (International Telecommunication Union–Radio) recommendations for DAB specify MPEG audio coding at rates of 192 Kbps and less [Noll95]. This coding rate is sufficient for broadcasting two-channel stereo audio but not for 5.1-channel surround sound. For further discussion of MPEG audio compression, see Section 5.3.

8.8 Summary

This chapter examined communications applications where data compression is used for efficient transmission. We learned the following:

- Profound changes are taking place in broadcasting with broadcasters lining up to provide more personal, more customized delivery of home entertainment and information services, all of which depend on data compression for economical delivery of voice, data, images, and video.
- MPEG compression is an integral part of the standard for HDTV and SDTV digital television.
- Direct broadcast satellite television became an overnight sensation, thanks in part to MPEG compression that allows four to eight times more channels.
- Cable television is transforming itself to provide a host of new interactive services that depend on digital television and MPEG compression.
- Telephone companies have similar objectives and look to MPEG data compression as a key technology for enabling video dial-tone service over existing phone lines.
- Wireless cable systems are moving to digital, MPEG-compressed transmissions to become competitive with other video services.
- Digital radio, a new technology that will allow broadcasters to provide CD-quality audio (and text), depends on MPEG audio compression to squeeze digital audio into available radio broadcast channels.

9

Consumer-Electronics
Applications

In this chapter, we examine consumer-electronics applications where, primarily, data compression is used for efficient data storage. This comes as no surprise because many consumer-electronics products for entertainment and information use personal storage media, discs and tapes today, with solid-state storage a future possibility. Data compression will also be important for future, communications-oriented consumer-electronics products, like HDTVs, where it will be part of the transmission standards. Lossless compression is used for text and other symbolic data, whereas various combinations of lossless and lossy compression are used for speech, audio, image, and video data.

9.1 Industry Overview

Were they living today, Thomas Edison and Guglielmo Marconi, the 19th-century inventors of the phonograph and radio, would surely be amazed by the variety of products on the shelves in 1990s electronics superstores. Beginning with record players and radios, and then television, an ever increasing diversity of consumer-electronics products provide home entertainment and information. The definition of what comprises consumer electronics is a bit fuzzy. Once, consumer electronics meant audio gear, radios, and television receivers, but today the range of products is much broader. Many of today's consumer-electronics products were first introduced for industrial or office applications and then migrated into the mass consumer market only after technology advances reduced their cost and features were added that improved their ease of use. The personal computer is but the latest example of a product making the transition from office to home. For our purposes, we will keep it simple: A consumer-electronics product is something sold by Best Buy, Circuit City, and other electronics retailers.

The rapid growth of consumer electronics can be traced to technology advances—low-cost, integrated-circuit semiconductor electronics, lasers, improved visual displays, smaller and more accurate audio reproducers, and advances in scanning and printing techniques to name a few. Low-cost mass production techniques for small electromechanical devices also play a role. Without a doubt, no factors are more important than the introduction of digital technology, the convergence of computers and communications, and the integration of audio, video, and computer-based equipment. Text, graphics, speech, audio, image, and video data all play starring roles in consumer-electronics products. The ability to store, process, and communicate all types of digital information is revolutionizing consumer electronics. This translates to improvements of existing products and to totally new products. Sometimes, it positions new, digital consumer-electronics products to eclipse older products based on analog technologies—film cameras, for example.

Every day it seems there are announcements of new, digital consumer electronics that will relegate today's analog products to join vinyl long-playing records and black-and-white television sets in the museum of old-fashioned, formerly dominant technologies. However, gee-whiz technology and amazing features do not always assure success. Consumers do not always assume new is better and, often, they are not easily motivated to pay more for it. Then, too, consumers may not be ready to give up on the products they already have, quashing sales opportunities for replacements, or they may not be interested in making revolutionary advances in how they are entertained or work. Simply pinning the digital label on a product does not influence consumers to buy it. Similarly, declaring that data compression is used in a product may not have much influence on consumers either, unless its advantages are obvious.

Earlier in the book data compression was said to be an essential ingredient in the digital revolution taking place in consumer-electronics products—and it is—for it is needed to tame the storage and transmission demands of digital data. However, in consumer electronics, data compression is neither totally transparent nor always a benign servant. Sometimes, but not always, data compression adds significant product cost when measured in additional logic chips and storage buffers. If so, its use may be constraining to high-end products, where cost sensitivities are not so great, but this is a double-edged sword because consumers expect higher quality when they pay more. The problem with today's data compression, at least for audio and video, is that it can compromise quality. Technologists may argue that the degradation can only be measured with sophisticated instruments, but consumers with keen ears and sharp eyes can (or think they can) spot the differences. This, along with high prices, has slowed sales of some compression-based digital products, particularly when those products are forced to compete with entrenched products that consumers consider to be satisfactory, if not superior.

Data compression standards for consumer-electronics products come from sources within and outside the industry. Historically, the industry has created its own unique, de facto standards—and this now includes data compression standards—for its storage-based products and convinced other industries to produce media that conform to those standards. In contrast, HDTVs and other communications-based consumer-electronics products must conform to standards set by the communications industry.

This chapter describes consumer-electronics products for which, with varying degrees of success, data compression is used for text, graphics, speech, audio, image, and video to provide entertainment and information. Additional compression-based products found at electronics retailers such as telephones, FAX machines, and some computer equipment were described in Chapter 7.

9.2   Digital Audio—Stereo Gear and Home Theater

By the early 1990s, the digital audio compact disc (CD) had displaced analog playback media. Vinyl long-playing records had all but disappeared, and sales of prerecorded cassette tapes continued their long decline. For various reasons, be it superior sound quality, durably, or whatever, the CD became and remains the largest-selling consumer audio storage media. About the same time, a new concept—home theater—was beginning to emerge. Home theater, the combination of large-screen television receivers and multichannel audio, allows home viewing of movies and other entertainment with all the impact once reserved for commercial theaters. In this section, we will look at home audio products that, for storage and transmission efficiency, use psychoacoustic audio compression techniques of the type discussed in Section 5.3. See Figure 5.4 for a block diagram of the encoding and decoding processes and Table 5.3 for specifications of the perceptual coders mentioned in this section.

Stereo players and recorders

Audio CDs, excellent as they are, have some limitations: They are not recordable, at least not the versions in consumers' hands. They are not ideal for portable applications—the discs are larger and harder to handle than cassette tapes, and when bumped, CD players are prone to skipping tracks. Analog cassette tapes, long dominant for recording and portable listening applications, are limited, too, in that they cannot match the audio quality of CDs. Steadily declined sales led market analysts to conclude that a replacement was needed for the venerable analog cassette, a replacement that would combine the audio quality of CDs and the recordability and ruggedness of cassettes, all within a compact package. This section looks at three digital audio products that stake a claim on the portable CD and analog cassette marketplace. All use data compression. Their media are depicted in Figure 9.1.

The Sony™ MiniDisc™ (MD) system was introduced in 1992. It is recordable

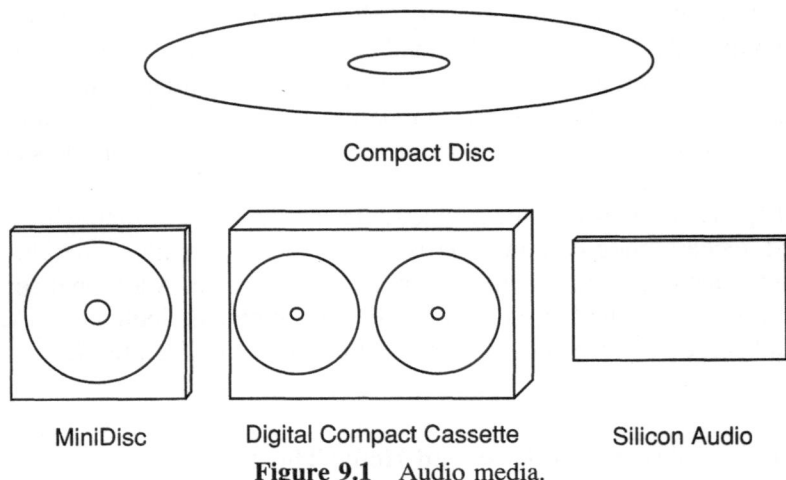

Compact Disc

MiniDisc   Digital Compact Cassette   Silicon Audio

Figure 9.1   Audio media.

(allowing it to replace the analog cassette tape), smaller than a CD (allowing lightweight portable players), and, with the same portable applications in mind, it is shock resistant. The new technology in MD is extensive: Magneto-optical discs provide recordability, whereas conventional read-only optical discs are used for music and software distribution. A half-size disc (64-mm-diameter MDs versus 120-mm-diameter CDs) encased in a hard shell provides small size and durability. Buffer memory for the bit stream coming off the optical pickup allows MD players to mask bump-induced interruptions, a technique which, later, was added to portable CD players. MDs and CDs are alike in other ways too: Both use prerecorded discs made of polycarbonate, whereon tracks of information are recorded as microscopic pits in an aluminum reflective layer. Both the prerecorded and recordable versions of the MD use track widths, track spacings, and data-encoding methods that are similar but not identical to the CD. For a full discussion of MD technology, see [Rana93, Nish94, Yosh94C].

An important difference between MD and CD is that the smaller MD holds only 140 MB of data, about one-fifth as much as the standard CD. To provide the same 74-minute playing time that CDs offer, audio data compression is a necessity. Starting with the 16-bit quantization and 44.1-KHz sampled stereo audio signal used for CDs, Sony engineers developed ATRAC (Adaptive TRansform Acoustic Coding), a proprietary psychoacoustic audio compression method. It is a hybrid coder: The encoding process begins with bandpass filters that break the audio spectrum into three subbands. Then a modified discrete cosine transform is applied to generate 512 spectral components. The output bit stream is generated by quantizing the spectral values and assigning bits according to psychoacoustic principles [Yosh94C]. ATRAC was designed to provide a 5:1 compression ratio, just the amount needed for making up the capacity difference between the MD and CD disc formats.

Philips introduced the Digital Compact Cassette™ (DCC™) system to the marketplace in 1992, positioning it as an extension of the Compact Cassette™ (analog cassette). It improves upon analog cassettes with sound quality that approaches the CD, and it offers better track-search cueing, text information for song titles, and a cassette that is less vulnerable to damage. Playing time, up to 120 minutes, is identical to the analog cassette because both use the same width tape and move it at the same speed. DCC tape transports differ in minor ways from analog tape transports, but either cassette may be loaded in DCC machines because their external dimensions are nearly identical. This makes DCC machines backward-compatible, providing playback for the large inventory of analog cassettes now in the hands of consumers. Internally, DCC technology is quite different, beginning with the tape itself, which is made of high-performance, video-grade material. New, thin-film, magneto-resistive tape heads can play back two tracks from analog cassettes and lay down and play back nine much narrower tracks for DCC. These tape heads increase the data rate for digital recording, but, still, the raw data rate is only 768 Kbps. System information—error correction, synchronization, and addressing symbols—uses half the bits, leaving only 384 Kbps available for audio recording, far short of the 1.4112 Mbps needed for CD-quality stereo. For a full discussion of DCC technology, see [Rana92, Hoog94].

To squeeze CD-quality stereo onto DCC, Philips engineers developed Precision Audio Subband Coding (PASC), a proprietary psychoacoustic audio compression algorithm. As the name implies, it is a subband coder. The encoding process begins with bandpass filters that break the audio spectrum into 32 subbands. Then the compressed output bit stream is generated by quantizing the filter output values and assigning bits according to psychoacoustic principles based on the hearing threshold and signal masking[1] [Hoog94]. The compressed output bit stream is then combined with system data and distributed over eight of the nine magnetic tracks. (The ninth track is used for recording auxiliary information that provides time, text, and control signals which contribute to the improved cueing function.) PASC was designed to provide a 4:1 compression ratio, just the amount needed to make up the difference between DCC and CD data rates.

In 1995, NEC Corporation demonstrated Silicon Audio™ technology, an audio-data storage system that uses semiconductor flash memory cards. Although no products are yet available—and none will be until electronic memory costs decline dramatically—audio players (and recorders) no larger than a deck of playing cards are envisioned for future products. Not only will Silicon Audio players be a fraction of the size and weight of current cassette tape and CD players, they will also be rugged and reliable because there are no moving parts. For a full discussion of Silicon Audio technology, see [Sugi95].

The storage technology for Silicon Audio is shared with computer applications that use electronic memory storage devices. (See the description of solid-state

---

[1] Up to this point, PASC coding is identical to MPEG-1 audio coding.

files in Section 6.6.) The problems with using this technology in consumer-electronics products are packaging density—stuffing sufficient memory into a small package—and cost. For a solution, NEC engineers turned to MPEG-1 layer II audio compression operating at 96 Kbps per channel (providing slightly more than 7:1 compression), a rate sufficient for near CD-quality sound. This allowed them to load 12 minutes of stereo music onto a 16-MB card. But for playing time equal to one CD, six of these cards are needed, and at mid-1990s prices, they would sell for about $6000! Thus, major advances must be made for solid-state storage to be a serious contender for home audio media.

Home theater

Multichannel sound for home theater recreates the conditions found in a movie theater by placing left, center, and right channel speakers across the front of the room near the television screen and surround channel speakers at the sides of the room, as shown in Figure 9.2. The sixth speaker, a subwoofer for low frequencies, is usually placed at the front too.

Initially, analog matrixing techniques were used to squeeze multichannel audio into the two stereo channels provided by laser videodiscs, VCRs, and stereo television. With matrixing, the center channel and a monophonic surround channel were encoded atop the left and right audio channels. During playback, they were extracted by decoding logic in the home audio/video receiver that amplified all four channels and directed low frequencies to the subwoofer. Various matrix-surround sound techniques were invented—Dolby Surround™, Dolby Pro Logic™, and others—but none could overcome the fundamental limitations of matrix encoding; namely channel separation between the left and right channels was high, as was the separation between the center and surround channels. But

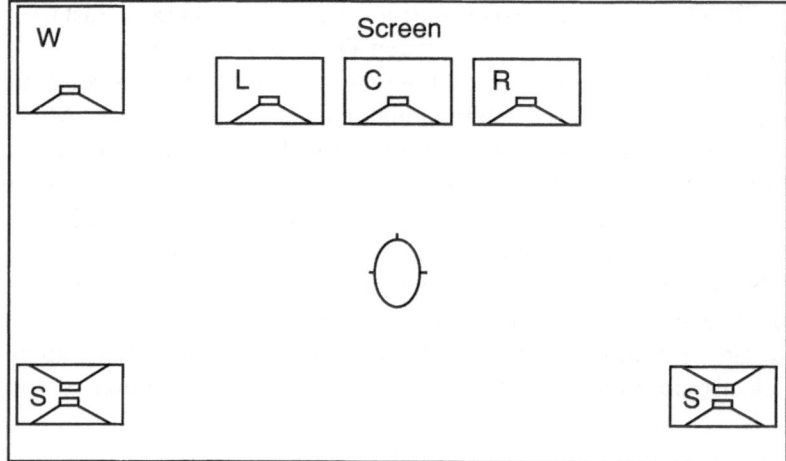

Figure 9.2   Home theater speaker placement.

between the center and left or right channels and between the surround and left or right channels it was quite low. Even with careful encoding, there was channel bleed-through, the dynamic range was limited, and not all combinations of sound could be reproduced. All these limitations detracted from the illusion of 3-D (three-dimensional) sound.

The solution is, of course, to provide discrete channels, but the basic problem is fitting the extra channels into existing disc, tape, and broadcast audio/video media. Using perceptual audio coding, a discrete-channel system known as 5.1-channel digital surround sound provides that solution. Five full-range channels for the left, center, right, and two surround channels, and a sixth channel for the subwoofer, which is limited to frequencies below 120 Hz, are provided. This allows 5.1-channel digital surround systems to reproduce a much more accurate 3-D soundfield. One perceptual audio coder, Dolby AC-3 encoding, has been adopted for all media to provide multichannel audio transmissions that accompany video [Rigg95, Taki95B]. As learned in Chapter 5, AC-3 incorporates an advance transform coder that can encode and transmit 5.1 channels in just 384 Kbps, a compression ratio approaching 11:1. It does this by using psychoacoustic principles and exploiting the correlation between individual channels. All channels are compressed and combined into a single composite signal; this signal can be recorded on all existing stereo media and on new media such as digital video discs and can also be transmitted by conventional television and HDTV. Products enabled for AC-3 began appearing in 1995.

Compressed digital audio in the marketplace: is it a winner?

Since the introduction of MiniDisc and Digital Compact Cassette and, later, with digital surround sound, psychoacoustic audio compression has been a subject for microscopic examination and, at times, heated debate. Some see it as a leading-edge technology to be used in innovative new audio products of all kinds, whereas others believe it to be a colossal blunder. To oversimplify the controversy about psychoacoustic audio compression, videophiles seem willing to accept the minor aberrations it introduces, whereas audiophiles definitely remain unconvinced.

There are some marketplace factors that may help to explain why the reactions to psychoacoustic audio compression are so varied. To begin with, the criteria for sound quality are different for audio/video versus audio-only products. For the home theater market, which is young and continues to grow wildly, technology and consumer expectations are still evolving. Surround sound, whose primary goal is realistic 3-D soundfield imaging, is acknowledged to be vastly improved by Dolby AC-3's fully discrete channels, stereo surround channels, and increased dynamic range. The quality of home theater sound is judged by more than the fidelity of music. Both experts and consumers appear willing to accept the slight imperfections that perceptual coding may add to their favorite movie soundtracks in favor of improvements to 3-D soundfield imaging. In contrast, the home audio market is saturated with products that offer extremely good stereo sound at very low prices. For several decades, stereo sound quality has improved, with audio professionals and consumers, alike, coming to expect the next generation of products to be even better. This is not an easy task, especially when the accuracy of stereo reproduction of music is the major or only factor (other than price) for judging goodness. But the search for higher levels of perfection continues; techniques such as higher sampling rates and 20- or 24-bit samples are being considered for improving on CD-quality sound [Pohl95C]. The introduction of perceptual coding to this environment violated the expectations for higher quality. Audiophile publications were quick to point this out, and they continue to warn that MD and DCC sound quality does not meet CD standards. In fairness, because MD and DCC aim to replace analog cassettes, perhaps neither should be judged by CD standards, but they are. However, both MD and DCC products currently are far more expensive than the analog cassette tape or CD products they intend to replace; so, applying higher standards may not be unreasonable.

There are some technical factors too. Not all perceptual coding algorithms are created equal. In praise of Dolby AC-3, experts often point out that it uses a highly efficient, sophisticated second-generation perceptual coder (an earlier version is used extensively in broadcasting) which can hide or reduce the sonic imperfections of perceptual coding [Taki95B]. What they are talking about is that AC-3 simultaneously encodes all channels and can exploit the correlation that exists between channels, an effect that grows with more channels. The encoder looks at what is happening in all channels and allocates to each of them bits from a shared pool. The channels with the greatest needs get larger proportions of the total bits available in the combined pool. This results in greater coding efficiency (higher compression ratios), and the overall sound quality can be much better than could be obtained with multiple, single-channel encoders. In contrast, ATRAC, in MD, and PASC, in DCC, encode each channel independently. Each channel receives a fixed number of bits, which may be more or less than needed for the highest sound quality. However, if simultaneous encoding were used in these applications, it would likely be less effective as there are only two stereo channels with which to work.

Another technical factor is that MD and DCC products can both decode and encode audio, unlike home theater equipment that only decodes. Audiophiles—and broadcasters who have devised demonstrations to prove the point—are concerned with the degradation that occurs when compressed media or compressed broadcasts are copied. Due to decoding and reencoding, minor sonic aberrations introduced by perceptual coding can be magnified in unpredictable ways[2]

---

[2] Both MD and DCC, like all digital audio recorders intended for U.S. consumer applications, incorporate circuitry that prevents making a direct digital copy of a source that is, itself, a direct digital copy of an original. When a compressed source is copied, it must first be decompressed before a copy can be made.

[Rana94]. Thus, at its present stage of development, perceptual audio coding may be quite satisfactory for playback-only applications but far less viable for home recording.

9.3   Digital Television

Without thinking much about it, we have all used "digital" television. Starting somewhere in the 1980s, manufacturers began incorporating digital functions in millions of "analog" NTSC, PAL, and SECAM broadcast-standard television receivers. Digital technology is used for everything from channel selection, to picture processing, to feature enhancements both spectacular, as is picture-in-picture, and mundane, as is displaying the time of day. The new wrinkle is that television receivers must be prepared to receive digitized, compressed broadcasts—what in the nineties we choose to call digital television.

As learned in Chapter 8, by the mid-1990s standards for terrestrial broadcasts of digital television in standard-definition television and high-definition television formats were close to completion. Meanwhile, NTSC standard television receivers were already receiving digital pictures and sound from direct broadcast satellite systems and, soon, would be from wired and wireless cable systems and telco video systems. All digital television broadcasting methods use MPEG (or Dolby AC-3) audio compression (described in Section 5.3) and MPEG video compression (described in Section 5.5). This and immediately following sections look at how data compression applies to the consumer-electronics products for receiving, reproducing, and recording digital television.

Drop into any electronics store today and you will find a wide choice of television receivers and peripheral devices including set-top boxes, VCRs, video camcorders, videodisc players, and other audio/visual products. As illustrated in Figure 9.3, all can interoperate thanks to the NTSC (PAL or SECAM) transmission standard for analog television.

Now, fast forward to the year 2000—when digital television is in full bloom—and visit the same store. Will you find digital television receivers and digital peripheral devices that interoperate using the SDTV/HDTV transmission standard for digital television transmission? Silly question; of course you will, because this is *the* standard for digital television, right? Actually, you may find something quite different. One reason is that digital set-top boxes, VCRs, video camcorders, videodisc players, and other audio/visual products are reaching the market today without the benefit of a crucial industry standard—a standard for a digital interface between peripheral devices and television receivers. These products all work with analog television receivers, but how they, or their successors, will interoperate with digital television receivers is unclear. The fundamental problem is that the consumer-electronics industry has not come to grips with how to handle data compression in peripheral devices. The problem is exacerbated when those devices must interoperate with digital television receivers that in themselves incorporate data compression, receivers which conform to the SDTV/HDTV transmission

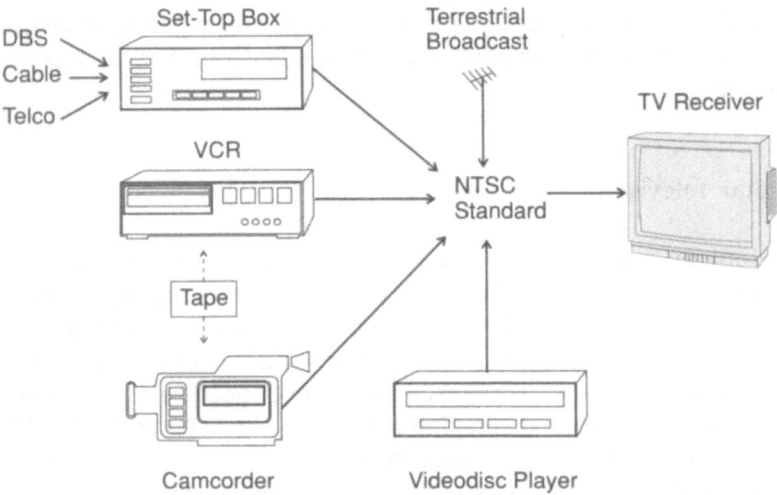

Figure 9.3   Television reception.

standard for terrestrial television broadcasts. To understand the difficulties that compressed digital television creates, let us explore what is happening in peripheral devices.

9.4   Digital Set-Top Boxes

A set-top box similar to that shown in Figure 9.4 is needed to receive digital television broadcasts on a standard analog television receiver. Digital set-top boxes are widely deployed for DBS and soon will be for cable television and telco video systems. While still in the formative stages, a digital set-top box may provide the solution for receiving digital SDTV on analog television receivers.

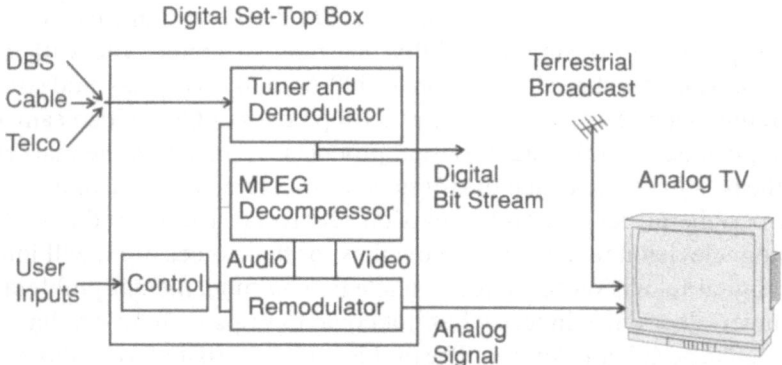

Figure 9.4   Digital television reception on analog television receivers.

Today's digital set-top boxes build on the capabilities found in convertor boxes used by (analog) cable television systems. To oversimplify the process, a channel is selected and the signal is demodulated. MPEG decompression is applied. Then the audio and video signals are remodulated to analog NTSC (PAL or SECAM) format for output on an unused television channel. Picture and sound appear when the television receiver is tuned to that channel. (The DSS set-top box for DBS television also outputs a compressed digital bit stream; more about this is coming up shortly.) A remote control for the set-top box allows users to select the digital channel for viewing and to control whatever interactive features are available.

A point often overlooked is that the tuning function in the analog television receiver is used only for receiving terrestrial broadcasts. A set-top box takes over the tuning function, nullifying or essentially bypassing the receiver's tuner, but that is not of much consequence with analog television.[3]

Now, consider how digital television sets of the future will receive digital television broadcasts. To *directly* receive SDTV/HDTV transmission-standard terrestrial broadcasts, without the aid of an external set-top box, digital television receivers will need a built-in tuner and an MPEG decompressor. But will they also receive digital broadcasts from DBS, cable, and telco networks in a way similar to that shown in Figure 9.3? The answer probably is "no," and here is why: When digital television sets are used with an external set-top box, which is needed to adapt to the differing broadcast standards of DBS, cable, and telco networks, the (tuning and) decompression function built into the television set must be nullified or bypassed—if the set-top box delivers a decompressed signal. Therein lies a problem that the consumer-electronics industry has yet to solve. Here are some possible solutions:

- A simple approach is for the set-top box to deliver a MPEG-compressed digital bit stream that the digital television receiver can decompress. To make this happen, a standard for compressed digital bit-stream inputs for television receivers must be developed. However, digital television service providers may be uninterested in this approach, for it reduces the set-top box to a simple digital version of the old analog cable television convertor box, potentially robbing the set-top box of interactive features.

- Digital set-top boxes of the future could include MPEG compressors, allowing the television signal to be remodulated to the SDTV/HDTV transmission standard for terrestrial broadcasts. Although fully supporting interactivity, it is not very cost-effective because MPEG compressors are complex and expensive. In addition, stacking lossy MPEG decoders and encoders can degrade sound and picture quality.

- Another possibility is to integrate the set-top box function into the television receiver.

---

[3] The only time anyone notices that the tuning function is done in the set-top box is when a VCR is used to record programs and channel-selection logic in the VCR cannot control tuning in the set-top box. Fortunately, ingenious but kludgy solutions have been devised.

This raises a host of marketing and technical issues: Whose set-top should be built-in, or should all of them? How will the set-top box dataflow be integrated? The industry has struggled with these issues for years and has not yet found a solution [Cici95].

- Probably the cleanest choice is that digital television receivers have inputs to accept decompressed audio and video signals, effectively bypassing the tuning and decompression functions. To make this happen, a standard for interoperating with decompressed signals must be developed.

9.5   Digital VCRs and Camcorders

As shown in Table 9.1, over the years an unending series of videotape recording formats has been introduced for professional and consumer applications. Some

Table 9.1   Digital videotape recording formats.

Recorders[1]	Format[2]	Year	Tape Width	Playing Time
Professional:				
Analog	Various	1961	2 in.	60 min
	Various	1967	1 in.	60 min
	U-matic	1969	¾ in.	60 min
Digital	D1[3]	1986	¾ in.	94 min
	D2	1988	¾ in.	208 min
	D3	1991	½ in.	245 min
	D5	1993	½ in.	123 min
	Digital Betacam™	1993	½ in.	125 min
	Ampex DCT	1993	½ in.	208 min
	D6	1994	¾ in.	60 min
Consumer:				
Analog	Betamax™	1975	½ in.	2 - 5 hr
	VHS	1976	½ in.	2 - 8 hr
	8 mm	1985	8 mm	2 - 4 hr
	S-VHS	1987	½ in.	2 - 8 hr
Digital	D-VHS	1995	½ in.	7 hr[4]
	DVC	1995	½ in.	4½ hr[4]

Notes:
[1]   Sources: [Hama95, Roth95, Warn96].
[2]   All are compliant with NTSC, PAL, or SECAM standards except D6 which is intended for HDTV.
[3]   D1 - D6 are SMPTE digital formats.
[4]   Playing time will be cut by one-half for a future HDTV mode.

formats appeared and quickly disappeared, having been supplanted by better technology or having met the fate of superior marketing at the hands of their competitors. Today, digital recording systems have largely replaced analog in professional videotape recorders, and newly introduced digital formats are looking to doing the same in consumer VCRs and camcorders.

In the broadcasting industry, the advantages of digital recording, namely fault-less reproduction of the video signal even after multiple copying and unerring timing stability for video and audio, are widely recognized. Starting in 1986, these advantages were provided to professional videotape recorders by the SMPTE (Society of Motion Picture and Television Engineers) D1 format and others soon to follow [Hama95]. Digital video demands recording at data rates far higher than analog, and, initially, high-quality pictures were achieved by purely electro-mechanical means—wider tape, multiple stacked heads, and parallel recording channels, for instance. More recently, advances in head and tape technology and data compression has been exploited. Not only do the latest products offer the same or higher-quality pictures, but their size and complexity have been reduced, and portable professional digital camcorders are now available. Compression ratios in today's professional videotape recorders are only 2:1 or slightly more. This modest reduction is achieved by using frame-by-frame, spatial discrete-cosine transform (DCT) intraframe coding similar to that found in JPEG (described in Section 5.4). Recent announcements suggest that more powerful MPEG-based compression will soon appear in professional gear [Hara95A].

With this background, let us turn our attention to data compression in consumer video recording. At the time of this writing, the consumer-electronics industry is deeply divided on how digital technology should be deployed in consumer VCRs and camcorders. Data compression is the central issue—should digital VCRs and camcorders use data compression/decompression and, if so, what kind? Unfortunately for consumers, incompatible products are reaching the marketplace. Here is a brief overview of what is available:

In 1995, JVC (Victor Company of Japan) introduced the D-VHS™ (Data-Video Home System) format. D-VHS VCRs record a compressed digital bit stream obtained from a peripheral device, such as the set-top box shown in Figure 9.4, and play it back through the same device. Because the bit stream is compressed, the data rate is sufficiently low for existing analog recording technology to be used. D-VHS recorders essentially are standard S-VHS (Super-VHS) machines to which error correction and digital signal processing logic has been added. Currently, digital bit streams from the DSS DBS set-top boxes are accepted, but, in the future, interfaces to other set-top boxes, digital television receivers, and computers are possible [Krau95A]. The first generation of D-VHS machines record SDTV-quality signals at 14.1 Mbps, providing up to 7 hours of recording on a standard S-VHS cassette. When HDTV signals become available, the D-VHS specification includes a high-definition mode that will allow future machines to record at 28.2 Mbps, providing up to 3½ hours of recording on one tape. The chief advantage of recording compressed bit streams is that digital VCRs can be much simpler and cheaper, for they contain no compression or decompression hardware. The downside, beyond requiring multiple interfaces because there is no standard yet for digital bit streams, is that digital camcorders cannot follow the same path. D-VHS compatible camcorders, should they become available, will need compression hardware to generate a compressed digital bit stream.

Also entering the marketplace in 1995 were products that conform to the Digital Video Cassette (DVC) standard. In 1994, a consortium of over 50 companies reached agreement on specifications for standard-definition and high-definition DVCRs (Digital VCRs) and camcorders that *do* incorporate compression and decompression. The DVC standard allows uncompressed video to be recorded digitally and, initially, decoded to analog for playback through NTSC-standard television receivers. Digital outputs also are available for making digital-to-digital copies with DVC-compliant VCRs and camcorders. In the future, digital outputs to personal computers will allow for DVC products to be part of computer-controlled video editing and production facilities [Hara95B]. First-generation DVC products provide over 500 lines of horizontal resolution, far better than the best analog VCRs which are limited to about 400 lines. SDTV-quality signals are recorded at 25 Mbps on a new ¼-inch format tape cassette that provides up to 4½ hours of recording time. When HDTV signals become available, the DVC specification includes a high-definition mode that will allow future machines to record at 50 Mbps, providing up to 2¼ hours of recording on one tape. The data compression found in DVC products is not MPEG but, rather, a frame-by-frame, DCT coding technique similar to that found in professional video gear. In the first-generation DVC products, the compression ratio is about 5:1.

Which solution will consumers embrace, D-VHS, DVC, or yet another alternative? Some industry observers assert that the D-VHS VCR will be just an interim device and all-digital VCRs that have the technology to decode compressed video signals will prevail. By the time you read this, the industry or the marketplace may have settled on a single solution. If not, welcome to a digital version of the Beta-VHS format war of the 1980s! Whatever the outcome, data compression will be part of the solution. Now, let us explore in greater depth the need for and the kind of data compression appropriate for digital VCRs and camcorders.

Video recording places different requirements on data compression than any of the video transmission applications that we have examined. An ideal data compression algorithm for video recording would:

- Provide symmetrical encoding and decoding time since video recorders must both record and playback
- Cause no (or very little) loss of image quality as video recorders are intermediate storage devices and tapes are often copied
- Allow each frame to be easily reconstructed for frame-by-frame access and allow moving forward and backward in the video stream during editing
- Allow decoding at varying speeds to provide a viewable picture during multispeed playback (slow-motion and high-speed picture search modes)

- Operate with widely-fluctuating bit error rates (caused by tape dropouts) encountered in magnetic recording channels
- Compress video sufficiently to overcome the limited data rates in the recording channel and the limited capacity and recording time of the recording media.

Clearly, none of the video compression algorithms examined so far meet all these requirements. The leader in transmission applications, MPEG, is not an ideal coding scheme for video recording: It is an asymmetric algorithm that requires sophisticated encoding hardware to achieve high compression ratios, which translates into expensive, power-hungry camcorders. It also makes extensive use of interframe coding, which makes frame-by-frame operations in VCRs difficult and expensive. The DCT techniques used in professional videotape records and DVC products, essentially the same as found in M-JPEG (motion-JPEG), come closest. (M-JPEG, as described Section 5.5, compresses video frame by frame as a sequence of still images.) But, can M-JPEG or any simple intraframe coding technique provide sufficient compression? To address this question, consider the following:

The recording mechanisms in consumer VCRs and camcorders must be simple to produce low-cost, small-sized devices for portable applications, and consumers expect ever-smaller tape cassettes to provide several hours of recording time. These two factors limit the recording rate and, essentially, determine how much compression is needed [With92]. Without going into great detail, the recording rate for today's consumer gear is limited to about 25 Mbps, with 50 Mbps projected for the future, and the maximum storage capacity of cassettes is about 50 GB for VCRs and 11 GB for camcorders [Hama95, Roth95]. This translates into the playing times and compression ratios shown in Table 9.2. Note that in computing compression ratios, the overhead for recording channel error correction is assumed to be 20% [With92].

Table 9.2 Digital VCR and camcorder playing times and compression ratios.

Recording Rate	Playing Time		Compression Ratio	
	50 GB cassette	11 GB cassette	SDTV @ 100 Mbps	HDTV @ 1.2 Gbps
25 Mbps	4.44 hr	1.0 hr	5:1	60:1
50 Mbps	2.22 hr	0.5 hr	2.5:1	30:1

Recording SDTV obviously poses few problems; the moderate compression ratios needed can be obtained with DCT intraframe coding with little if any compromise in image quality. Recording HDTV is more difficult. Higher compression ratios are needed, and whatever method is chosen—DCT intraframe, MPEG interframe, or something else—image quality degradation becomes a concern. Higher recording rates, which depend on future advances in head and tape technology, may provide an alternative.

9.6   Digital Video Disc

If predictions come true, the digital video disc (DVD) will soon be the medium of choice for in-home playback of rented movies and direct-to-video productions. DVD promises a revolution in home video. Consumers will enjoy far-higher picture quality than provided by tapes played on their analog VCRs, with the ease and convenience of a CD-sized disc. DVDs will play on multimedia computers, sparking production of media for both entertainment and education. Media producers will also benefit with lower production costs and better control over unauthorized duplication. With immense digital storage and future potential for recording, DVDs may replace VCRs and become the mass storage media of choice in multimedia computers.

A bit of history: The DVD is not the first attempt to sell consumers on optical storage for video. The analog LaserDisc™, the lone survivor of videodisc format wars fought in the 1970s, has never won much public support, with LaserDisc players in fewer than 1% of U.S. households. Long the choice of serious videophiles seeking the highest-quality pictures, LaserDiscs continue to be relatively expensive, and the availability of new and rental titles remains limited. The plight of LaserDisc can be attributed partly to marketing and partly to its ungainly 12-inch size, acceptable in the era of vinyl records but not today.

The Video CD, the first generation of digital videodiscs, came to market in 1993. Using CD-ROM disc technology, MPEG-1 data compression, and modified CD players, it allows up to 74 minutes of full-motion video and stereo sound to be recorded on a standard 120-mm CD. The Video CD was originally created for video karaoke machines but much broader uses were envisioned [Yosh93B]. Its backers strongly promoted it as the new media for distributing movies, but the movie deals never got off the ground. Hollywood turned thumbs down, being duly unimpressed by a media that provided marginally acceptable video quality for big-screen productions and could not contain a feature film on a single disc. Today, Video CD lives on as the storage media for video karaoke, video games, and limited production of movies for the Philips CD-I™ (Compact Disc-Interactive) multimedia player. Also, there has been a recent resurgence of interest in using Video CD for computer multimedia.

The influence of Hollywood media producers (and the computer industry) helped to define today's DVD. Hollywood was looking for a media that not only provided high-quality video for full-length feature films but included videophile features such as 16:9 wide-screen display formats, multilanguage audio tracks, and surround sound, and included other features such as copy protect and parental lockout. The challenge to manufactures was to come up with a high-density CD that had the storage capacity to make this possible. And that they did—in duplicate! In 1994, teams led by Sony/Philips and by Toshiba/Time-Warner developed competing high-density CD formats that used different encoding and recording techniques for placing data on 120-mm discs. With the Sony/Philips format perhaps having some advantages for the computer industry and its need for high-density CD-ROMs, both proposed formats were equally adept for video, provided the storage capacity, image quality, and features for which Hollywood was looking. For a time, it appeared that both formats would be launched in the marketplace. Sony/Philips lined up CD-ROM drive makers and computer industry support for its offering; not to be outdone, Toshiba/Time Warner garnered the support of some major Hollywood film studios. What followed was a marketing blitz by both groups, each showing their format could handle both computer and entertainment applications. However, there soon were strong signals from the marketplace urging a merger. Key players in the computer industry realized it is impossible to separate PC-based multimedia applications from television-based video applications, and they would be stuck with supporting both formats [Yosh95B]. Important members of the film production and distribution industry, eyeing prospects for launching a lucrative DVD movie-rental business, realized that having two groups of consumer-electronics companies slugging it out in the marketplace was not in their interest, and reportedly threatened to embrace neither format [Yosh95F].

In 1995, a merger deal was struck, creating today's DVD. Data encoding and recording technologies were merged and a jumble of patent cross-licensing issues was resolved to produce a single standard. Actually, the standard specifies several disc formats, a multimedia CD for computers, the DVD for use in consumer video players, and future higher-density discs and recordable formats.

DVD specifies MPEG-2 video and Dolby AC-3 audio compression. Both video and audio are decompressed by VLSI chips incorporated in consumer DVD players. For now, their output conforms to either NTSC or PAL standards, with HDTV to be addressed sometime in the future. An interesting aspect of DVD is how more than 2 hours of high-quality video is squeezed onto the disc and the role MPEG-2 plays. Part of the solution is the increased storage capacity realized by reducing the physical dimensions for storing each bit and using a shorter-wavelength laser for readout. Another part relates to using highly efficient encoding and (in the future) recording on dual-layer and dual-sided discs. MPEG-2 data compression contributes too; for unlike MPEG-1, which operates at a fixed rate, it supports variable-rate encoding. This allows the bit-stream rate to be increased during high-action sequences and decreased at other times. Somewhat akin to the variable transmission rate for channels in the DSS direct broadcast satellite system, this feature of MPEG-2 is exploited by variable-bit-rate technology in DVD. By adding a variable-bit-rate-controller function to the MPEG-2 encoder and varying the DVD playback bit rate, data can be efficiently encoded and placed on the disc at a lower average transfer rate, thus extending the playing time.

A summary of past, present, and future videodiscs discussed in this section is provided in Table 9.3.

9.7 Digital Photography

If you are looking to polish your image, try digital photography! It is still not inexpensive, and the picture quality is not yet the equal of film. But digital

Table 9.3 Videodisc specifications.

	Capacity (GB)	Data Rate (Mbps)	Playing Time (minutes)	Picture Resolution (pixels)	Audio/Video Compression
LaserDisc	32 / 64[1]	71.7[1]	60 / 120	415 x 480	None
Video CD	0.65	1.2	74	352 x 240	MPEG/MPEG-1
DVD	4.7	3.5-11 (avg-max)	133 (typical)	720 x 480	AC-3/MPEG-2
HD-DVD (future)	18	3-11 (avg-max)	Video format dependent	HDTV format	AC-3/MPEG-2

Notes:
[1] LaserDisc is an analog storage media. Digital capacity and data rate are estimated equivalents.

photography allows images to be processed in ways that film can never hope to do, and do it with greater speed and ease. There are consumer products and tools for digitally capturing, processing, printing, and displaying photographs, whether just for making snapshots or for more serious entertainment, photojournalism, and desktop publishing activities. Let us begin by exploring the selection of equipment available. Figure 9.5 depicts how photographs can be digitally captured, processed, and viewed. For those still using conventional cameras, or having a backlog of film-based images, scanners can digitize negatives, slides, and photographs for storage and processing. Digital cameras directly digitize images (how they do this will be examined in Section 9.8) and provide the

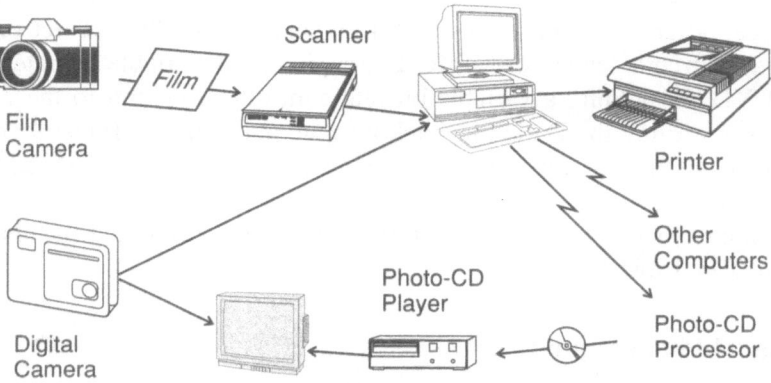

Figure 9.5 Tools for digital photography.

quickest means for getting them into a computer. The computer is a vital element of digital photography. Image processing software allows digital photographs to be manipulated easily and edited as needed, included in documents, or simply to be printed. Digital photography increases the number of options for viewing photographs. Printers attached to personal computers can produce color prints that range in quality from good to excellent, roughly in proportion to the cost of the printer. But there are other options, one being that in the future, local photofinishers can easily go online, allowing them to receive digital pictures from customers and make high-quality prints to be picked up at the customer's convenience. Another choice is to display, not print, pictures. Photographers can display digital pictures on their computer monitor or transmit them on a network to other personal computer users. Some digital cameras have built-in LCD displays and, besides sending images to computers, where they can be displayed and manipulated, provide connections for displaying images on television receivers or recording them on VCRs. Yet another option is to send digital images to a photofinisher and have them recorded on a Photo CD™, a technique that has been available for some time. Photo CD technology will be examined in Section 9.9.

Despite all the advantages of digital imagery, which photographic and electronics companies are eager to exploit, technical problems have kept digital photography stalled in low gear for many years. The problem with digital images—we have said it before—is they require immense numbers of bits to represent them. Today, with advances in image sensors, storage technology, digital electronics, and data compression, digital photography is becoming affordable for professional photographers, small-office entrepreneurs, and well-heeled consumers.

9.8 Digital Cameras

Electronic still-video cameras were first introduced to the consumer marketplace in 1981 [With92]. These cameras operated like video camcorders but were designed to capture one frame at a time. They were expensive and, because they borrowed analog technology from video camcorders, their images were no better than television quality and could not be digitally processed. Today's totally digital electronic cameras are still expensive, but the image quality has improved greatly. All models, high-end and simple digital cameras, alike, offer much more function. The latest versions of digital cameras fall into three categories: There are professional digital cameras that seek to duplicate the image quality, look, feel, and operation of high-end, single-lens-reflex 35-mm film cameras. They are intended and priced for serious commercial photographers. The middle ground is held by far less costly semiprofessional digital cameras that offer many professional camera functions but with less image resolution. These cameras have proven attractive to small businesses such as car dealers, real-estate agents, insurance agents, and others who need small photos for advertising and record-keeping purposes. They are also attractive to large organizations, who can sometimes offset the cost of digital cameras by film savings alone, such as insurance companies that have millions of digital photos as part of their underwriting and claims systems. At the low end, the "snapshot" digital cameras intended for amateurs, betraying their technical heritage, look, feel, and function like video camcorders, from which much is borrowed. Although the image resolution is (still too) limited, they include features that address the consumer market such as built-in liquid-crystal display (LCD) screens for image composition and review, NTSC outputs to television receivers, VCRs, and video color printers, and digital outputs to home computers.

There is still a ways to go before digital cameras can hope to match the image quality produced by film cameras. Table 9.4 provides a comparison of the resolution limits for 35-mm film and typical digital cameras marketed in 1996. Although inexpensive 35-mm cameras assuredly do not provide the full resolution of 35-mm film, they do set a high standard that only the most expensive digital cameras have yet to approach. However, ultrahigh resolution is not very important for amateur snapshots or even commercial applications where only small-size prints are needed. For these applications, digital camera manufacturers can point to features such as the ability to instantly view pictures, to digitally manipulate images, whether for making exposure adjustments, cropping, or some-

Table 9.4   Digital imaging specifications.

Still-Image Products[1] (Typical)	Image Resolution (megapixels)	Image Color Representation (3 x bits / pixel)	Image Size (Uncompressed)	Storage for 100 Images (Compressed 15:1)
35-mm film - max. resolution	18M = 5320 x 3550	36 bit	85 MB	567 MB
35-mm film - hi-resol. scanning	6M = 3072 x 2048	36 bit	28 MB	189 MB
Professional digital camera	1.5M = 1536 x 1024	36 bit	7 MB	47 MB
Semiprofessional digital camera	0.375M = 756 x 512	24 bit	1.2 MB	7.7 MB
"Snapshot" digital camera	0.125M = 512 x 256	24 bit	0.4 MB	2.6 MB

Notes:
[1]   For descriptions of 1995-1996 products see [Anto95, Busc95, Scha95, Port96]. Prices range from less than $700 for snapshot digital cameras to $30,000 for professional models.

thing more sophisticated, and to electronically transmit pictures and incorporate them in printed documents.

The block diagram for a digital camera is shown in Figure 9.6. Operating under microprocessor control, images are captured by a CCD (charge-coupled device) image sensor, processed, and converted to digital format. The digital image is temporarily stored in the frame buffer while it is being processed. The digital image processing block performs several functions: It first compresses a newly captured image and sends it to the on-board image storage. Later, under user control, it retrieves compressed images from image storage and decompresses them. The reconstructed images can be routed to computers via the digital output function and (depending on the camera design) to the camera's LCD screen, a television receiver, or a VCR via the analog output function.

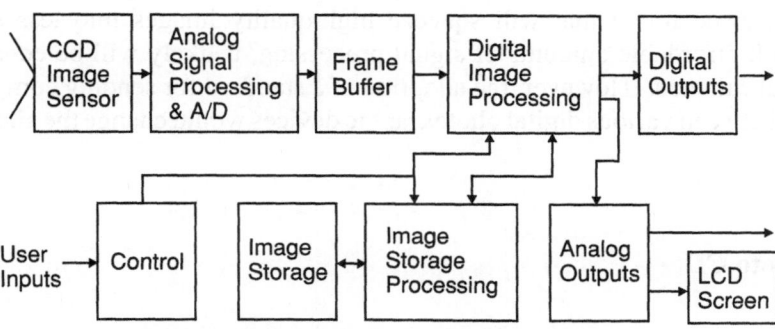

Figure 9.6 Digital camera block diagram.

Data compression provided the breakthrough needed for making totally digital electronic cameras feasible because, for portability, the camera must store up to 100 images. Reducing the amount of on-board storage is crucial, in that storage capacity largely determines how bulky and power hungry—and expensive—the camera will be. (The amount of on-board storage also contributes to setting limits on the allowable resolution, but this is largely controlled by the size and expense of the CCD array.) Compressing huge image files into smaller and smaller storage space allows using compact magnetic or solid-state storage media, either removable or fixed within the camera body. Today's high-end digital cameras use removable, large-capacity PCMCIA-format (credit-card-size) hard disk cards or flash memory cards. (See Section 6.6.) Less pricy models must make do with smaller amounts of nonremovable flash memory with removable, compact-format flash memory cards being an extra-cost option.

JPEG is now an accepted compression method for digital cameras. Simpler compression algorithms were used in early digital cameras—not because JPEG was unknown or unavailable—but for a quite different reason [With92]. One constraint in digital cameras is the size and power consumption of the electronics, which must be battery powered. Therefore, the adoption of JPEG was delayed until small-size, power-efficient integrated circuits for its implementation became available. Compression ratios are typically 15:1 (or less) as indicated in Table 9.4.

Digital cameras are still-evolving products, sitting on the leading edges of several technology curves. Their success is most assuredly linked to higher-resolution and lower-cost CCD arrays, more compact and higher capacity storage, increased VLSI processing speed with lower power consumption, and better data compression. Marketplace demands for increased resolution at lower cost will continue to drive digital camera design. Whereas advances in CCD array technology define the front-end (image capture) function and cost, data compression essentially defines the back-end (image storage) function and cost. JPEG may now be the best possible image compression method, but one should not rule out other techniques. Being a closed process (see Section 3.4), there is no real requirement that standardized data compression be used in digital cameras. If a method can be found that will squeeze high-quality images into less storage space with affordable amounts of signal processing, it likely will be considered for digital cameras. (However, the adoption of a standard for sending compressed pictures between various digital photographic devices would change the situation.)

9.9   Photo CD

Although digital cameras may be priced out of the reach of amateur photographers, with the Photo CD system everyone can experience the advantages of electronic imaging using their existing 35-mm cameras. The Photo CD system was jointly developed by Kodak™ and Philips. It allows photographers to simply take an undeveloped or developed roll of 35-mm film to a photofinisher who, by using a special imaging workstation, can transfer their photos in digital form onto a write-once CD-ROM. Each disc can hold over 100 images and may be updated, so new photos can be added to a partially filled disc. In 1992, Kodak began marketing consumer and professional Photo CD products that allow stored digital images to be displayed on television receivers or computer monitors or to be printed by photofinishers. Consumers can load the discs into a specially modified CD player and view high-quality images on conventional television receivers. The consumer Photo CD player might be thought of as a digital replacement for the slide projector—one that allows viewers to sequence through the pictures in any order, to do fades, dissolves, and wipes, and to rotate, enlarge, and crop images during viewing. Whether a technology ahead of its time or whether consumers (who like the author) have relegated their 35-mm slides and slide projectors to the storage closet in favor of prints, the Photo CD player has not yet captured much attention in the consumer market.

Other uses for Photo CD are doing much better. Many consumers and professionals are into desktop publishing. Using a personal computer equipped with a CD-

ROM XA[4] compatible drive, and Photo CD software, which is now a part of even modestly priced desktop publishing packages, they can view their photographs and include them in documents. Another option, called Photo CD Portfolio II, which has a more professional orientation, allows 35-mm photographs to be combined with audio, text, and computer-generated graphics on a single disc [ElTi92, Seyb95A]. Whether to liven up a slide presentation, develop a multilanguage tutorial, or produce photo-filled publications, authors can create high-quality audio/visual discs, either by sending their material to a professional lab or by using a disk writer attached to their computer. The resulting disc may be played on personal computers, the Kodak Photo CD player, or CD-based multimedia gear such as the Philips CD-I™ player.[5] Prints may also be made from the images stored on disc. In addition, professional versions of the Photo CD support applications such as storing images captured on 4 × 5-inch film and storing X-ray images captured by medical imaging modalities.

Let us explore the role data compression plays in the consumer Photo CD system. To capture 35-mm images, the Photo CD process begins by scanning each image at 3072 × 2048 pixels with 24-bit color. This provides the high-quality digital images needed for printing; it also produces a lot of data—nearly 19 MB for each image! If uncompressed, only 30-some images could be stored on a CD, far short of what a typical slide projector tray contains. Kodak and Philips engineers may or may not have had this comparison in mind when they designed the Photo CD system, but write-once optical discs are quite expensive, and packing more images on each disc makes the concept more attractive. Also, reading an uncompressed image from a CD would be a slow process—requiring about 30 seconds even with a 4X-speed CD-ROM player. Consumers would surely grow impatient while waiting for their favorite vacation slide to be painted on the television screen, and desktop computer users trying to scan through picture libraries could not tolerate this rate. Then, too, the resolution of conventional television receivers and computer displays is far lower than the Photo CD scanning resolution, so much of this data is not needed for display purposes. Obviously (we say with confidence), data compression is the answer, but what type?

The solution chosen for Photo CD is a multiresolution technology that loads the disc with an Image Pac™ file containing compressed images stored at *five* different resolutions.[6] This range of image sizes is intended to make the Photo CD system more useful to consumers and professional users alike. As Table

---

[4] CD-ROM XA is an extended CD-ROM format that provides the ability to interleave sound, images, and text on the same disc.

[5] The Philips CD-I player and other interactive multimedia set-top boxes are discussed in Section 9.10.

[6] A sixth format, scanned at 6144 × 4096 pixels with 24-bit color, and not included on the consumer Photo CD disc, is available for professional applications using 4 × 5-inch or other large-format film [ElTi92, Koda94].

9.5 shows, each image resolution is intended for a different application and, interestingly, differing compression techniques are used to support these applications. Photo CD image coding and compression operate as follows: To code an image, the Photo CD process always begins with a positive image (i.e., negatives are converted to positive images). Through a series of transformations, the digital image is represented in a special PhotoYCC™ (luminance, chrominance, chrominance) color component format. This format differs from standard digital television YC_BC_R coding in that it uses primary RGB color values which preserve the extended dynamic range of film images, supporting both printing and video display [Rich91, Koda94].

Table 9.5   Photo CD image resolutions.

Image Component	Image Resolution	Application
Base/16	192 x 128	Thumbnail index images
Base/4	384 x 256	¼ SDTV
Base	768 x 512	SDTV
4Base	1536 x 1024	HDTV, Small prints
16Base	3072 x 2048	Hardcopy prints (≤ 16-in. x 20-in.)

Compression for the three lowest-resolution images consists of no more than subsampling the chrominance components by a factor of 2 in each direction. This technique, which is commonly used in image and video compression, provides a 2:1 compression with little, if any, visible loss of image quality. This method was chosen because the three lower-resolution images represent only a small fraction of the total data and because it allows these images to be quickly made available for viewing. For example, consumers who view photographs on television receivers or desktop publishers who use tools such as small thumbnail images for scanning image libraries can do so with simple hardware or software and without waiting for images to be decompressed.

To fit over 100 images on a single disc, all five different resolutions must fit into about 6 MB of storage. By itself, chrominance subsampling cannot sufficiently compress the two higher-resolution images to achieve this goal.[7] This means these images must be further compressed, and, to do so, a pyramid coding technique is used. Because this coding method has not been encountered previously, let us take a few moments to understand what it does.

---

[7] A detail of the Photo CD process is that the 16Base image is chrominance subsampled, but the 4Base image is not [Koda94].

When a set of successively smaller images is created by "downsampling" (low-pass filtering and subsampling) the preceding larger image in the set and these images are conceptually stacked one atop the other, they form a pyramid like the one shown in Figure 9.7. This method is also known as hierarchical coding (the stack forms a hierarchy of images) because the image is coded in a way that allows it to be used at different quality levels or resolutions. It is also a form of progressive coding, yet another term used to describe this technique [Penn93]. A progressive encoder is one that successively scans an image with each scan producing finer and finer detail. This allows the image to be progressively transmitted to a receiver in stages; at first, a low-resolution image is sent, followed by more detailed information that allows higher and higher resolution images to be reconstructed [Rabb91]. This approach is useful for operating across a slow network, where users can work online with a lower-resolution version of an image, downloading a higher-resolution version only when necessary. The same is true for Photo CD users who must retrieve images from relatively slow CD-ROM drives.

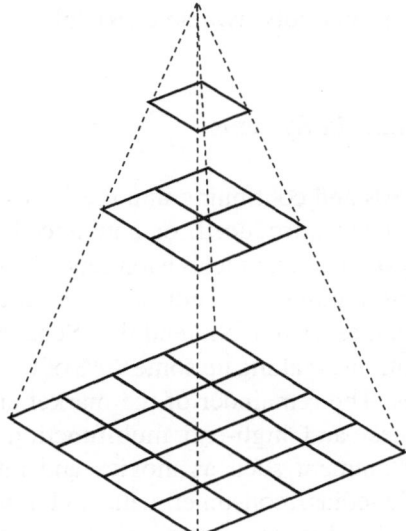

Figure 9.7 Pyramidal multiresolution coding.

The pyramid coding process begins with the original image that is low-pass filtered and subsampled, usually by a factor of 2 in each direction. This creates the first reduced-resolution image. Then that image is downsampled to produce the next image. This continues until the lowest-resolution image in the pyramid is formed. The actual compression process begins with the lowest resolution image that is upsampled (scaled up) to the next higher resolution and subtracted from the next higher resolution image to get a difference image. The difference image is then encoded (compressed) using an appropriate image compression method (such as JPEG's DCT, quantization, and entropy coding techniques).

This operation continues until all higher-resolution images in the pyramid have been coded.

As previously stated, pyramid coding is used for storing only the two highest-resolution Photo CD images. These images contain the bulk of the total data, but, because (today) they are not used for television display, they do not have the same "real-time" decoding requirements as do lower-resolution images. Therefore, more complexity and longer decoding times are acceptable. Reconstructing the 1536×1024-pixel 4Base image involves the following: The compressed 4Base difference image is retrieved from storage and decompressed. The 768×512-pixel Base image is retrieved and upsampled to 1536×1024 pixels. These two images are added, pixel by pixel, to obtain the full 1536×1024-pixel image. Essentially the same steps are followed to reconstruct the 3072×2048-pixel image, using both the 4Base and 16Base difference images.

As to the exact compression method used for storing the difference images, it is not JPEG. At the time the Photo CD system was being developed, the JPEG specification was still being drafted. Kodak engineers chose, instead, to develop an algorithm based on quantization and variable length Huffman coding. Being proprietary, few details are publicly available [Rich91, Koda94].[8]

9.10   Interactive Multimedia Systems

Beginning in the mid-1980s and continuing into the 1990s, a multitude of intelligent set-top boxes have been introduced, or announced, all aimed at building interactive multimedia systems around television sets. These products are primarily intended for home entertainment and education but are found in schools and businesses too. Video games (from Nintendo™, Sega™, and others) are the leading consumer applications, making up some 90% of the market for interactive, multimedia set-top boxes. The remainder of the market encompasses Photo CD players, karaoke machines, and high-end multifunction boxes. In-home uses include interactive entertainment such as movies and music videos, reference material such as encyclopedias, consumer data and transactions, educational software, and more. School and business uses include education, training, interact-

---

[8] However, JPEG is the compression method chosen for the FlashPix™ digital photo file format recently developed by Kodak [Cost96, Koda96]. Whereas Photo CD is intended for storing and archiving digital images, FlashPix is designed for sharing them on computers and across networks. It allows images to be stored at multiple resolutions, similar to Photo CD, and in either RGB or Photo YCC color component format. A unique feature of FlashPix is that the original image is divided into tiles, each containing 64×64 pixels. For lower resolution images, adjacent tiles are combined, with the smallest image consisting of only one 64×64 pixel tile. JPEG compression is an option. Each tile is compressed independently, which does not result in the most efficient compression, but has the advantage that individual tiles may be decompressed to access, display, or print part of the image.

ive kiosks, and other business-oriented multimedia-based applications. Multimedia data types include text, speech, audio, graphics, animation, still images, and motion-video.

Today's consumer multimedia systems are stand-alone players that range in price from less than $100 to somewhat more than $500. These price points— for products that are essentially computers without keyboards, displays, and hard files—are far lower than any multimedia home computer.[9] Low prices are achieved by using a television set for video and still-image display and for audio playback, and by using low-cost storage media. Some consumer multimedia systems store information in ROM cartridges, but, increasingly, the chosen storage media is CD-ROM, and future products will likely use DVD. These systems are interactive, allowing the viewer to control what is seen and heard with simple hand-held controllers for games or TV-like remote controls for higher-function players. Future interactive multimedia set-top boxes are likely to go online; at least that is what cable television, telco networks, and others (see Chapter 8) are planning as they eagerly eye the opportunities for interactive multimedia.

The marketplace reception for these products is decidedly mixed. Millions of videogame machines have been sold, whereas other products that can do more than play games face stiff competition and have not done as well. Today, the territory staked out by high-end stand-alone multimedia players has largely been overrun by multimedia PCs which, despite the difference in price, both consumers and businesses are turning to for multimedia entertainment and education applications. Part of the reason is many advanced interactive multimedia applications really require a keyboard, not a TV remote, to control them. Then, too, PCs are increasingly becoming capable multimedia platforms. Although no one will mistake a multimedia PC for an arcade-quality videogame machine, PCs are getting much better at running games, and they run almost all the applications for which high-end stand-alone multimedia players were created. Other advantages are that PCs allow more creative uses of multimedia and PCs can be connected to online information services to find more of it. Another factor favoring PCs is that a far broader range of multimedia applications is available for either IBM-compatible or Apple computers than for any one high-end stand-alone multimedia player. Largely incompatible products, these stand-alone multimedia players observe no interchange standards (except audio CDs, and perhaps Photo CDs, but definitely not the contents of CD-ROMs). This places stand-alone multimedia players at a disadvantage because software developers prefer "open" architecture PCs, of which there are only two targets, to proprietary architecture stand-alone multimedia players, of which there are many. Software developers may be easily enticed to videogame machines, which have huge distributions, but not to limited-distribution, high-end stand-alone multimedia players.

---

[9] The price of PCs, although still much greater than $500, is dropping. The $500 PC continues to be a target of the computer industry, but that is another (long) story.

Historically, interactive multimedia set-top boxes have been trendsetters, being the first to introduce new, innovative multimedia technologies for consumer and business applications. These products use high-performance 16-, 32-, and 64-bit VLSI including RISC processors, DSPs, 3-D graphics accelerators, and data decompressors. They were first with leading-edge features such as video on CD-ROMs and 3-D graphics—technologies that later migrated to multimedia PCs. Figure 9.8 shows the components to be found in an interactive multimedia set-top box. This hypothetical high-end system is organized around a shared bus and an RISC processor executing a real-time operating system that controls the operation of several specialized coprocessors and dedicated functional units. Lesser set-top products will not include all these components, but a challenge for all interactive multimedia set-top boxes, beginning with the very first and continuing to the present generation, is to include enough high-performance audiovisual elements to attract consumers and, yet, maintain a reasonable price.[10] An essential part of this effort is the processing and decompression of audio, image, and, particularly, video data.

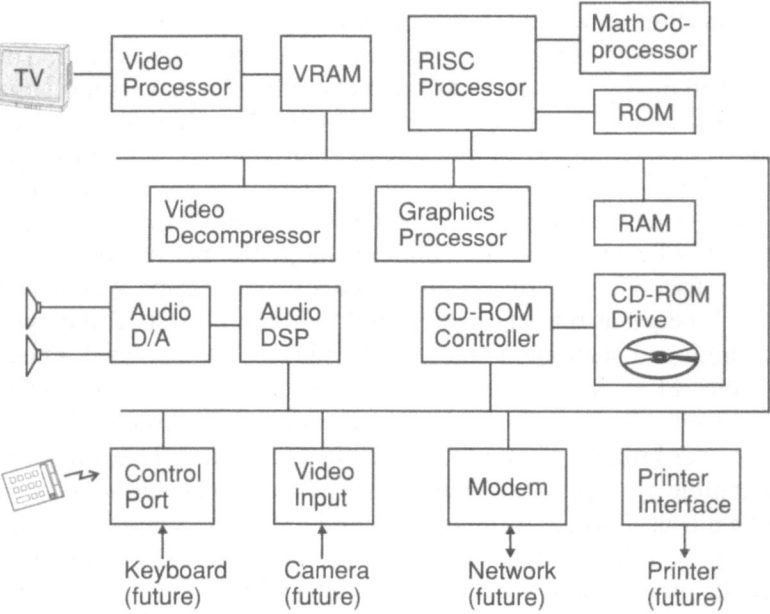

Figure 9.8   Interactive multimedia system.

For audio, the major challenge existing interactive multimedia players face is providing different levels of quality for various applications. For instance, the Philips CD-I (Compact Disc -Interactive) player, an early high-end entry in this

---

[10] A recent trend is to add keyboards, modems, and printer interfaces to interactive multimedia set-top boxes, equipping them to be Internet browsers [Gros95].

field, offers four audio quality levels ranging from 16-bit PCM-coded CD-quality stereo to 4-bit ADPCM-coded speech-quality audio [Luth91, Mcco94A]. Future interactive multimedia products will be called on to handle Dolby AC-3 format compressed audio and, for game-oriented applications, 3-D interactive audio [Yosh95A]. A DSP (digital signal processor) is an economical solution for processing audio because it can be programmed for differing coding formats and decompression techniques.

Still images are relatively easy to deal with—that is, in comparison to video. Nowadays, most high-end set-top boxes have the bandwidth and processing power needed for video—and, therefore, for images too. The major challenge that images present, beyond handling differing image-encoding formats, is fetching them from the CD-ROM and displaying them quickly. The still images that interactive multimedia players must handle do not contain all that much data, even when stored in uncompressed format. Images containing about 720×480 pixels at 12 bits per pixel, or less, are all that is needed for television display. Therefore, they may be retrieved and moved through the system relatively quickly. Often the performance issue is not the CD-ROM speed, or the system bandwidth, but, rather, the processing time for decompressing compressed images. There are several solutions: One is to just avoid the problem and store uncompressed images, as does the Photo CD system described in Section 9.9. For approaches that begin with compressed images, the question is what format to use and how to quickly decompress an image. Early interactive multimedia players, such as the Philips CD-I announced in 1985, chose to store still images in (proprietary) formats that could be decompressed by the on-board video decompression hardware running in single-frame mode [Meer92]. Now, there are other choices. One is to use JPEG compression and a dedicated JPEG coprocessor, although, JPEG has yet to establish itself in this market. A more economical solution is to do decompression (JPEG or otherwise) in software running on the RISC processor; today's RISC processors are powerful enough to make software decompression acceptable for many image-based applications.

Video was and still is the most demanding of all digital multimedia data types. The first generation of interactive multimedia set-top boxes, designed in the mid-1980s when digital video for consumer electronics was definitely leading-edge (some wags would say bleeding-edge) technology, had limited video capability. Designers were constrained by CD-ROM storage capacity limitations, by the cost (and availability) of decompression hardware, and by not having effective decompression algorithms that would run on this hardware. Increasing CD-ROM storage capacity was not an option. So, instead, they concentrated on data compression techniques that would squeeze video into ever-smaller amounts of storage and that would allow it to be decompressed with the available hardware. What resulted was a bevy of proprietary compression algorithms that, to put it charitably, produced video of less than broadcast quality. Partial-screen video, low-to-medium resolution, limited color depth, and substandard frame rates were the norms. Consumers were not impressed.

The second generation of interactive multimedia products, at least second generation in video capability, began to take shape in the in the 1991-1993 time frame. An effort led by Philips and JVC produced the Video CD standard, initially for karaoke systems that show moving pictures and lyrics, and since adopted for a variety of set-top boxes and multimedia PCs. (See the Video CD discussion in Section 9.6.) The Video CD uses MPEG-1 compression, and, thanks to advances in VLSI, single-chip decoders are available and affordable to interactive multimedia set-top boxes. The result is these products deliver full-screen, medium-resolution (352 × 240 pixels) video with full color depth at 30 fps.

The next generation of interactive multimedia set-top boxes, still on the drawing boards but likely to reach the marketplace by 1997, can be expected to offer even higher-quality video. Industry observers expect these products to be based on the DVD[11] [Krau95B]. This means increased storage capacity will be available for all types of multimedia, video included. Also, by leveraging the low-cost MPEG-2 decompression chips that DVD players will use, interactive multimedia set-top boxes will deliver full-screen, high-resolution video (up to 720 × 480 pixels) with full color depth at 30 fps.

9.11 Multimedia PCs

Nearly all home personal computers and many intended for businesses carry the Multimedia PC (MPC) trademark. This means they include CD-ROM drives, sound cards, speakers, microphones, data compression features, and more.[12] Multimedia PCs are all-purpose tools for entertainment, education, and business. Not surprisingly, in 1995 they accounted for nearly 40% of sales by large electronics retailers, and by 1997 nearly 50% of U.S. homes are expected to have at least one PC [Mcwi95]. In Chapter 2, we began to learn of the problems that all computers face in delivering interactive multimedia, and in Chapter 6, we learned of the progress that mobile and desktop computer designers have made in addressing this challenge; that is, by surrounding the basic PC with the trappings of multimedia, and by improving the internals—adding storage capacity, bandwidth, CPU power, VLSI for graphics and compression, and better software for real-time processing—and by improving the externals—higher-resolution monitors and connections to higher bandwidth networks—PCs are becoming creditable multimedia machines.

Turning the humble PC into a bold multimedia warrior has not been easy. Finding the right strategy for handling compressed multimedia data has proven

---

[11] One observation is that essentially the same VLSI components are needed to build advanced game-playing systems and DVD players.

[12] The MPC trademark is administered by the Multimedia PC Marketing Council, an industry group that maintains an ever-changing standard which defines minimum requirements for multimedia PCs [MBR95].

a most difficult task, a struggle that is still in progress. When multimedia PCs handle speech, audio, image, and video data, they face all the same limitations encountered by interactive multimedia set-top boxes (storage capacity, processing speed, and bandwidth)—and more! The reason is PCs must deal with a far wider range of multimedia applications including the following:

- Interactive multimedia playback from CD-ROM
- Multimedia serving and interactive applications from hard disk storage
- Networked multimedia applications
- Desktop multimedia production and authoring applications
- Desktop videoconferencing
- Analog television audio and video capture, digitization, and display

In fact, some people both outside the computer industry and insiders (who should be more realistic) expect PCs to do no less than flawlessly run every multimedia application that anyone could program. This blissful state of affairs has not been reached yet, in part, because effective, universal data compression technology still eludes PC system designers.

Our study of data compression in multimedia computers will focus, as has the PC industry, on video compression. Handling speech and audio is straightforward, with the electronics reduced to a single chip on the motherboard of most PCs [Wils95E]. However, as will soon be evident, coordinating audio and video is a challenge. Also, compressed multichannel audio has yet to appear in PCs, so there still may be some lessons to be learned. As to images, handling images has scarcely raised a blip on any PC designer's radar screen; software has proven adequate. PCs have sufficient processing power to manipulate images stored in JPEG, Photo CD, or any other miscellaneous image format, and images have no real-time processing requirements. Although, today's image processing activities mostly involve decompression, display, and simple editing tasks (cropping, scaling, and rotation), so the requirements may change if future applications demand more complex image processing. Handling video (with synchronized audio) is not so easy.

The problem with video on PCs, other than the high data rates, is no one representation of digital video or no one compression method is right for all applications. Over the years, the PC industry has produced a gaggle of video compression algorithms, mostly executed in software, mostly proprietary, and primarily intended for video playback. In 1995, with the adoption of the MPC Level 3 specification, MPEG-1 decompression became a standard feature for multimedia computers [MBR95]. Most observers concede that for full-screen, full-rate video playback MPEG-1 produces unquestionably better results than any of the proprietary algorithms.[13] However, when MPEG-1 encodes data in

---

[13] The accepted standard for full-screen, full-rate PC video is 640 × 480 pixels at 30 fps.

its most compact format, it is essentially unusable for multimedia authoring applications where frame-by-frame access is required. For videoconferencing, even with full hardware implementation, none of the video playback algorithms—the proprietary algorithms or MPEG-1—are ideal. Therefore, multiple different PC video compression (and decompression) algorithms are needed to cover the range of PC video applications.

Video requirements for multimedia PCs

Which video compression algorithms are right for multimedia PCs and what makes them right? Video coders and decoders (codecs) are traditionally judged by the image quality they produce and how effectively they compress video to meet storage and bandwidth limitations. Video codecs for multimedia PCs must also be measured by the resources needed for compressing and decompressing video data, by their suitability for the intended applications, and by their support for PC graphics displays. All these criteria interact, and, often, the term "scalability" is used to describe the merits of a video codec. Codecs that can cover a wide range in any one or more of these criteria are said to be scalable. Let us examine more closely what scalability really means for multimedia PC video compression.

The first element is computation load. Any compression or decompression algorithm can be run in software—in theory. Practically speaking, some algorithms do require hardware, but discount that for the moment. Successful software video compression and decompression algorithms are those that produce quality images and leave resources available to run the application(s). They do not consume too many CPU cycles, nor do they consume too much memory, and they produce compact data representations that PC displays can handle. Software-only algorithms that rely exclusively on the PC's CPU to do video decompression must be designed to avoid its limitations: To accommodate base-level PCs, integer arithmetic is favored over floating-point arithmetic. To simplify and speed up the decoding task, because CPUs are better at manipulating data in a multiplicity of bytes, a byte-oriented video stream syntax is used by many software-only algorithms. Unfortunately, it results in loss of storage efficiency when compared to the typical compressed bit stream definitions employed for communications-oriented video applications, because it prohibits applying lossless variable-length coding at the tail end.

To date, software-only algorithms have proven nearly useless for broadcast-quality work. They do not offer real-time encoding, thus excluding video production applications. They do offer low-complexity, scalable video playback, but often at the expense of image quality. Reduced image spatial resolution, aggressive color subsampling, reduced pixel depth, and reduced frame rates or dropped frames are compromises made by software-only PC video (de)compression algorithms in the name of reduced computation work load. When these trade-offs are not acceptable, compression hardware, hardware assists for software-only algorithms, or better algorithms are required.

That brings us to the second element, the applications. For multimedia playback, whether done in software or hardware, ease of decoding is the most important issue, as a multimedia CD-ROM that can be played on low-cost PCs without expensive video features has the greatest sales potential. For other applications, those where both encoding and decoding must be done on the multimedia PC, different codec criteria apply. In multimedia production and authoring, where editing is required, it is important that the coder produce a data stream that supports frame-by-frame access. This means interframe coding, which can produce the highest compression ratios, is not a wise choice. For videoconferencing, as learned in Chapter 5, it is important that the encoding and decoding time be symmetrical and the time delays for either be low and well controlled. Techniques that can be executed in real time, such as those used by the H.261 algorithm described in Chapter 5, are needed. Table 9.6 summarizes application requirements for PC video codecs.

The third element is support for PC graphics displays. PCs are blessed or cursed with tremendous display flexibility, perhaps similar to future HDTV

Table 9.6 Application requirements for multimedia PC video codecs.

Video Codec Characteristics	Multimedia Playback Applications	Video Production and Authoring Applications	Videoconferencing Applications
Scalable image quality	Trade-off for software-only playback	Trade-off for frame-by-frame access (I-frames only)	Trade-off for communications bandwidth
Scalable compression ratio	Trade-off for minimum storage size or data rate Trade-off for software-only playback	Trade-off for frame-by-frame access	Higher is better
Low memory consumption	Important for low-cost, software-only playback	Important, but high-end PCs are used for these applications	Important for low-cost, hardware-assisted codecs
Simple decode (playback speed)	Software-only decode for low-cost applications	Desirable	Hardware
Simple encode (asymmetry)	—	Desirable but not required	Hardware
Editability (frame by frame)	Some applications require frame-by-frame playback	Required	—
Low delay (real-time video)	—	—	Required

receivers. In conventional television receivers, a single color representation scheme, a single spatial resolution, and a fixed frame rate apply, but all these parameters can vary for PC displays and all interact with PC video compression. PC displays use an RGB color system, different from YC_BC_R or any broadcast video representation. Furthermore, there are various RGB formats; the highest-quality representations use 24 bits for each pixel, but 16-bit, 8-bit, and even 4-bit color is available to PC applications. It should come as no surprise that the software-only algorithms created by the PC industry tap this capability as a simple form of video compression [Luth91]. (Some would say data reduction, but we will call it compression.)

PC displays are driven with 24-bit RGB color. So, as Figure 9.9 shows, color format conversion is necessary when the video compression algorithm uses another encoding. The simplest conversion is upscaling 16-bit RGB color, restoring the low-order bits truncated during the compression process. (Typical 16-bit RGB color formats encode each color component in 5 bits, leaving 1

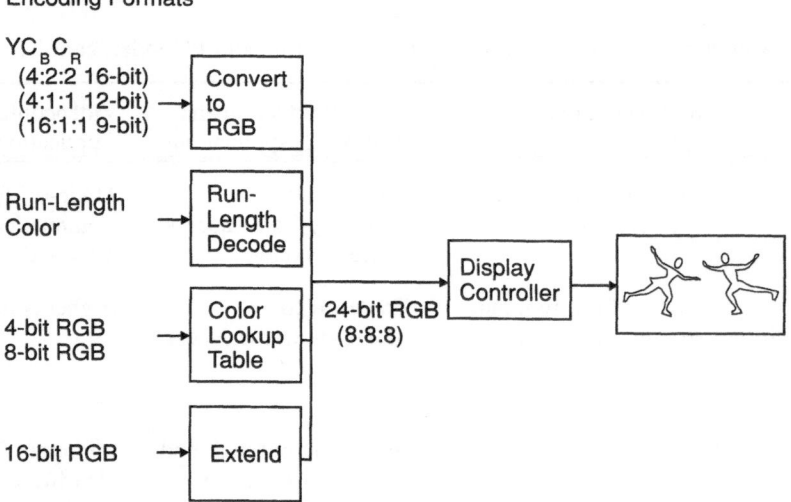

Figure 9.9   PC color format conversion.

bit unused.) Although 16-bit color produces realistic images, it affords little compression; consequently, some algorithms use 8-bit or even 4-bit color. These encodings are converted by accessing a color-lookup table that contains the 24-bit equivalent for each 8-bit or 4-bit pixel value. The color-lookup table is created during encoding, a process which can grow quite complex if the color-lookup table is dynamically changed to track color changes. Neither 8-bit nor 4-bit color can deal with color shading in complex scenes; so, these formats are best reserved for simple computer-generated images and animations where only a few colors are needed. The same is true for run-length color, the third encoding format shown in Figure 9.9. The idea here is to compactly represent runs of like-colored pixels, again, an idea that works well for computer-generated images and animations where large areas contain the same color. For complex images, YC_BC_R or some other form of luminance-chrominance representation provides greater compression because the chrominance components can be subsampled. The advantage of a luminance-chrominance format is, besides producing better color quality in full-motion images, that it uses less bandwidth and memory than any of the RGB schemes. Some software-only PC compression algorithms aggressively subsample the chrominance components to drive down bandwidth and memory to the lowest possible values. Using 4×4 blocks of pixels, they create, in effect, a 9-bits-per-pixel representation. Other PC video compression algorithms conform to less drastic subsampling strategies, the ones found in communications applications. In any event, video encoded in a luminance-chrominance format usually is not converted into RGB format until needed for display. The conversion process proves to be straightforward, using well-known color-space transformations [Penn93] and is implemented in modern PC display controllers [Cole94].

Another aspect of displaying video on PCs is scaling the image size. One might argue this has nothing to do with video compression, but there is a close connection, and some compression algorithms are better able to support image-size scaling than others. Algorithms that provide data at multiple resolutions, somewhat like the multiresolution technique used by the Photo CD system (although its TV-displayable images are not compressed), make image-size scaling easier. However, practically speaking, no compression algorithm could provide all the image sizes needed for PCs, so display scaling techniques still must be applied.

Here is what must be done to scale image size: Figure 9.10 shows a decoded but unscaled MPEG-1 video image as it might appear on a VGA-resolution or

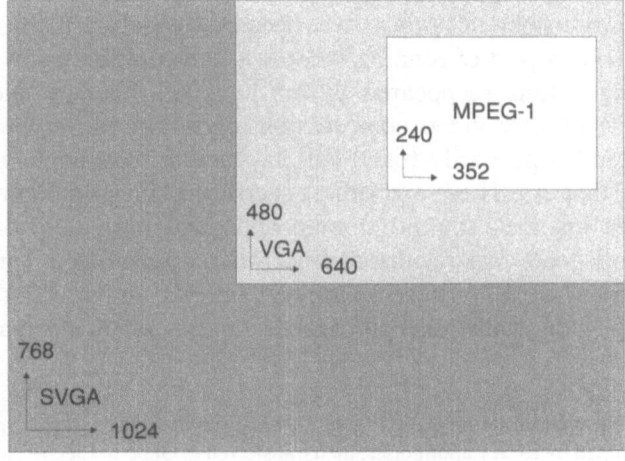

Figure 9.10   PC display screen.

SVGA-resolution PC screen.[14] The MPEG-1 video window may be positioned anywhere on the screen. The unscaled window occupies about one-fourth of the VGA-resolution screen but would occupy a much smaller fraction of the SVGA-resolution screen. To control the window size, making it either larger or smaller, each pixel in the MPEG-1 image must be scaled. Making the window smaller is the least difficult. To do so, rows and columns of pixels within the MPEG-1 image may simply be dropped (decimated); or, for better image quality, each pixel in the smaller image may be created by averaging neighboring pixels in the original image. Making the window larger requires more care because the results will be more visible. One might simply replicate pixels in two dimensions, but the scaled-up image is likely to be blocky, exhibiting a type of artifact known as pixellation. Pixel interpolation provides a better solution in that each pixel in the scaled-up image is created by applying a color smoothing or dithering algorithm to pixels in the original MPEG-1 image [Netr95].

PC video software compression

For many years, highly influential hardware and software forces within the PC industry have promoted the idea that video compression should be run in software, just as are other processing tasks. Advocates for software video compression cite it as the only sensible choice for an era when the algorithms and the applications themselves continue to evolve, and no standard algorithm(s) exists that can be safely committed to hardware. Software video compression, they argue, allows PC costs to be kept low and a variety of algorithms to be run in support of all video-oriented applications.

Historically, PC video compression software owes much to DVI™ (Digital Video Interactive), a pioneering technology effort that in 1986 demonstrated full-motion video running on PCs[15] [Luth91]. DVI technology included video software compression algorithms that ran on a programmable coprocessor. (Recall that the 1980s PC processors were way underpowered for video, or anything but text processing.) More robust PC processors became available in the early 1990s, which offered the prospect of running video without coprocessor assistance. The DVI-inspired algorithms reappeared under the Indeo™ name and were soon joined by a slew of new video compression algorithms developed by the PC industry, all intended primarily for video playback at reasonable speeds on the low-cost PCs of that era. These algorithms sacrificed video quality and compression (i.e., increasing the required storage and data rate) in favor of reduced computation work load. The results, at least when applied to full-motion video, were disappointing—small postage-stamp-size images, and often jerky, questionable quality color video with unsynchronized sound, or no sound at all. Typically,

---

[14] MPEG-1 is used to illustrate display scaling. Other algorithms have similar requirements.

[15] DVI was developed by RCA Laboratories, then transferred to General Electric, and subsequently sold to Intel.

the best of this generation of software video algorithms delivered 320 × 240 resolution pictures at 15 fps on a dedicated Intel i486™, values that scale with processor speed [Wolf93A, Rodr94]. However, most applications using these algorithms were forced to make do with much lower resolutions and frame rates, being constrained by storage size and data rate and by being unable to dedicate all the processor resources to video decompression. Nevertheless, the novelty of seeing video on a PC screen had a tremendous impact on everyone. A whole generation of CD-ROM multimedia playback applications for PCs and game machines was built on these algorithms, applications where less than broadcast-quality video met with some degree of consumer acceptance.

Table 9.7 lists some of many PC software video algorithms created during this era. Although primarily applied to video playback, all these software algorithms also can compress video but do so very slowly on standard PCs. However,

Table 9.7   Examples of proprietary PC software video algorithms.

Codec Manufacturer	Compression Technique	Coding Methods	Data Rate Control Method
Captain Crunch™ Media Vision Inc.	Wavelet transform subband	Intraframe	—
Cell™ Sun Microsystems Inc.	Vector quantization	Intraframe Interframe	—
Cinepak™ SuperMac Technologies (acquired by Radius Inc.)	Vector quantization	Intraframe Interframe	Quality-level scaling
Fractal Video Pro™ Iterated Systems Inc.	Fractal transform	—	—
Indeo™ 4.0 Intel Corp.	Vector quantization	Intraframe Interframe	Frame dropping
Indeo 4.1 Video Interactive Intel Corp.	Wavelet transform subband	Intraframe Interframe	Quality-level scaling & frame dropping
TrueMotion-S™ Horizon Technologies and Duck Corp.	Non-DCT transform subband Arithmetic coding	Intraframe	Quality-level scaling
Video 1™ Microsoft Corp. (developed by Media Vision)	Vector quantization (motive)	Intraframe Interframe	—

essentially all manufacturers back them with hardware cards that provide real-time compression (and decompression) for applications such as authoring and videoconferencing. All these algorithms are considered proprietary by their manufacturers, so public information about their inner workings is limited (as blank entries in Table 9.7 suggest). Their external operating characteristics are well known, nevertheless, having been subjected to extensive field testing. As a class, many observers judge them to provide about the same overall picture quality, but there are measurable differences [Ozer94, Brya95, Ozer95A]. For example, some are better at handling complexities such as scene-to-scene transitions, and some achieve higher compression ratios (i.e., smaller storage sizes and lower data rates) than others. The picture quality of these software algorithms is often said to be much lower than what hardware-assisted codecs like MPEG can provide. But, in fairness, the observed results depend greatly on the PCs on which they run, and the best of these algorithms can deliver full-screen, 30-fps performance on modern PCs [Ozer95B].

The software environment for desktop multimedia application development is built upon tools such as Apple QuickTime™ and Microsoft Video For Windows™ [Hoff92, Beer93, Pere95]. These operating system extensions allow developers to perform operations such as video capture, editing, and compression and to create data files that contain integrated audio and video. They support many of the software algorithms listed in Table 9.7 and various adaptions of M-JPEG, MPEG, and other standard video compression algorithms available in software and hardware. This dizzying array of algorithms presents multimedia application developers with a problem; namely, which algorithm should they choose? Circa 1995, Indeo 4.0, Cinepak, and TrueMotion-S are ascribed to be among the most widely used [Somo95, Turl95], but other algorithms dominate application niches. For instance, fractal compression is the leader for CD-ROM encyclopedias. Some of these algorithms also have been used for videoconferencing (with hardware assistance). For a time, Intel promoted Indeo 4.0 as a standard for PC videoconferencing but, bowing to compatibility, in 1995 endorsed H.320, an international standard for videoconferencing. Any algorithm that uses only intraframe coding is a clear-cut choice for video editing. Interframe coding *may* provide more compression (and this depends on many factors), but intraframe-only coding allows frame-by-frame access. Also, sometimes intraframe-only video algorithms are applied to still-image applications.

By 1993, it was painfully evident that PC video compression was in disarray. With multimedia software vendor loyalties split among many choices, not one of the proprietary algorithms listed in Table 9.7 (or any other algorithm) could claim to be a clear industry leader. Then, too, the compromises in picture quality and data rate that all the software-only algorithms made to reduce the computation burden on base-level PCs were regrettably apparent. Application developers, and the PC industry too, knew that PC video needed to be improved—quickly! PC users were soon to be (or were being) exposed to other home entertainment products that offered higher-quality digital video. It was simply a matter of time before they would walk away from multimedia PCs that delivered less.

What was needed was a "standard" PC video compression algorithm, one that would provide all PC video applications with high-quality video, one that would operate in software on low-cost PCs, not just in hardware on high-end systems. But what should that algorithm be; should it be a new algorithm, or if an existing video algorithm, which one? In the 1993 time frame, various PC industry groups, committees, and consortiums were linked with efforts (or rumors of efforts) to select a standard PC video compression algorithm [Coll93, Wolf93A]. Alas, all those efforts led nowhere, which is not unexpected because they faced an impossible task: No one vendor had the marketplace presence to convince others that its proprietary algorithm should be the standard; and, more telling, no one known algorithm, proprietary or standard, could handle all PC video applications.

Now move the clock forward to 1995 when, as stated earlier, MPEG-1 decompression was included in the MPC Level 3 specification for multimedia computers—in effect, creating the new "standard" PC video algorithm. How did that come about? First, MPEG-1 technology can play back full-screen, full-motion video with much clearer pictures and synchronized sound at low data rates and at a quality level that the proprietary algorithms are hard-pressed to match. The catch is that the DCT-based intraframe coding and sophisticated interframe coding needed to accomplish this are compute intensive, and encoding is even more difficult. Conventional wisdom says MPEG-1 is a hardware-only algorithm, not suitable for low-cost PCs, and is intended for broadcasting (or multimedia playback), not video production or authoring. Between 1993 and 1995, three events occurred that changed conventional wisdom: A new generation of more powerful Pentium™ and PowerPC™ processors hit the marketplace. Becoming the engines for essentially all PCs, they allow MPEG-1 encoded video to be played back at reasonable frame rates in software (but on 100% dedicated processors). Hardware MPEG-1 decoders became affordable for PCs, having been reduced to a single, low-cost chip for widespread deployment in DBS and other consumer applications. Software for MPEG-1 *encoding* (and decoding) was developed that, using only I-frames, allows frame-by-frame access for video editing. The turning point for MPEG-1 that pushed it over the top came in 1995 when Microsoft included MPEG-1 decompression software in Windows 95 and several PC manufacturers introduced MPEG-1 decompression hardware as a standard feature [Turl95].

So, MPEG-1 won out in the multimedia PC video compression standards battle and, finally, there is *a* standard algorithm, right? Not quite. As discussed in Section 7.8, desktop videoconferencing is still a technology in transition, and it remains to be decided what compression algorithm it will use. Reasons were suggested why H.320-compliant H.261 or H.324-compliant H.263 may be winners—namely, they are standards designed specifically for videoconferencing and do have market presence. One would not expect MPEG-1 to be used for videoconferencing (because it is an asymmetric algorithm not designed for low delay time, and so on). Nevertheless, if most future PCs have built-in MPEG-1 decoding hardware, and with the cost for MPEG-1 encoding hardware dropping rapidly, someone will surely try using MPEG-1 for videoconferencing. Stranger things have happened!

Then, too, we must look forward and consider that multimedia PCs will continue to be influenced by other consumer-electronics hardware and applications. One event almost sure to occur is that players for DVDs (see Section 9.6) will be attached to PCs. At some future time, the allure of vastly increased storage capacity and higher data rates will prove irresistible to PC multimedia developers. If they choose to follow entertainment-industry standards, MPEG-2 encoded video and Dolby AC-3 encoded audio must be handled by multimedia PCs. MPEG-1 is hardly the final solution for PC video compression.

PC video hardware compression

PC manufacturers have found many ways to integrate multimedia processing, video compression included. Software-only video compression is one solution, but it is not a problem-free solution; namely a lot of processing muscle is required to decompress video and even more to compress it and dedicating the CPU to video processing may leave insufficient resources for running video together with anything else. More to the point, video processing demands continue to run ahead of CPU growth as visually better but computational more complex video compression algorithms invade the marketplace. Another factor that argues against a software-only solution is that most multimedia video applications demand both audio and video be compressed or decompressed together. Not only must audio and video be synchronized, but audio processing is CPU intensive. Also, audio and video data streams must be continually processed, which is difficult to do in the CPU, given the interrupt-driven nature of the PC. When interrupted, say by an I/O device, the CPU must suspend video processing, or whatever task it is doing, and go off to handle the interrupt. The result is pauses and gaps in audio and video delivery. Finally, a large amount of bandwidth is needed to move uncompressed video around inside the PC. What this means will be examined momentarily, but the end result is that the CPU may be starved for data, leaving it with nothing to compress or decompress, and, thus, interrupting the video (and audio) data stream.

When software-only processing is not enough, specialized hardware can provide the resources needed for processing audio and video. It can assure continuous processing of the data streams and, when properly placed, assure uncompressed video will not overwhelm the PC dataflow. With the aid of Figure 9.11, we will explore several options for placing hardware in the PC dataflow to accelerate audio and video processing. Ideally, to get the most out of data compression—to aggressively reduce storage and bandwidth—video should be compressed in the video subsystem and decompressed in the graphics controller. In this way, video is compressed when captured and remains compressed until needed for

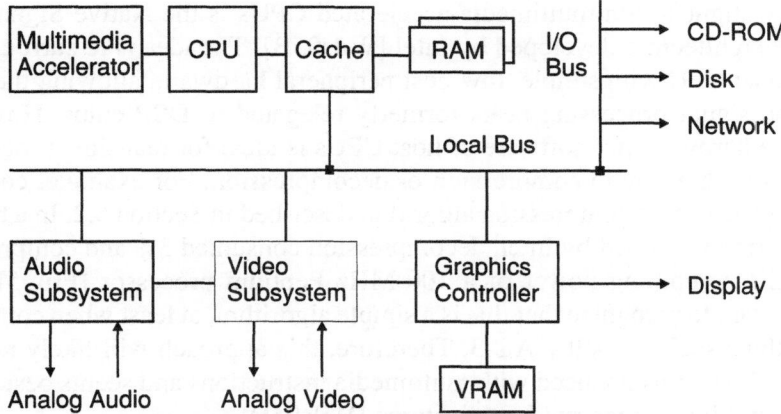

Figure 9.11   Multimedia PC organization.

display. It is always stored in compressed format, and no internal PC data path ever carries uncompressed video. For audio, ideally, both compression and decompression should be placed in the audio subsystem. Audio is compressed as it is captured and remains compressed until sent to the output devices. So much for what is ideal; here is reality:

First, there are multimedia-accelerated CPUs. PC manufacturers and silicon designers have devised several schemes for turning the CPU into a more efficient software engine for graphics, image, audio, and video processing. Included are the following:

- CPU chips that incorporate specialized multimedia instructions. Companies including Intel, Hewlett-Packard, and Sun Microsystems have announced multimedia CPU chips [Wils94A, Lee95, Ocon95, Wolf95B]. The new instructions in these processors comprise core operations needed to more efficiently manipulate pixels and other complex diffuse data. The performance gained by this approach is limited. For any given level of silicon integration, only a certain number of new instructions can be accommodated on-chip, and the CPU dataflow remains attuned to symbolic (text, numbers) data processing.

- Multimedia coprocessor chips. Several semiconductor companies have announced chips which act as companions to the host CPU chip [Clar95, Wils95C, Wils95G, Yosh95G]. These chips handle only multimedia data and are appropriate when the highest levels of performance are needed. They forego conventional dataflows in favor of parallel architectures that promise up to 50 times the performance of conventional CPUs.

- Other approaches that use a combination of chips. The intent is to allow the CPU to take on some multimedia processing tasks while offloading others to achieve lower costs or greater integration for cost-size-power-sensitive products such as notebook computers. One example is MPEG-1 decompression as implemented by IBM Aptiva™ PCs. Video decompression is run in software on the CPU and audio decompression runs in its programmable Mwave™ DSP chip [Ozer95C].

Closely aligned with multimedia-accelerated CPUs is the Native Signal Processing™ architecture developed by Intel [Wils95B]. The idea is to surround the conventional CPU with simple, low-cost peripheral hardware, allowing the CPU to take on signal processing tasks formerly relegated to DSP chips. However, neither the hardware nor software of host CPUs is ideal for real-time processing operations such as audio compression or decompression. For example, consider the Truespeech voice compression algorithm described in Section 5.2. In a benchmark reportedly devised by Intel, decompression consumed 3% and compression 32% of the computing power of a 100-MHz Pentium processor [Frit95]. It is also important to recognize that this is a simple algorithm, at least when compared to algorithms such as Dolby AC-3. Therefore, this approach will likely need to employ a CPU chip enhanced with multimedia instructions and seems best suited to low-cost, highly integrated applications [Wils95D].

Multimedia-accelerated CPUs can compress and decompress data faster but do nothing to address the bus bandwidth needed for moving uncompressed video data around inside the PC. Consider MPEG-1, by today's standards a moderate-resolution video format. When uncompressed, MPEG-1 video consumes a significant portion of local bus bandwidth and exceeds the bandwidth of typical I/O buses.[16] Thus, moving compression and decompression out of the CPU makes sense for better performance when PCs must do more than just playback video, and for higher-resolution video applications, or for compressing video of any resolution. Referring again to Figure 9.11, there are two locations for dedicated video compression and decompression hardware—in the video subsystem and in the graphics controller.

Video subsystems provide the most flexible, highest-quality video processing and they offload all uncompressed video traffic from the PC buses. Originally, PC video subsystems were implemented as add-on boards (because the internal dataflows of 1980s PCs were totally incapable of handling video). Today, there are two choices: add-on and integrated video subsystems. Whether add-on or integrated, a video subsystem dedicates silicon to doing nothing other than video processing. In this way, it can be assured that 30 fps of uncompressed video will be delivered to the graphics controller (and synchronized, uncompressed audio to the audio subsystem). For compression, it is assured that analog video can be captured and compressed to whatever resolution and frame rate required.

Add-on boards still are the only real solution for compressing video, and they are popular options for high-quality video decompression. The original add-on video subsystem boards were programmable, allowing a variety of compression algorithms. Some still are, but the trend is to offer just one standardized compres-

---

[16] Uncompressed MPEG-1 video in 24-bit RGB-displayable format requires 7.6 MBS. The data rate for the ISA (Industry Standard Architecture) bus, a widely used I/O bus, is 5–8 MBS. The typical data rate for the PCI™ (Peripheral Component Interface) bus, a widely used PC local bus, is about 35–40 MBS.

sion algorithm—some variation of MPEG. The second choice, an integrated video subsystem, is an affirmation of the power of standardization too. Decompression-only (MPEG-1) video subsystems are beginning to be integrated on the PC motherboard [Frit95]. Not only is the cost for dedicated MPEG-1 decompression hardware comparable to that for a faster CPU needed to handle decompression in software, but, given the state of the art, the video quality is better.

The graphics controller is the ideal site for video decompression (but only for decompression, not compression) because for playback, no other PC component needs to handle uncompressed video. (Uncompressed audio must be routed to the audio subsystem via a direct path not shown in Figure 9.11.) A cost advantage of doing decompression in the graphics controller is that the VRAM (video random access memory) may be shared by the decompressor and the graphics accelerator chips. The ultimate low-cost solution for MPEG-1 video playback (or any other video format) is an integrated video-compression-and-graphics-accelerator chip. Circa 1995, these functions were on separate chips, and industry observers thought they would remain that way [Turl95]. The reasons they cited were that MPEG-1 decompressors and graphics accelerators each require a large number of logic circuits that cannot be shared, making the chip very large in 1995 silicon technology, and no one could be certain how long MPEG-1 would be the "standard" for PC video. However, the PC industry does not stand still. In 1996, some MPEG-2 decompression functions began appearing in graphics controller chips, this in anticipation of DVD playback becoming a standard PC function [Wils96].

PC video summary

PC video can roughly be divided into three eras: the formative years, when nonstandard video compression and playback in software on standard PC hardware dominated; the mid-1990s, when MPEG-1 video playback in software or hardware on multimedia-enabled PCs became a standard and videoconferencing was still a future application in search of a standard; and the future, when (if predictions come true) MPEG-2 video playback and H.320/H.324 videoconferencing will be standards. Table 9.8 summarizes characteristics for the variety of software and hardware implementations discussed in this section.

9.12 Multifunction Office Machines

The digital Swiss Army knife for home and office seems a fitting description of multifunction office machines. Major manufacturers are producing all-in-one multifunction office machines priced within reach of small or home offices. These products combine the function of a FAX machine, a scanner, a printer, a copier, and a telephone. They can operate as a stand-alone copy machine, and when connected to a telephone line, they can be used as a FAX machine or simply as

Table 9.8   Cost-benefits analysis of PC video compression.

Location	Decompression	Compression
CPU software	A - Low-cost if CPU performance is adequate A - Flexible—programmable D - Uncompressed video on PC buses D - CPU load D - Video quality depends on CPU load	A - Flexible—programmable D - Uncompressed video on PC buses D - CPU load D - Low performance
Multimedia-accelerated CPU	A - Faster CPU software	A - Faster CPU software
Video subsystem	A - Flexible if programmable A - Compressed video on PC buses A - High-quality video playback D - Cost	A - Flexible if programmable A - Compressed video on PC buses A - High-quality video capture
Graphics controller	A - Low-cost with shared VRAM A - Compressed video on PC buses A - High-quality video playback D - Inflexible if not programmable	Not applicable

Notes:
A - advantage; D - disadvantage.

a telephone; or they can be connected to and controlled by a PC and operated as a scanner, printer, or PC FAX. For larger offices, manufactures have gotten on the bandwagon, too, with networked midrange, multifunction printers and copiers. Copier manufacturers, seeking to leverage their high-speed printers, scanners, and paper-handling systems, have added FAX and printer function. Printer manufacturers, not wanting to be left behind, have added FAX, scanner, and copier function. Consequently, multifunction products span a wide range of functionality and performance ranging from two-page-per-minute faxing at 200-dot-per-inch resolution to 100-page-per-minute printing and copying at 1200-dot-per-inch resolution [Rens95].

Consumer-oriented all-in-one products best illustrate the multifunction nature of these machines. These products essentially are reengineered FAX machines infused with PC-inspired I/O devices and heavy doses of digital technology; that is, the major components of a FAX machine are a scanner, a printer, a telephone, and a modem. All-in-one multifunction office machines substitute low-cost, compact, high-function PC printer and scanner mechanisms, add a PC interface, and interconnect all components via digital intercommunication protocols. As shown in Figure 9.12, a shared memory is used to store image data awaiting transfer to an I/O device or the PC interface. The shared memory is a key element of these products, for it promotes multifunction operation by allowing all the I/O devices and interfaces to work concurrently. For instance, an outbound FAX document can be scanned and transmitted while a PC document is being printed; or, if the scanner and printer are tied up with copying a document, the pages for an incoming FAX transmission can be buffered in memory until the printer becomes available.

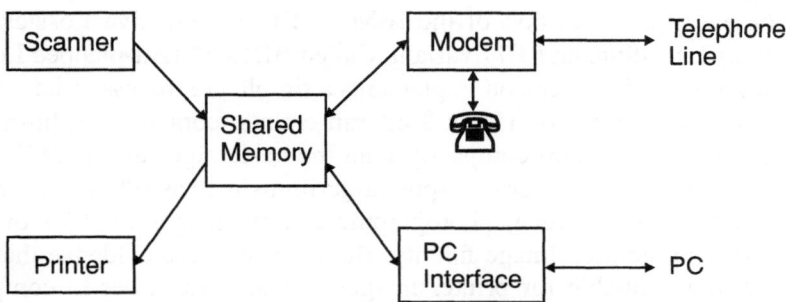

Figure 9.12   Multifunction office machine dataflow.

The shared memory is also one of the most costly components because so much capacity is needed to maximize performance. To deliver the functions that multifunction office machines advertise, large amounts of bit-mapped image data must be stored and flow through the shared memory. Even the simplest machines provide buffering for more than 20 incoming and 20 outgoing FAX pages which, at ½ MB per (uncompressed) page, requires tens of megabytes. Printing and copying are big memory consumers too. The trend in both home and office equipment is to move to higher-resolution printing, which dramatically increases the amount of bit-mapped information that must be stored. Nearly 17 MB is needed to store each rasterized page for the most demanding printing tasks run on high-function printers.[17] To assure a smooth work flow for printing or copying (and faxing and scanning too), more than one page must be buffered. For multi-function printers and copiers that support duplex (back-to-back) printing, and yet more complex functions such as collated-copy printing and out-of-order printing, the memory requirement is even greater.

The price-sensitive office peripherals marketplace demands a design that minimizes cost, and, therefore, all multifunction office machines use compression technology to pack more page images into less memory. A variety of compression algorithms are used. There are no standards here, nor need there be, as these are

---

[17] An 8½ × 11-inch page scanned at 200 × 200-dots-per-inch for faxing ≅½ MB. The same page scanned at 1200 × 1200-dots-per-inch for a laser printer ≅17 MB.

closed processes. All products support shared memory with some type of lossless compression, whereas some may also use lossy compression for large, bit-mapped photographic images. General-purpose lossless compression algorithms such as Lempel-Ziv dictionary algorithms (or almost any of the algorithms discussed in Chapter 4) will reduce the memory required by approximately 2 times. Expect somewhat more from application-specific lossless algorithms intended for bit-mapped images. AHA™, a manufacturer of high-speed compression coprocessor VLSI chips, advertises a typical compression ratio of 4:1 for its customized lossless algorithm [AHA95]. Another example of an application-specific algorithm is based on an extension of the IBM ALDC™ (Adaptive Lossless Data Compression) algorithm, an LZ77 variant. Called BDLC™ (Bit-mapped Lossless Data Compression), the extension implements a simple preprocessor that encodes strings of consecutive 0's or 1's as 8-bit run counts, compressing bit-mapped data some 1.5–3 times more compactly than the basic algorithm [Craf95].

For lossy compression, general-purpose algorithms such as JPEG can compress continuous-tone, natural-scene, photographic-quality images by 10:1 or more, depending on the required image fidelity. But there is some evidence that other codings are more suitable for printer images—or at least easier to compute—and, as a result, customized proprietary lossy algorithms are popular. One example is an algorithm developed by Mitsubishi that uses block truncation coding (BTC) [Oka92]. BTC attempts to preserve image quality by breaking the page into small blocks, computing the gray-scale mean and variance within each block, and quantizing individual pixels with respect to those values [Netr95]. During decoding, approximate gray-scale values for each pixel are reconstructed. Typical compression ratios range from about 3:1 to nearly 5:1 for BTC, much lower than JPEG, but significantly reducing the shared memory required for high-function printing. Another example of a customized proprietary lossy algorithm for printer images is the Image Adapt™ technique used by some Hewlett-Packard printers [Seyb93]. Image Adapt compresses large, bit-mapped photographic images by breaking the page into small sections, counting and storing the number of dots in each section, but not saving the exact position of each dot to conserve memory. To reconstruct the image, each section is filled with the same number of dots, scattered in a fixed pattern. The effect is a less detailed image, but one that preserves shades of gray.

Maintaining a compressed, shared memory in a multifunction office machine presents some unique challenges in that independent data streams must flow in and out concurrently—for instance, out to the printer and in from the scanner during copying. This requires both compression and decompression to be active simultaneously. There are several implementation choices that cover the wide range of functionality and performance found in these products[18]: RISC CPUs

---

[18] The uncompressed data rate for faxing two pages per minute at 200-dots-per-inch resolution is 0.017 MBS and for printing 100 pages per minute at 1200-dots-per-inch resolution is 28 MBS.

can run multiplexed compression and decompression operations in software sufficiently fast for entry-level products, but not for high-function products. Hardware codecs are the solution for high-speed operation. One design option is to use two chips, one for compression and a second for decompression, but this adds to product cost. Another approach is to use a single-chip codec that contains independent engines for simultaneously compressing and decompressing data. One example is a dual-function application-specific coprocessor from AHA [AHA95]. For high-speed operations such as copying, it can maintain a 25-MBS decompressed dataflow to the printer while receiving and compressing data from the scanner at the same rate. No matter how the compression and decompression functions are implemented, they must present a constant flow of information to timing-sensitive I/O devices.

9.13   Digital Speech Products

With telephone answering machines and personal memo recorders leading the way, digital technology is popping up in a variety of consumer products for recording the human voice. These products use memory chips to store digitized speech. Until digital technology became available, microcassette tapes were the only storage media choice for these products. The advantages of digital technology over tape are obvious to consumers—smaller, more efficient, and more reliable products with no moving parts, instant access and playback of messages in any order, and more. But tape-based speech-recording products are tough competitors. They are mature, low-cost products that can record lengthy messages—up to 45 minutes on each side of the tape. The strengths of tape are, unfortunately, the greatest weaknesses of digital recording in that many memory chips are needed to store lengthy messages, and for these products memory chips are expensive components. If digital-based products are to compete, they must match the recording time and cost of tape-based products. Data compression is the solution.

Nowhere else are the advantages of data compression more clearly illustrated than by this application. The product design trade-offs are simple: One choice is to continue using more and more memory chips to increase recording time, thus driving up product cost. The other is to add a DSP chip running speech compression, thus driving down product cost by allowing each memory chip to store speech 10–25 times more efficiently. Every increase of compression algorithm efficiency increases the minutes of speech stored, whatever the amount of memory available.

A simplified dataflow for recording compressed digital speech is shown in Figure 9.13. Under microprocessor control, incoming speech is digitized, compressed in the DSP, and stored in memory. For playback, the process is reversed.

Table 9.9 shows the recording times that can be achieved with algorithms that code telephone-quality speech at the rates described in Section 5.2. Memory

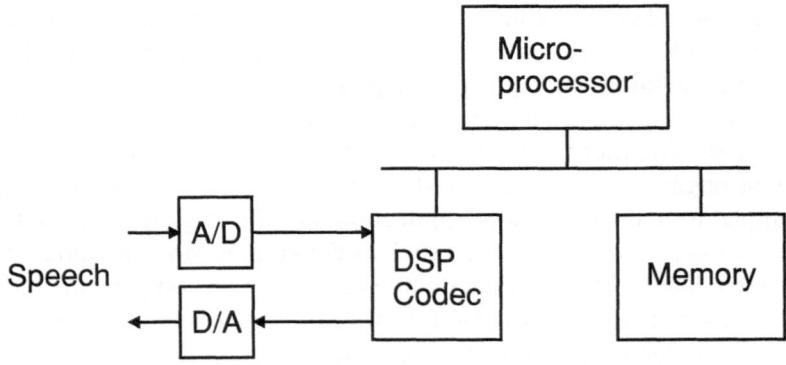

Figure 9.13   Digital speech recording.

sizes are based on 4-megabit chips, typical of 1995-era technology found in these products [Edge95C].

Table 9.9   Recording time (minutes).

Encoded Bit Rate (Kbps)	Memory Capacity		
	4 Mbits	8 Mbits	16 Mbits
64[1]	1	2	4
4.8	15	29	58
3	23	46	93
2.4	29	58	116

Notes:
[1] Uncompressed telephone-quality speech.

9.14   Summary

This chapter examined consumer-electronics applications where, primarily, data compression is used for efficient data storage. We learned the following:

- The digital revolution in entertainment and information has unleashed a torrent of speech, audio, image, video, and computer consumer-electronics products that depend on data compression.
- Data compression can contribute to the success of a consumer-electronics product by adding value that consumers can appreciate.

- Data compression allows using more compact storage media for stereo audio gear, but in some recently introduced products, it compromises sound quality and contributes to higher prices.

- For multichannel home theater, Dolby AC-3 data compression improves sound quality with fully discrete channels, stereo surround channels, and increased dynamic range—all carried on existing media and with little increase in cost over previous products.

- All digital television transmission methods use data compression; the problem for consumer-electronics gear is how digital television receivers and peripheral devices will interoperate with compressed digital signals.

- No industry standard yet exists for handling data compression in television peripheral devices such as set-top boxes, VCRs, video camcorders, and videodisc players.

- SDTV/HDTV receivers can be expected to include built-in MPEG-2 decoders.

- Trend-setting set-top boxes both decode MPEG-2 to NTSC-standard video and provide a compressed bit stream.

- Digital VCRs and camcorders are being marketed, some without and some with built-in data compression. Those that do compress, use a frame-by-frame, DCT coding technique defined by the DVC standard.

- A standard for digital videodiscs has been forged, and DVD players will include MPEG-2 decompression.

- Digital photography products include digital cameras and Photo CD players. To reduce image storage requirements, both use data compression—JPEG for digital cameras and a proprietary multiresolution technology for Photo CD.

- Interactive multimedia systems ranging from set-top videogame players to Internet browsers use a variety of proprietary and standard data compression technology, primarily to reduce multimedia storage requirements.

- Multimedia PCs handle a wide range of applications, some requiring both compressing and decompressing multimedia data.

- PC video has proven most difficult, necessitating hardware and software redesign to support its high data rates and real-time processing needs.

- Following a long struggle to establish PC data compression standards and develop cost-effective implementations, MPEG-1 is today's choice for playback. PC videoconferencing appears to be settling on H.261/H.263. In the near future, with the introduction of DVD devices, MPEG-2 is sure to become yet another PC video format.

- Multifunction office machines require concurrently operating data compression and decompression. The task is to minimize the amount of shared memory, the key component for multifunction operation and one of the most expensive, by reducing the amount of data flowing to and from it.

- Nowhere else are the advantages of data compression more clearly illustrated than for digital speech products such as telephone answering machines and personal memo recorders. Replacing a large number of memory chips with a DSP chip running data compression defines a lower-cost product that can record much longer, a win-win situation for manufacturers and consumers.

10

Publishing Applications

In this chapter, we examine publishing applications for which data compression is used for efficient data storage and to reduce bandwidth for information transmission. In publishing, various combinations of lossless and lossy compression are needed to support a multiplicity of multimedia data types.

10.1 Industry Overview

The concept of publishing is simple: Take an idea, describe it in words and pictures, and distribute the product in some physical form. As a business venture, publishing is far more complex. Publishing, one of the world's oldest enterprises, is a large, highly diversified industry. It is also an industry experiencing a total and rapid transformation unlike any before in its long, rich history. In a few short years, traditional publishing has been revolutionized with computer-based technology replacing centuries-old production and distribution methods. Monolithic publishers have been replaced by new, distributed business models where production, publishing, printing, and distribution often are separately owned businesses, all interconnected to communicate electronically created information. At the same time, electronic publishing has become more than a buzzword with electronic documents taking their place alongside print media. Within the industry, digital replication, storage, and transmission facilities are replacing printing presses and paper. For delivering information to readers (or should we say viewers), CD-ROM drives and Internet connections are replacing trips to libraries and bookstores, mail, and newspaper delivery. Paper documents certainly are on no one's endangered species list, but their production costs have continued to climb while just the opposite is true for electronic documents. This factor, in combination with lower reproduction and distribution costs, and the ability to target an audience, no matter how small or scattered, assures continued growth for electronic documents. Table 10.1 introduces the publishing media described in this chapter.

Table 10.1   Publishing media.

Industry Segment	Production Elements	Distribution Media	Delivery Vehicles
Traditional Books Magazines Newspapers	Text, graphics, and images	Paper and microfilm	Retail stores Mail Home delivery services
Electronic CD-ROM	Text, graphics, images, animation, audio, and video	CD-ROM	Multimedia PC TV and set-top box
Online	Text, graphics, images, animation, audio, and video	Electronic network (e.g., Internet)	Multimedia PC

Current applications for data compression in the publishing industry are mostly concerned with efficiently storing all types of data, including text, graphics, speech, audio, image, and video. Providing source material on CD-ROM for multimedia applications is an established part of the industry. Encyclopedias and other reference materials are widely available on CD-ROM. Other opportunities for data compression are emerging too. Two examples are efficiently storing digital text-based products and efficiently storing and transmitting online, communications-based publications.

Many different data compression schemes are employed; standards are not yet prevalent. Examples in this chapter clearly show this situation is quite acceptable for many storage-based products because they are closed applications where the application-provider produces and controls the product from media creation to distribution and playback. Online publications can fall into this category, too, but the Internet is setting de facto standards for all online publishers.

10.2   Traditional Publishing

Figure 10.1 provides a simplified view of traditional book, magazine, and newspaper publishing. The process begins with authors and advertisers who have informa-

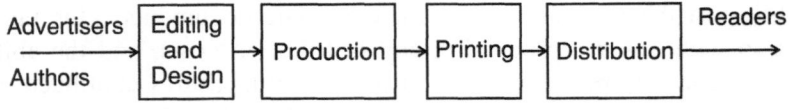

Figure 10.1   Publishing process.

tion they wish to see in print. The first step is editing and design to prepare the raw material; activities include editing text, selecting photographs, generating graphics, and creating advertising layouts. During production, the visual elements are brought together in preparation for printing. Here, formatting operations including size selection, layout, and pagination take place. Following printing, copies are distributed to readers. Today, each step in the process is accomplished with computerized digital publishing facilities. Word processing, digital graphics, digital imaging, and computerized phototypesetting are tools of the trade. Whether for publishing in print or electronic media, preparing a document in electronic format is far more efficient than previous methods, if for no other reason than it simplifies repeated updates and reprints.

There are two important applications for data compression in this process—digital delivery of documents between sites and maintaining a digital image archive. Digital publishing generates very large data files. High-resolution page images are needed for printing and, especially for newspapers, the page format is large, which means many bits are needed for each digitized page image. Most important, these files must be transmitted over networks because the individual steps of the publishing process may be done at separate physical locations, often by separately owned businesses. Then, too, publications often require extensive graphics and images that must be stored in digital format.

Digital delivery is used to transmit ad copy from advertisers and advertising agencies to newspaper and magazine publishers. It is also used to send print-ready page images from publishers of national newspapers and magazines to remote printing plants. For instance, the *Wall Street Journal* is published in New York City and regional editions are printed at Des Moines, Iowa and at other sites across the country. These applications set no new trends or requirements for data compression technology, but the reduced costs and shorter times for transmitting compressed data are significant. Typically, text, graphics, and print-ready page images are compressed with LZW or other lossless algorithms. Photographs are compressed with lossless or lossy JPEG or Photo CD algorithms. Vendors of software for delivering documents to multisite publishing operations routinely incorporate these data compression technologies in their products [Edwa94].

Digital image archiving is an important new publishing tool. Photo archives have long been a staple element of wire services, newspapers, and magazines. As any movie-goer knows, when reporters refer to the *morgue*, they do not always mean a place where dead bodies are kept but rather a stockpile of old photos. Digital image archiving updates the morgue of old, making it far more manageable, far more useful, and far more valuable. Far larger collections of photos can be stored digitally in less physical space and thoroughly searched much faster. Not just photos, but graphics, artwork, and all types of images can be stored. Existing libraries of newspaper clippings or any paper documents, now held in either hard copy or on microfilm, can be scanned into the digital image archive too. Probably the most significant aspect of digital image archives, at least for the publishers and service firms that own them, is that their content is a marketable commodity. For a fee, many organizations are now quite willing to open their digital archives to customers seeking particular types of images [Bens94].

The publishing industry actually uses digital image archiving in two ways, as a repository for information needed during production and as a true long-term archive, which leads to questions about what information to store and its storage format. The basic conflict is balancing the requirements of a lean, mean repository that can service immediate production needs versus an archive that contains everything which might be important for future reference. Although digital storage technology (see Section 6.2) addresses both needs—by storing immediate material in electronic storage and on magnetic disk online storage, and by storing long-term archived material on optical disc nearline storage—there are cost and performance penalties for maintaining a large archive. Thus, in the real world, publishers must decide what information to store and in what form to store it.

Consider a newspaper photo morgue, which, in the past, was a library of photos stored on film. An advantage of film is that the storage cost is essentially the same whether a picture is a large, full-color print or a small, black-and-white mug shot. The disadvantages are cataloging and retrieving photos is labor intensive and a film library takes up ever-growing amounts of physical space. Digital archiving is exactly the reverse. Physical space needs are much less. Cataloging is simpler and retrieval is much faster and more effective. Selecting the right photo from dozens of thumbnail images that can be displayed almost instantly requires nothing more than a few keystrokes or mouse clicks. But the cost for storing digitized photos and the access time depends on their resolution and whether they are color or black-and-white. Therefore, newspaper archivers must carefully choose from among assorted storage formats that include those shown in Table 10.2.

The conflicts between access time, usage requirements, electronic data storage cost, and information content are obvious. Fortunately, data compression alters the equation. Both JPEG and Photo CD image compression are widely used in publishing archival systems with vendor products equally split between these formats [Seyb95C]. Essentially, there is no one correct resolution for storing images, and images are typically stored at multiple different resolutions to accommodate various usage requirements. Because both JPEG and Photo CD can store color images in luminance-chrominance display format (YC_BC_R and PhotoYCC,

Table 10.2   Newspaper image archive storage formats.

Image Format	Resolution (typical)	Uses
Thumbnail	192 x 128 or less, 8-bit pixels	Quick access for image selection during production
Full screen, full color	640 x 480, 24-bit pixels	Image display during production
Cropped and screened	Varies	Pertinent historical information (e.g., column wide, black-and-white close-up shots in as-printed format)
Full resolution, full color	3072 x 2048, 36-bit pixels	Hi-resolution originals scanned from 35-mm film with no perceptible information loss

respectively), image management software typically provides for converting to CMYK format for printing.[1] Other color conversions for printing include 12-bit to 8-bit range compression, tonal compression (for setting white and black points), color management, and unsharp masking [Seyb95B].

10.3   Electronic Publishing

Sometime during the PC revolution of the 1980s, the term *software publisher* was coined to describe a business that developed and marketed computer programs and, in that era, distributed them on floppy disks. Only a little imagination was needed to recognize that any form of machine-readable (i.e., digitized) information could be distributed in the same way. Today, with almost all information processed by computer-aided (mostly desktop) publishing tools, and with far better distribu- tion media, nearly anything distributed in print is a candidate for what is now called electronic publishing. Even documents that might never have been prin- ted—because they are too massive, too specialized, too short-lived, or for what- ever reason—can be economically distributed via electronic media and reach their intended readers, no matter how large or how small the audience may be. Translating existing documents into an electronic format is also a good way to find an audience for what may have been an underused, inaccessible, or expensive resource. One of the most exciting aspects of electronic publishing is that multime-

---

[1] CMYK format represents color as cyan (a blue-green), magenta, yellow, and black, the ink colors used for printing [Penn93].

dia enhancements can be added to existing documents, making them attractive to a new and potentially much wider audience.

There are two forms of electronic publishing: CD-ROM publishing and online publishing. Both will be examined shortly, but, first, some general thoughts about electronic publishing. Traditional book publishers have made the transition from print to electronic media with varying degrees of success. Electronic publishing is not a replacement for paper, and a good electronic book is not simply a copy of a printed book. Then, too, the audiences for paper and electronic books may not be the same. Making a good electronic book, one that takes full advantage of electronic publishing and will sell, demands more work and more investment—in the product itself and in marketing the product. Electronic books are computer searchable, and they can include animation, audio, and video. For these reasons, massive reference books including encyclopedias, dictionaries, and technical volumes, are rapidly moving to CD-ROM. Another advantage is that electronic books are far cheaper to replicate than paper. Also, they weigh next to nothing and take up precious little shelf space. Granted, a multimedia PC is needed to "read" an electronic book, but there are millions of users with PCs, and all are prospective customers. This makes the audience for specialized reference material far wider than ever before, and with a large potential market, prices can be kept low.

Electronic publishing is about more than just porting books and reference materials to electronic media. Magazines and newspapers are published in electronic formats, as are educational and training materials; so is computer software—the original electronic publishing application. Besides materials intended to inform readers, entertainment is a part of electronic publishing, too, in the form of interactive games, movies, audio, and image products. If this diverse collection of products can be said to have anything in common, it is that all are produced with the same digital publishing tools and distributed on the same media.

Electronic publishing involves steps that parallel those found in traditional publishing, but reordered, and with important differences. Figure 10.2 shows what is involved. As in traditional publishing, electronic publishing begins by processing the information (editing, design, composition, formatting, and so on) to create the document. In contrast to traditional publishing, the publisher then distributes the document and the user, not the publisher, reproduces it. For those

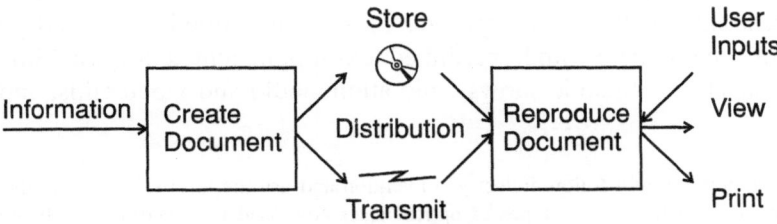

Figure 10.2 Electronic publishing information flow.

familiar with desktop publishing tools, it is as if the tool is split in two parts, with the publisher in control of the front-end processing steps and the user in control of the back-end processing (display or printing) steps. Alternatively, those with a network-centric view of the world may view this as a client-server process, where the publisher serves up electronic documents for the user clients.

Whatever your view, there are dozens of desktop publishing tools for creating electronic documents and nearly as many electronic document formats, the form information takes during intermediate publishing steps [Rose95]. With print media, the choice of publishing tools or electronic document format is of little concern to anyone other than the publisher, as they only affect the processing stages leading to a paper output. Not so with electronic publishing, where readers are intimately involved in the publishing process. User PCs contain the software for unformatting and viewing or printing the document. Therefore, publishers must choose tools and formats that are compatible with the reader's software (as for online Internet distribution) or provide readers with compatible software (as for CD-ROM distribution). But perhaps the most important aspect of tools and formats for electronic distribution is how efficiently they store information, as this determines how much information can be packed on a CD-ROM and how long a network transmission will take. In one sense, most electronic document tools and formats are alike—they use data compression to compactly store text and graphics or whatever multimedia data types they handle. What they fail to do is agree on the type of compression to use, as we will see shortly.

CD-ROM publishing

Distributing information and entertainment via electronic networks is attractive, but today and for some time to come network infrastructure sets limits on what is possible. Although today's CD-ROMs[2] lack the ability to instantaneously access the huge volumes of data to be found on networks, they can provide access to about 650 MB of information at several times the rate of the fastest telephone-line modems. This makes CD-ROM publishing an attractive compromise. The advantages and limitations of CD-ROM publishing are perhaps best illustrated by encyclopedias. In terms of sales and technology, encyclopedias rank among the most successful electronic publications [Bane95]. There are numerous publishers, millions of copies have been sold, and the best of these products allow readers to do things that the paper versions cannot. Natural-language search tools and multimedia presentations make it easy to find and comprehend information. The paper versions, being limited to text and graphics, cannot hope to compete with hyperlinked text supplemented not just with images but also narrated with slide shows, animation, audio and video clips, and more.

---

[2] In this section, we will follow industry convention and use the term *CD-ROM* in its broadest sense to cover all of the various types of optical discs now used for electronic publishing—CD-ROM, CD-ROM-XA, CD-I, and Video CD.

An emerging trend is to hyperlink the CD-ROM contents with online information sources, providing access to the latest information about a subject or providing access to related reference materials. The strength of these and other CD-ROM publications is greatly enhanced by their interactive, television like capabilities, which also highlights the major limitations of the CD-ROM media. This becomes particularly evident in that current CD-ROM publications contain only token, highly compressed video clips, played back in software with all of the restrictions described in Section 9.11.

CD-ROM publishers face many challenges. One set of issues relates to their inventiveness in learning to use the media and its production tools to maximum advantage, along with learning how to market their products. Then, too, the technical limitations of CD-ROM media itself constrain what their products can do. Today's CD-ROM drives are slow to randomly access data, their playback data rate is low (when compared to magnetic disks or fast networks), and their storage capacity is too limited for some applications. These technical limitations have been and are being addressed in the following ways: Smart programming can partially hide the random-access speed limitations, by caching data on magnetic disk, or simply by carefully planning data access patterns. CD-ROM playback speed has been increased by 2, 4, 6, and now 8 times. While this improves the playback rate for video and other linear presentations, it shrinks the playing time since the storage capacity remains unchanged. The storage capacity, which has proven quite adequate for applications with little video content, limits applications such as interactive education and training where there is little but video content. Data compression can only partially alleviate the storage capacity limitations. MPEG-1 compressed video is limited to 74 minutes and even more complex algorithms such as fractals pack no more than 2 hours of quality video on today's CD-ROMs.[3] The only real solution for video-based electronic publishing applications lies in the future with DVD-ROM that, as shown in Section 9.6, can pack much more data onto the disc and deliver it at higher data rates.

Online publishing

Few could appreciate the explosive growth in online publishing to follow when the World Wide Web hypertext system was added to the Internet in 1990. What the Web provides is a public, globally accessible, Internet-wide distributed hypertext system that operates on a client-server computer model. Using client software known as a browser, a user can download information from Web servers and display or playback text, graphics, audio, video or any other type of multimedia information. Although online information services like CompuServe and America Online™ have provided electronic delivery of information to consumers

---

[3] More telling, this assumes there will be nothing but video on the disc, which for most electronic publishing applications is unlikely. For example, the *Encyclopaedia Britannica* CD-ROM is reported to contain about 300 MB of text (uncompressed) [Bane95].

for several years, as have Internet bulletin-board systems, none have captured the public's attention quite like the Web with its graphical interface. Actually, the Web did not become a real phenomenon until about 1993 when the number of network-connected, multimedia-enabled personal computers began to skyrocket. One measure of the Web's popularity is the number of Web servers connected to the Internet. As shown in Figure 10.3, beginning in 1993, in 3 short years the

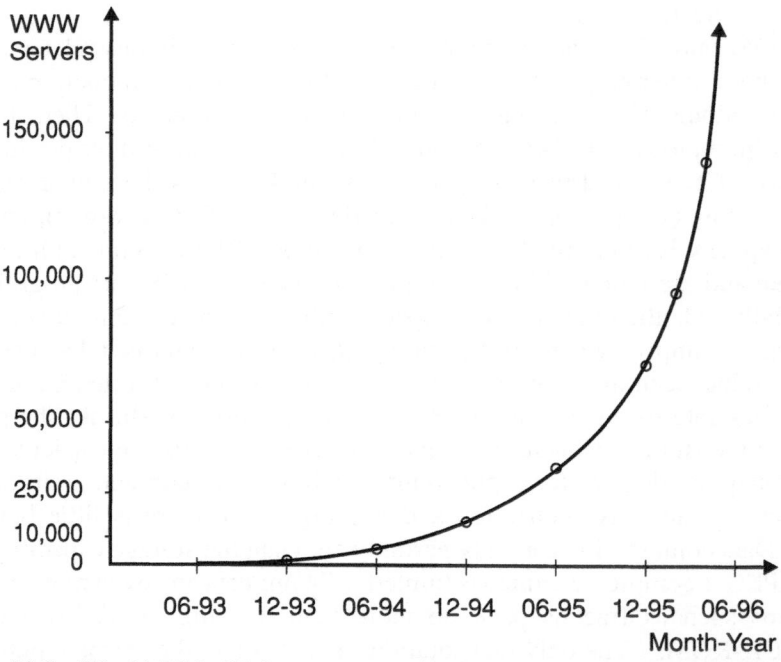

Figure 10.3   World Wide Web server growth. (Source: WebCrawler™ [WEBC96].)

number of Web servers exploded from essentially nothing to six-digit values.[4] By the mid-1990s, it seemed almost everyone had something to tell or sell the world. Being part of the Internet, the Web imposes few if any restrictions on who may provide what information content. To ardent Web surfers, this means nearly unlimited opportunities to spend endless hours searching for and viewing information from almost uncountable Web servers owned by individuals, organizations, and businesses.

Online newspapers, perhaps, best illustrate what is attracting so many to online publishing. One of the advantages of going online is that it allows local newspapers

---

[4] A Web server is a computer that contains the home page (the first page) and related information for one or more organizations or individuals. Many widely varying estimates of the Web size have been reported, differing in the counting techniques employed. An even less reliable measure is the number of people using the Web. Some estimates of Internet users (of which Web users are but a fraction) range upward of 50 million in 1996 [Bour95].

to deliver local content that print media cannot; in-depth coverage of neighborhood sports, school activities, and community politics are some examples. Then, too, online newspapers can provide frequent updates to news of interest, late-breaking stories, and more extensive photo coverage than their paper-based counterparts. Another advantage of an online newspaper is that it can provide features that print media cannot; searchable classified ads is a good example, as is providing detailed local television listings that are searchable, customizable to viewer preferences, and can be enhanced with codes for automatically programming VCRs. Online newspapers can take advantage of computer-based features to heighten reader interest and encourage them to explore. Allowing readers to access and search an archive of back issues is one possibility. On a more global scale, it may mean providing readers with hyperlinks to related or background information from national newspapers or global news services. In the future, online newspapers may choose to supplement words and graphics with audio and video clips.

For those who are now publishing on the Web, or are planning to publish on it or on any online service, there are many yet-unresolved questions about online publishing. The most important business-related question is how to make money with online publications [Goul95, Seyb95D]. Whether the publication be a newspaper or anything else, how to publish online, what information to publish, how to protect it, and how to deliver it are issues that must be addressed. Most of these issues go far beyond the scope of this book, but to understand how data compression enters into online publishing, we must address two technical limitations online publishers face—storage capacity and bandwidth. Storage capacity is an issue that anyone maintaining a digital archive must address, online publishers included. The availability and cost of network bandwidth affects both online publishers and readers. It limits the services that online publishers can offer, and, most important, it has a lot to do with reader satisfaction. Anyone who has spent what seems like an interminable amount of time waiting for graphic images to be downloaded will testify to this.

The role of data compression

There are an endless variety of text, graphics, audio, and video compression algorithms that all electronic publishers can use to address storage and bandwidth limitations. First, consider CD-ROM publishing: CD-ROM publishers have enjoyed great flexibility in their choice of data compression technology and they have been innovators, being the first to use a variety of advanced compression techniques. CD-ROM publishing is a closed process with publishers not only creating the content but also providing the software for playing back the CD-ROM. This means they are free to choose the data compression that is best for their product. Here, "best" implies a high compression ratio and sensible decode time because compression speed and compatibility are unimportant. To aid publishers in selecting a compression technique, one manufacturer provides an automated software tool that uses an array of compression engines to analyze an electronic document file and select the compression technique(s) that will shrink data into the least amount of space. Along with the compressed file, the capaCD™ tool also provides the decompression programs that users will need to read the file [Karn95].

An example of the advanced compression techniques used by CD-ROM publishers is fractal compression. Fractal algorithms are very effective for squeezing high-quality, natural-scene images into the fewest number of bits, but at the expense of slow and complex encoding. However, the upside is that decoding is fast and simple. What makes fractal algorithms attractive to CD-ROM publishers is that these are exactly the right characteristics for electronic media distribution. The time spent encoding a high-quality, compactly stored image is of little consequence to anyone but the publisher, whereas the results benefit the product and its readers. Another example is the evolution of CD-ROM video. In 1991, QuickTime movies measured 160 × 120 pixels and played at about 10 fps on single-speed CD-ROM drives. Today, MPEG-1 coded movies measure 352 × 240 pixels and can play at 30 fps. In the future, with faster, higher-density discs, CD-ROM publishers will undoubtedly include MPEG-2 video in their products.

Now, consider online publishing: As mentioned previously, CD-ROM publishers are joining ranks with other online publishers by linking their products with online information sources. In so doing, they face a different set of data compression requirements and paradigms that affect all online publishers. Here, text compression options abound, with some form of LZW probably being most common, but with few important differences in efficiency for any of the lossless algorithms (and no quality differences). Many graphics compression algorithms are used by online publishers, with great differences in both efficiency and quality. One example is GIF that has been a leading format for online information services and Internet transmissions but, as discussed in Section 3.5, licensing and royalty fee questions contribute to its uncertain future. Then, too, GIF is a lossless algorithm, and its image files are relatively large with long download times. To control file size, GIF images are limited to 256 colors. To make the downloading time less objectionable, CompuServe developed a hierarchical form of GIF that first sends a low-resolution image which can be viewed while waiting for the full-resolution image to download. In contrast, lossy compression algorithms are far more effective for creating compact image files of any resolution, and media developers are beginning to put 16-bit color JPEG-compressed images on the Internet [Gibb95].

As to audio and video compression, online publishers who hope to reach large audiences must wait for the online services and Internet to develop standards and technology for transmitting real-time data on their networks. The basic problem is that existing networks are not geared to guarantee bandwidth and assure on-time delivery of data packets. Internet-based audio and video transmissions have been demonstrated, and growing numbers of users are experimenting with an Internet virtual network known as MBONE (Multicast Backbone), but the transmissions are plagued with out-of-sync audio and jerky video [Kobi95B].

Several companies are working to overcome these limitations with proprietary data transmission (and compression) schemes for both audio and video [Fren95, Lang95B, Mokh95, Come96]. Then, too, MPEG audio and video compression and the H.324 videotelephony standard may be the solutions for which everyone is looking.

10.4 Summary

This chapter examined publishing applications for which data compression is used for efficient data storage and for reducing transmission bandwidth. We learned the following:

- The publishing industry has undergone total and rapid transformation, with electronically created information being distributed on paper and electronic media.
- Traditional publishers must transmit very large data files between sites and must maintain large digital image archives. Data compression allows both to be done more effectively.
- LZW and other lossless algorithms are used for transmitting text files, graphics, and print-ready page images, whereas lossy JPEG and Photo CD algorithms are used for storing and transmitting digital images.
- Digital image archives are used for both production and long-term storage, requiring images to be stored at several resolutions.
- Almost all information processed by computer-aided tools is a candidate for electronic publishing, distributed either on CD-ROMs or on networks.
- In electronic publishing, the choice of tools and formats used to create the document and the choice of data compression affect how efficiently information can be delivered to the reader.
- CD-ROM publishers extensively use data compression to alleviate the data rate and storage capacity limitations of today's discs, but totally video-based electronic publications must wait for future DVD-ROM discs.
- Online publishers extensively use data compression to alleviate network bandwidth and server storage capacity limitations, but existing networks are not yet up to the challenges of distributing audio and video data.
- CD-ROM publishers have been free to choose the compression algorithms that are best for their product as they provide the playback software. As they begin linking their products with online information sources, it will be necessary to conform to the de facto compression standards and technology that is evolving for all online publications.

11

Entertainment Applications

In this chapter, we examine entertainment applications for which data compression can be used for efficient data storage and to reduce bandwidth for information transmission. Various combinations of lossless and lossy compression are needed to support the multiplicity of multimedia data types encountered in these applications.

11.1 Industry Overview

Over the years the definition of entertainment and the entertainment industry has changed. Once, entertainment meant the performing arts—live theater, dance, and music, primarily. Sometime in the 1880s, entrepreneurs began commercialized these once-serious and unprofitable art forms, making them no-so-serious and creating the first entertainment businesses. Stage shows, circuses, sporting events, and even early-day theme parks were part of the new entertainment world. In the early 1900s, motion pictures and phonographs added a whole new dimension to entertainment, for now the performance need not be live but could be recorded and distributed for profit. With radio in the 1930s, and television in the mid-1950s, electronic media created new forums for mass entertainment, *electronic* entertainment. Now, in the 1990s, the entertainment industry is a leading U.S. exporter, a leading employer, and, a role model for mass marketing. It also is a driver of new technology with, for instance, high-powered computers and the latest software techniques being applied to making movies and video games. With the intermingling of media, computer, and communications technologies, yet another radical transformation of the entertainment industry is underway.

Old paradigms for entertainment production and distribution are fading as media moguls make alliances with computer makers and the communications industry, maneuvering to create global info-entertainment conglomerates that control both production and distribution. At the root of the upheaval, of course, is digital technology and the new ways it presents to produce and distribute entertainment.

The entertainment industry presents a large, relatively untapped opportunity to exploit all the virtues of data compression for storage efficiency, transmission bandwidth conservation, and transmission time reduction. This industry does it all: it produces the products; it stores, archives, and distributes the media, and, with movie theaters, even provides the facilities to deliver its products to consumers. Earlier chapters of this book describe how data compression is used by the storage media and transmission channels that the entertainment industry relies on for distributing its products (excluding film-based movies). Also described is how data compression applies to the consumer-electronics gear that viewers and listeners use to playback these products. Consequently, this chapter concentrates on how data compression is used for producing movies, television and radio programs, audio recordings, and video games. It will also examine the role of compression in preparing these products for distribution and for archiving them. Table 11.1 introduces the electronic entertainment products discussed in this chapter.

The entertainment industry deals almost exclusively in audio and video—audio and video tapes, compact discs of all kinds, movies, television and radio programming, and video games are among its most important products. Digital data processing opens many new opportunities for data compression in media production, storage, archiving, distribution, and reproduction. The entertainment industry is rapidly adopting digital data processing tools for all phases of its operation. Data compression might seem the only practical means of managing the huge volumes of data generated during production, but there are quality issues associated with processing original source material, delaying its adoption. Data compression is, however, recognized as the key to cost-effective storage, perhaps for archiving, and certainly for distribution of digitized music, movies, games, and other software.

Data compression standards are important for entertainment applications, and the industry is actively involved in setting those standards. It has and continues to work with the consumer-electronics, computer, and communications industries in formulating standards for digital audio, image, and video. The JPEG (Joint Photographic Experts Group) and MPEG (Motion Picture Experts Group) standards bear witness to this effort.

11.2 Media Production and Distribution

A simplified view of the production and distribution process for electronic entertainment products appears in Figure 11.1. It begins with people—actors, advertis-

Table 11.1   Entertainment media.

Industry Segment	Production Elements	Distribution Media	Delivery Vehicles
Movies	Moving images and audio	Film Videocassette Video CD DVD Electronic network	Film cinema TV and VCR TV and set-top box TV and DVD player Electronic cinema
Television programs	Video, audio, and text	Terrestrial broadcast Satellite broadcast Cable network Telco network	TV TV and set-top box TV and set-top box TV and set-top box
Radio programs	Audio	Terrestrial broadcast Satellite broadcast Cable network	Radio receiver Radio receiver Radio receiver
Recordings	Audio	CD Cassette tape MiniDisc DCC	CD player Tape player MiniDisc player DCC player
Video games	Graphics, animation, images, audio, and video	ROM cartridge CD-ROM	Game player Multimedia PC

ers, authors, producers—who have ideas for entertainment.[1] Images, sound, and other data are captured (on film, tape, or computer disk), after which follows editing and, often, many terribly complex production steps. The end result is a product that can be printed (in movie film terminology) or copied on electronic media and distributed.

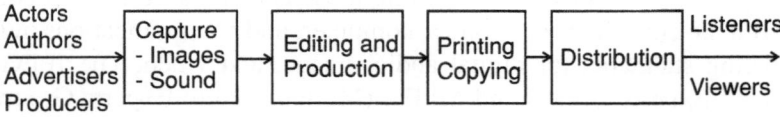

Figure 11.1   Electronic entertainment production and distribution.

An inescapable fact in this age of digital media is that, in some ways, the electronic entertainment media business is much like electronic publishing. From

---

[1] Who is to say that advertising is not entertainment?

a marketing perspective, the two are often difficult to distinguish in that both distribute their products on the same media, and home-bound customers use the same equipment to view or listen to the results. Moreover, both share many of the same production tools and technologies. Without exception, all branches of the entertainment industry have totally embraced digital production technology, even for film-based movies that are essentially the last bastion of a once totally analog empire. Today, entertainment producers transform real-world images and sounds into digital format almost immediately upon capture—by digitally scanning film, by digitizing video and audio—and maintain them in digital format throughout the editing and production steps. Furthermore, some entertainment products are created within a computer and are inherently digital. Modern-day animations (some of us still want to call them cartoons) and video games are digital from the beginning and remain that way. Whatever the initial format, conversion (back) to analog only happens when preparing the product for distribution, and then only when printing or copying to analog media.

Production

Let there be no doubt, the opportunities for data compression in entertainment media production are enormous. To illustrate:

- Movie film is digitized at high resolutions and pixel depths. Industry standards call for digitizing 35-mm format frames (known as Academy format) at not less than 3656×2664 pixels and a pixel depth not less than 12 bits for each RGB component (i.e., 36 bits per pixel). Larger film formats may use as much as 6144×4096 pixels at the same pixel depth [Brah95].
- Broadcast-quality television images are digitized at not less than 720×480 pixels and a pixel depth of 12 or 16 bits for each SDTV frame, and much more for HDTV frames. (See Table 5.8.)
- Graphics images are digitized at resolutions up to and equaling 35-mm film format.
- Audio channels are digitized, often at CD-quality levels (44.1 KHz, 16-bit samples).

Here is one example of how this translates into storage capacities and data rates: One minute of digitized Academy-format motion-picture film (nearly 44 MB per frame at 24 fps) requires some 63 GB of storage. This results in a data rate of more than 1 GBS for full-rate playback. In practice, even with the high-end workstations and servers that major film studios employ, rarely can more than a few minutes of full-resolution digitized film be manipulated online. Other examples are less extreme, but the point is that in entertainment media production, there are huge volumes of data to be stored and transmitted.

Obviously, data compression is needed, but the question is, Can it be used—safely? Product quality is the central issue. All audio, image, and video compression algorithms that use lossy compression—the ones that can significantly reduce storage capacities and data rates—degrade quality. Lossless compression algorithms do not, but the reduction they provide may be totally inadequate. It would appear that within the entertainment industry, there is general agreement that digital technology, compression included, must in no way compromise the end product; its quality level must be as good or better than with analog technology. This leaves much room for interpretation about where and how in the production cycle to use data compression to deal with storage capacity and bandwidth limitations.

Seemingly, the major film studios have elected to at least partially sidestep the issue by throwing money at the problem: buy more and faster disks, and the high-end graphics workstations and supercomputers to run them; use the fastest-available communications lines, or wait for new high-bandwidth communications technologies such as (155 Mbps) ATM. Consequently, data compression appears to have a limited role in mid-1990s movie production, as the following examples cited in the literature suggest [Brah95, Karv95, Cumm96]: Videoconferences are held with remote production sites. Overnight dailies, newly-shot footage to be reviewed by the director or other studio personnel, are sent over high-bandwidth communications networks. Compressed files are sent between sites during product development, for instance, when collaborating on changes to animated sequences. Some producers choose to use JPEG or other compression techniques during the development stages of a project, some do not [Coco95]. For those that do, compression reduces the storage needed to play back long animated sequences. Compressed images also speed up processing when testing ideas and concepts. However, once the final product has been determined, it is created from full-resolution digital files that have not been subjected to (lossy) compression, a strategy that is not unreasonable, as the primary means of distribution is high-resolution film.[2]

Video production is a different story. Although analog-based equipment is far from extinct, the availability of low-cost, digital desktop tools that can produce broadcast-quality video is rapidly making video production a cottage industry. Professional broadcasters, corporate video producers, and serious amateurs are turning to UNIX workstations and high-powered PCs for producing television programming, computer animations, educational materials, and interactive video games. These computers can be configured with motion-video capture cards, graphics accelerators, hardware compressor cards, sound cards, CD-ROM recorders, VCR controllers, and just about any piece of gear needed for desktop video production. The software menu is no less extensive with dozens of tools for video editing, animation, and special effects, for audio mixing, and for production. This is a cost-sensitive environment where minimizing storage capacity and bandwidth is important, and data compression is needed throughout all phases of the production process. As the discussion of multimedia PCs made clear (see Section 9.11), there are various proprietary schemes for video (and audio)

---

[2] Digital storage will replace film in future electronic cinemas where video projectors will show high-resolution, HDTV-format movies. Digital-format theatrical releases will be downloaded from satellites or wideband networks, stored, and played back from an on-site video server [Wolf93B].

compression, but they offer less than what is needed for professional or near-professional video production. The key here is to use data compression that can produce images and audio at the quality levels needed for television, meaning that the end product has an acceptable level of visible and audible artifacts. Today, editing and production tools that use M-JPEG are state of the art.

Radio programming, either live or recorded, is transmitted to broadcasters over various terrestrial and satellite links. The digital transmission links that replace their analog predecessors provide lower cost and higher fidelity. Data compression is used for transmitting digital radio programming, not because the data rates are impossibly high but to reduce transmission costs. Transmitting CD-quality stereo requires 1.41 Mbps, well within T-1 line rates (see Table 7.3), but wideband transmission is expensive. Then, too, many radio programs originate from remote locations where only standard phone lines and—just maybe—ISDN lines are available. Examples include the following:

- Radio talk shows from across town or around the world
- Remote live broadcasts of local, national, or global events
- Sending commercials from advertising agencies to radio stations

The production of commercials provides a good illustration of how digital technology (and data compression) has transformed radio programming. Producers once recorded commercials on tape and sent copies to radio stations by courier. Now, with digital technology and data compression, high-quality audio can be sent over standard voice-grade analog or ISDN phone lines, allowing commercials to be sent for much less cost. The transmission is 3–10 times slower than real time, but the added time is of little consequence because radio stations store the commercials—digitally, on computer disk or on MiniDisc, in compressed format—for later playback [Mcco94B]. The same approach is used for distributing the latest song releases, where in about 10 minutes a 3 minute song can be sent over IDSN lines simultaneously to hundreds of radio stations[3] [Dick95B].

As for compression technologies for radio programming, any of the perceptual audio codecs described in Section 5.3 might be appropriate. However, professional broadcasters are concerned with audio quality and the introduction of artifacts, as data compression may be used multiple times in the broadcast chain. (The consequences are described in Section 14.4.) MPEG-1 audio coding (see Table 5.3) is in widespread usage in studio and broadcast equipment audio channels. So, too, are proprietary digital audio codecs from various manufacturers, including AC-2™ [4] (Dolby Laboratories Inc.), APT-X™ (Audio Processing Technology

---

[3] Similar technology is used in television programming. Equipment is available that lets broadcast journalists send compressed videotaped news stories from the field via cellular telephone links [Mcco94C]. One Los Angeles television advertising distributor sends MPEG-2 encoded commercials over T-1 links to area cable system operators [Dick95A].

[4] AC-2 is a predecessor of the Dolby AC-3 multichannel coder described in Section 5.3.

Inc.), SEDAT™ (Scientific Atlanta Inc.), and others [Fors94, PrSo94]. In the interest of audio quality, moderate compression ratios are used, with 3:1–4:1 being typical.

Producing digital audio recordings presents yet another variation on the need for data compression. A recording session once was a simple undertaking. All that was needed was to bring together willing artists, assemble them in front of a microphone, and switch on the recorder. Most assuredly the recording process has grown far more sophisticated over the years with, for example, multiple-track recorders allowing individual instruments or voices to be recorded at different times or places and combined to make the final product. In the 1990s, the concept of a recording session takes on new dimensions, for with high-speed data communications, it is no longer necessary to assemble the artists in a recording studio. They may be located anywhere in the world, far from each other, far from the recording equipment, and linked only by communications lines. As incredulous as this may seem, multisite recording has its place within an industry that must accommodate high-profile artists with busy schedules [AmNe94, Pohl96]. On a more prosaic level, like radio broadcasts, recordings can be compressed and transmitted on communications lines between studio and production facilities.

Distribution

Once, distributing entertainment products meant making a master copy and then, using film printers, tape duplicators, or CD stampers, cranking out copies. It still does, but in today's marketplace distribution is more complex. As Table 11.1 suggests, most entertainment products are distributed on multiple media, and when those media are compressed, extra effort is needed to create the master copies. Here is what must be done: For each distribution medium, a master copy of the entertainment product is needed. Digital data must be converted to the format of the distribution media. For analog distribution media, digital-to-analog conversion is required; digitized movies must be scanned onto film, digitized video must be converted into NTSC, PAL, or SECAM format, and so on. For digital distribution media, the data may already be in the correct format, but with so many distribution media using compression, this is unusual. Each distribution media typically requires its own brand of compression. In Section 10.3, we learned that CD-ROM publishers often select an algorithm from among many, an example that hints at what may be involved. Here is yet another example showing how complicated things can get:

Motion picture films for theaters are printed with an analog stereo optical soundtrack that runs along the edge of the film. Over the years, various schemes have been used to augment the film to provide theaters with multichannel sound; first, analog magnetic soundtracks were added, and, now, digital optical soundtracks are recorded on the film in various formats [Pohl95A]. Figure 11.2 shows how three currently popular multichannel digital formats are squeezed onto 35-mm film along with the analog stereo optical soundtrack.

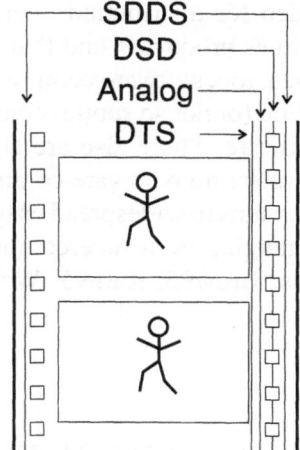

Figure 11.2 35-mm motion picture film format.

Not only is a different track layout used by each of these three multichannel audio systems but each uses a different form of data compression. If film studios choose to distribute multiformat prints, as they have done, their production facilities must be equipped with data compression equipment for each of these algorithms:

- The DTS™ (Digital Theater Systems) track contains a timing code used to synchronize the film with an external CD-ROM drive where six audio channels are stored in compressed format. The proprietary Coherent Acoustics™ coding algorithm compresses CD-quality audio data by 3:1, using 240 Kbps for each channel, for a total data rate of 1.44 Mbps [Mitc95, Taki95B].
- The DSD™ (Dolby Stereo Digital) track contains six AC-3 encoded CD-quality audio channels compressed to a total data rate of 320 Kbps. (Dolby AC-3 is discussed in Section 5.3.)
- The SDDS™ (Sony Dynamic Digital Sound) tracks contain eight ATRAC-encoded CD-quality audio channels. ATRAC, originally developed for MiniDisc, provides a 5:1 compression ratio. (See Sections 5.3 and 9.2.)

As for the data compression equipment needed when preparing an entertainment product for distribution, both hardware and software solutions abound, especially for video. Dedicated hardware is essentially the only practical solution for real-time video stream compression. Reasonably priced dedicated hardware compressors are available for most popular algorithms. A good example is MPEG video compressors. In 1993, MPEG hardware encoders were scarce commodities at any price. By 1995, silicon manufactures had jumped on the MPEG bandwagon and prices fell dramatically; PC-priced MPEG-1 encoder boards were available, with MPEG-2 encoders soon to follow. However, real-time operation is not a necessity when preparing video for distribution, merely a convenience (unless it is a live broadcast). Sometimes producers find that software compression is a more economical solution. Then, too, software compression can be more effective in that software can do the subtle (or not so subtle) compression operations which may not be affordable in hardware. There also are algorithms, too complex, or too uncommon, for which there are no hardware compressors. For these reasons, software video compression remains in widespread usage within the entertainment industry, running on systems ranging from supercomputers and high-end parallel processors to PC workstations [Brow95, Karn95, Wolf95C].

11.3   Media Archiving

Media archives for movies, television and radio programs, audio recordings, and video games fulfill several important roles in the entertainment industry: During the production cycle, short-term archives provide a repository for work in progress. This data is also used to create master copies for distribution. Now, with the entertainment, computer, and communications industries choosing to join forces, a different type of archive is emerging—audio and video servers. These specialized computers provide the repository for entertainment products to be distributed online. Media producers also maintain vintage material in long-term archives and use it in many different ways. For instance, they may incorporate stock scene footage or an old newsreel clip in a new film; or they may pull an old film or audio recording from their vaults (archives) and rerelease it. Not only is there historic value, but the entertainment industry realizes significant revenue from recycling its archived materials.

Not incidentally, counterparts to all these archiving applications are found in the (electronic) publishing industry. The primary difference is that entertainment archives are more complex, often storing a mixture of data types—audio and (film) images, audio and video, and sometimes text too. As in publishing, entertainment organizations must store data in varying formats, sampled at various rates or resolutions, and compressed as needed to meet differing application needs. The question is, What kind of data compression can safely be used for archiving?

From discussions earlier in this chapter, it is obvious that short-term, production-cycle archives must contain audio, images, and video of uncompromising quality. Either data must be uncompressed or, if compressed, only lossless compression or mild forms of lossy compression can be used. From discussions in earlier chapters, it is clear what type of compression is appropriate for audio and video servers; namely, data must be stored on the server in the compressed formats that broadcast and network standards dictate, MPEG-2, for example.

The compression issues for long-term archives are more complicated. To begin with, the amount of material that entertainment companies would like to store in long-term digital archives is huge. They have vaults filled with old movies and newsreels, warehouses filled with tapes of old television and radio programs, and vast catalogs of vintage 78 RPM and vinyl audio recordings. Despite the expense, entertainment companies are motivated to convert their existing archives to digital because all of this material resides on bulky, deteriorating analog media that are not terribly accessible or searchable—limitations which digital archiving on dense, durable media such as optical discs can undo. But transferring old material from analog media into a digital archive poses problems too. Decisions (read mistakes) made during the transfer process cannot be undone if the analog media is no more, either being lost through deterioration or by deliberate destruction. Essentially the same issues must be dealt with when newly produced digital media is to be archived: What scanning resolution and pixel depth should be used for (movie or video) images? What sampling rate and how many bits per sample should be used for audio? If the digital data will be compressed with a lossy algorithm, which algorithm should be used and how lossy should it be?

From a historical standpoint, everything should be saved at the highest quality appropriate for the analog (or digital) media and with absolutely no loss of information. From an economics standpoint, this may be impractical. There are no easy answers, and certainly none that fit all situations. A range of practical solutions has emerged, mostly based on the expected future uses for the archived material and the volume of material. For example, some 60 million feet of old Fox Movietone News™ newsreels (more than 11,000 hours running time) have been transferred to digital tape [BrCa93, Brah95]. The black-and-white images were scanned at a relatively low resolution of 1024 × 1024 pixels (using an anamorphic lens to translate the rectangular film image into a square). Despite the enormous volumes of data generated, no data compression was used in deference to possible future uses for this material. Recording companies have large collections too; they are digitizing their catalogs of analog material at CD-quality levels and storing them with no data compression in anticipation of future signal processing techniques that may become available to improve sound quality [Fost94].

Nevertheless, lossless data compression is a tool that long-term archivers need to consider. With absolutely no quality compromises, lossless compression can reduce the amount of archival storage with significant impact on archiving costs: Lossless JPEG compresses images by typically 2 times [Penn93]. Lossless M-JPEG will do the same for video. Huffman or dictionary algorithms compress audio by up to 1.5 times [Nels92], and they can compress text and graphics by even larger factors (as shown in Figure 4.6).

If lossy compression is used for archiving, it is important to recognize that not all lossy algorithms and their encoders are created equal; that is, a lossy algorithm which is right for data transmission may not be the one to use for archiving. Here, one may willingly choose to sacrifice compression ratio for quality. Some lossy algorithms allow their encoding parameters to be adjusted and trade-offs to be made between quality and compression ratio. With some algorithms, more investment in encoding complexity and time makes higher-quality possible at any compression ratio. An example is provided in the MPEG audio algorithm which allows more complex psychoacoustic models for high-quality lossy archiving [Pan95]. Similar trade-offs in encoder complexity are found in MPEG video encoders [Schä95].

11.4 Summary

This chapter examined entertainment applications where data compression can be used for efficient data storage and for reducing transmission bandwidth. We learned the following:

- The entertainment industry is rapidly adopting digital electronic media for production and for distribution.
- Media producers must manage very large data files. Concerns for product quality limit the applications for (lossy) data compression during the production cycle.
- Media distributors make extensive use of all forms of data compression for reducing the volume of data to be transmitted or stored.
- Media distributors must use various compression algorithms for different distribution media.
- Preparing an entertainment product for distribution need not be a real-time operation. Hardware encoders are used when available, but software provides more flexibility and opportunity for optimization.
- Media archives fulfill important roles in the entertainment industry: They act as the repositories for data during production and for entertainment products to be distributed online from media servers. They also provide long-term storage for vintage films, recordings, and other entertainment materials.
- The use of lossy compression for archived data must be carefully considered, weighing the savings in storage against possible loss of irretrievable information.

12

Healthcare Applications

In this chapter, we examine healthcare industry applications for which data compression is used for efficient data storage and to reduce transmission time. Both lossless and lossy compression are used to support complex electronic data management systems in an industry with exacting legal requirements and regulatory policies.

12.1 Industry Overview

Physicians have always depended on gathering information about their patients and using it for diagnosis, treatment, and cure of disease. They still do, and now much of that information is electronic. All forms of electronic information—text, sound, images, and video—are indispensable to the practice of modern medicine. Today's physicians not only gather information; they must share it too. In an era when medical institutions are growing larger, physicians rarely work alone. Often they must consult with fellow practitioners on the most effective forms of treatment, and as medical institutions are becoming geographically dispersed, more often than not their colleagues are far away. These practices demand effective, efficient digital data handling and communications. As in many other industries, whose primary businesses are neither, computers and communications are indispensable to healthcare. Their role in healthcare administration and management is well defined but, perhaps, overshadowed by their role in diagnosis and treatment. Here, computers and communications along with other electronic technologies come together in complex distributed systems for capturing, storing, communicating, and using electronic patient data. Now, as the U.S. healthcare system reorganizes and restructures itself to manage and contain healthcare costs, efficient storage and communication of electronic medical information is even more crucial. This chapter will explore the part that data compression plays in accomplishing this for medical imaging systems, an increasingly important healthcare tool.

Data compression allows high-resolution digitized medical images to be handled efficiently. These images are gathered by a variety of imaging modalities during patient exams. They must be accurately captured and, often, transmitted over great distances to the physicians who are most qualified to interpret the displayed images and provide accurate diagnoses. Medical images must be stored for many years according to stringent legal requirements and regulatory policies that govern the healthcare industry.

Standards for all aspects of medical imaging are extremely important, particularly communications standards that allow interoperation of equipment from various manufacturers. The healthcare industry has adopted a standard file format for medical images that specifies the algorithms which may be used for encapsulating and communicating compressed images. Lossless compression is used for archiving images, mainly because the medical community recognizes it as a safe choice, raising no quality or legal concerns. The issues surrounding the use of lossy compression for archiving are still under consideration.

12.2   Medical Imaging Systems

Digital images are increasingly important in medicine. Not only have digital image processing and enhancement provided new tools for extracting useful forms of diagnostic information, and continue to do so, but digital imagery is more efficient. Over the past years, various digital image collection, processing, transmission, and archiving systems have been developed for medical applications. Although initially applied to radiology and pathology (only radiology applications will be described in this chapter), the same technology is now used in other areas of medicine too. Radiological medical imaging devices use some form of energy to stimulate a patient's tissues and, by measuring the interaction, construct an image that gives information for diagnosing diseases and injuries. Conventional (projection) X-rays, the oldest form of radiological imaging, still are used in about 70–75% of the radiological examinations in the United States. The remaining radiological examinations use newer methods, including computed tomography (CT), magnetic resonance imaging (MRI), ultrasonography (US), digital subtraction angiography (DSA), and digital fluorography (DF), and several nuclear medicine techniques, including positron emission tomography (PET) and single photon emission computerized tomography (SPECT) [Chim92, Wong95]. These newer radiological methods capture images in digital form and then produce images on film. X-ray images can also be captured directly in digital form by computed radiography (CR) techniques. However, most X-ray images are still captured on film, and, therefore, these X-ray images must be scanned and digitized if digital format is required.

The healthcare industry spends huge sums to create, track, and store image data gathered during patient examinations. Traditionally, images for a radiological study are captured by a diagnostic imager (called an imaging modality) that produces a film which then must be developed. A radiologist analyzes the film and produces a diagnostic report. The film and report are then routed throughout the medical institution during treatment of the patient. At some point in time, both the film and report, along with other records created during treatment, will be archived. There are legal requirements for retaining medical information, usually for 3–7 years but in some instances up to 30 years [Dall90], and patient follow-up and medical research makes an archive indispensable. Medical records archives are both necessary and important, but they are expensive. Each year throughout the world, new warehouses are built just to hold patient records, and evermore people are needed to manage them. In some cases, it is true that long-established but people-intensive procedures for handling medical records have served well. But medical institutions, straining under the task of managing a growing deluge of film and paper, desperately need a lower-cost solution in keeping with the emphasis on improving the efficiency of the healthcare system.

Digital imaging contributes to that solution, as do computers and communications networks. Computers and communications networks can store, retrieve, and route digital images (or any other digitized diagnostic data) much more quickly and efficiently than people handling film and paper could ever hope to do, and with less chance of losing a patient's records. Digitized images can be handled in the same way that patient tracking, scheduling, and billing are now handled— by computers connected in medical institution-wide networks. The key to making this happen is an image management and communications system (IMACS) that accepts pictures or images in digital form, with associated text, and then distributes them over a network [Trev92].

Using computer and communications technology for handling medical images is hardly a new idea. In the mid-1960s, universities and some medical institutions began developing bits and pieces for what was called a picture-archiving and communications system (PACS). Worldwide, many major medical institutions began installing PACS prototypes in the 1980s.[1] Finding digital technology adequate for dealing with medical images and integrating PACS into the procedures and work flow of medical institutions proved challenging. After many years of development, PACS technology is now part of integrated solutions—IMACS— that are now being put into clinical operation. Design issues include the following:

- Digitized medical images consume vast amounts of storage and transmission times are long. A two-dimensional gray-scale radiological image may contain up to 4K

---

[1] Information on design, development, and PACS installations can be found in the *Proceeding on Medical Imaging: PACS Design and Evaluation*, edited by R. G. Jost et al., an annual publication of SPIE, and in [Valk92]

× 5K, 12-bit pixels. A single image consumes up to 40 MB of storage. Depending on network speed, its transmission time may be seconds, minutes, or even hours.

- Newly captured medical images must be available for display within seconds, and doctors often need to view several images simultaneously.
- The spatial resolution and pixel depth (number of gray levels) of medical images is often higher than what conventional computer displays can handle.
- Users within the medical community have differing requirements for image quality. Radiologists doing primary diagnosis require the image be displayed at its maximum resolution, whereas other users may make do with lower resolution and more economical displays.
- Image processing, such as data compression that introduces artifacts—details not present in the original image—is unacceptable if there is any chance the radiologists' diagnosis might be affected.
- The networks connecting IMACS components must handle text and multiple image types (and sometimes voice and video for consultations).
- A diversity of products must be integrated to build an IMACS. The installed base of medical imaging modalities requires special attention. Many imaging modalities are designed to deliver digital pictures only to film printers, not to computer displays, and, lacking standards, their digital outputs often are encoded in proprietary formats.
- A suitable replacement for film-based X-ray imaging modalities must be found to complete the transition to a "filmless" medical institution.
- Tens of gigabytes of images are collected each day at large medical institutions. This data must be available for immediate viewing and archived for long-term storage.

Except for conventional film X-rays, collecting digital medical images is usually not too difficult because imaging modalities have adequate local memory and dedicated hardware to efficiently acquire images and most have digital outputs.[2] The critical issues for IMACS are how to economically archive images and to transmit and display the archived images promptly when requested. Data compression is a key piece of the solution.

12.3 IMACS Operation

To understand how an IMACS operates, consider the model system shown in Figure 12.1. The components of an IMACS are tied together by networks. LANs provide links within a site. WANs provide links to the remote sites of a medical institution or provide links to different institutions for teleradiology consultation.

---

[2] No digital technology has yet been found to completely replace X-ray film. Computed radiography (CR), in which X-rays impinge on an imaging plate instead of film, is the most likely candidate. But CR imaging modalities currently provide, at best, only half the spatial resolution of those using film (which, in many cases, is compensated for by greater contrast resolution). The other choice is a film digitizer, but this does not eliminate the need for film. Among various types of film digitizers, the laser scanning digitizer is best able to preserve the resolution of the original film images.

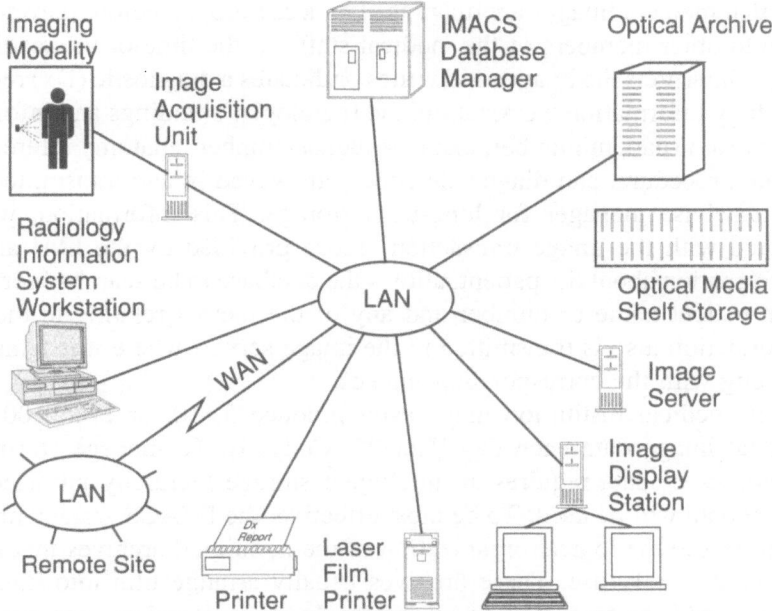

Figure 12.1 An Image management and communications system.

An IMACS database manager computer provides overall management of the IMACS, including the work flow, the data, and the devices connected to the network.

IMACS components perform the following functions: Imaging modalities capture, process, store, and display digital medical images, and most imaging modalities can make film copies. Imaging modalities are complex systems that make extensive use of signal processing technology to create viewable medical images. This includes image transformation and quantization techniques, which are compression methods in themselves, but that is another story. Our concern is with how the digital medical images that imaging modalities do create are stored, transmitted, and viewed within medical institutions. The first step is obtaining the images from the imaging modalities. The digital output of an imaging modality is interfaced to the IMACS by a gateway processor that we will call an image acquisition unit (IAU). There are many different types of imaging modalities. For each imaging modality, an IAU must be programmed to capture its image data, convert the data to a standard file format for archiving (for example, the ACR/NEMA DICOM V3.0 standard file format for medical images [NEMA94]), and transmit the data on the IMACS network. The IAU sends image data to the optical archive, where it is permanently stored, and to an image server for temporary storage. When the images have been successfully stored, the IAU forwards a record of these transactions to the IMACS database manager.

Besides images, an IMACS also must capture diagnostic reports. It is standard practice that medical images are diagnosed by a radiologist before they are made available to other members of the medical staff. At the time of the reading, the radiologist interprets the images and writes or dictates a diagnostic (Dx) report. At the radiology information workstation, the radiologist's findings and information about the exam (patient number, exam sequence number, anatomy reference and indication, procedure, and diagnostic codes) are keyed in and transmitted to the IMACS database manager for long-term storage. This information, which is coordinated with the image transaction record provided by the IAU and with other information about the patient, allows the database to be searched for images based on patient name or number and any of the factors relating to the exam. This information also is transmitted to the image server, where it is temporarily stored along with the corresponding images.

A large medical institution may easily produce 5, 10, or even 100 GB of radiological image data each day [Keiz92, Cody93]. To manage storing such large amounts of data requires an intelligent storage hierarchy knowledgeable of how the data will be used. To be most effective, the IMACS storage hierarchy must conform to the logical organization of the nondigital archives that medical institutions currently use. These archives usually arrange film into immediate, short-term, and long-term storage categories. In clinical applications, newly collected images must be available for diagnosis and review within a few seconds whenever a user at an image display station keys a request. In our model IMACS, these images are stored on image servers that use fast magnetic disks to cache the images for active patients, those whose treatment is in process. The images stored on the image servers must be continually replaced with newer images because storage is limited. After a few hours, days, or weeks have passed and a replaced image is needed, as it may be when the patient returns for additional treatment, it must be fetched from the optical archive. Data stored on optical jukeboxes can be retrieved in a few tens of seconds. In situations where the need can be anticipated, images can be prefetched, and optical jukebox access time is not an issue. Optical jukeboxes can contain several hundred gigabytes of data, but they cannot hold all the image data collected over time. Thus, images for inactive patient histories must be moved to long-term shelf storage, only to return to the optical jukebox when the patient checks in again or when the archive is used for historical research and teaching purposes. (Obviously, retrieving images from shelf storage takes much longer.)

Medical images and diagnostic reports are viewed on image display stations, and images are printed on laser film printers, whereas diagnostic reports are printed on conventional printers. Images stored in the IMACS database may also be viewed at imaging modalities, and, if requested, an IAU may retrieve images from the optical archive and send them back to the imaging modality it serves. Image display stations are high-powered workstations that drive large, high-resolution displays. For primary diagnosis, 19-inch screens with $2K \times 2.5K$ pixels at 8 bits/pixel, or greater, are typical. The workstation must have sufficient processing power, local memory, and disk storage to allow rapidly switching between and displaying the images and diagnostic report associated with a patient exam. Image display stations used by radiologists for making primary diagnoses require two or more displays, whereas those used by clinicians for reviewing images may need only one display. When images and the accompanying diagnostic report are to be viewed, they are obtained from the image server. The images must be formatted before they can be viewed. This process is more complicated than it might seem, because image display stations have resolution and pixel-depth capabilities (number of bits per pixel) that are less than the archived data format.[3] Similarly, should the user request printing the images, they too must be formatted to meet the differing capabilities of printing devices. Image formatting is a function that can be done either by the image server or by intelligent image display stations. Where it is done in our model IMACS, and the reasons for choosing one or the other, will become clear shortly.

12.4 The Role of Data Compression in IMACS

Data compression is a critical factor for success if IMACS is ever to fully replace film-based medical imaging. Because compressed images use fewer bits, they are less expensive to store and they can be transmitted more rapidly. This increases the appeal of IMACS by lowering storage and transmission costs and shortening response times. However, many early PACS prototypes operated successfully without compression, basically because they only handled small images produced by the "digital" imaging modalities such as CT and MRI (comprising but a fraction of the total opportunity). This all changes when IMACS must handle the full range of medical images. To appreciate why, consider Table 12.1, which provides typical sizes and transmission times for all types of uncompressed digitized medical images. The storage required for large images is a critical issue, obviously, because X-ray images comprise about 70–75% of the opportunity. Even more critical is the transmission time for large images, which is far too long for high-performance interactive image viewing, whether across a local LAN or across a WAN. For applications where images must be sent over telephone lines—in particular, on-call teleradiology, a leading-edge application—the transmission time for images of any size but the smallest is completely unreasonable.

Figure 12.2 shows the work flow for medical images in our model IMACS. The most effective way to use data compression in this application is to always store compressed images and, whenever possible, eliminate uncompressed image

---

[3] Image data is always archived at the spatial resolution and pixel depth provided by the imaging modality. For instance, if 6-, 8-, 10-, or 12-bit data is collected, it will be archived that way (with each pixel stored as 8 or 16 bits if uncompressed). Image displays usually cannot deliver more than 256 gray levels, requiring window adjustment to select 8 bits from each pixel for presentation. If the display's spatial resolution is less than that of the image, decimation or zooming must be done to select part of the image for display.

Table 12.1   Uncompressed radiological image sizes and transmission times.

Imaging Modality [1]	Image Spatial Resolution and Pixel Depth [2] (Typical)	Images per Exam [3] (Typical)	Storage for Exam Results [4] (MB)	Minimum Transmission Time for Exam Results [5]		
				LAN @ 10 Mbps	WAN @ 1.5 Mbps	ISDN @ 128 Kbps
CT	512 x 512 x 12	30	15.7	12.6 sec	83.9 sec	16.4 min
MRI	256 x 256 x 12	50	6.6	5.2 sec	35 sec	6.8 min
US	512 x 512 x 6	36	9.4	7.5 sec	50.3 sec	9.8 min
DSA	1024 x 1024 x 8	20	21	16.8 sec	111.8 sec	21.8 min
DF	1024 x 1024 x 8	15	15.7	12.6 sec	83.9 sec	16.4 min
SPECT	128 x 128 x 16	50	1.6	1.3 sec	8.7 sec	1.7 min
PET	128 x 128 x 16	62	2	1.6 sec	10.8 sec	2.1 min
CR	2048 x 2560 x 10	4	41.9	33.6 sec	223.7 sec	43.7 min
X-ray[6]	4096 x 5120 x 12	4	167.8	134.2 sec	894.8 sec	174.8 min

Notes:
[1] CT = computed tomography, MRI = magnetic resonance imaging, US = ultrasonography, DSA = digital subtractive angiography, DF = digital fluorography, SPECT = single photon emission computerized tomography, PET = positron emission tomography, CR = computed radiography.
[2] Resolution and pixel depth = pixels x pixels x bits/pixel.
[3] Sources for image sizes and number of images per exam include [Chim92, Cody93, Wong95].
[4] Imaging modalities output 6-bit and 8-bit pixels stored as 8 bits; 10-bit and 12-bit pixels stored as 16 bits.
[5] Timings assume the data transfer protocol is 100% efficient and there is no delay time waiting for the line to become available. Actual data rate on LANs may range from much lower to somewhat higher than 10 Mbps. On WANs, the data rate may be much lower than 1.5-Mbps T-1 link rates, whereas new WANs such as ATM operating at 155 Mbps will provide much higher data rates.
[6] Digitized 14-in. x 17-in. film.

traffic from the IMACS network. This requires that compression be located close to the image sources and decompression close to the displays and printers. The result: Storage is reduced by a factor equal to the compression ratio, as is network traffic. Doing compression and decompression at the locations suggested in Figure 12.2 accomplishes this goal. A few words of explanation will help to clarify our choices: Image display stations are assumed to have sufficient power to decompress data. If not, the decompression function moves back to the image server and the uncompressed network traffic increases. Printers cannot accept compressed medical images, even though some can accept compressed text. Therefore, Figure 12.2 shows decompression for image printers in the image server.

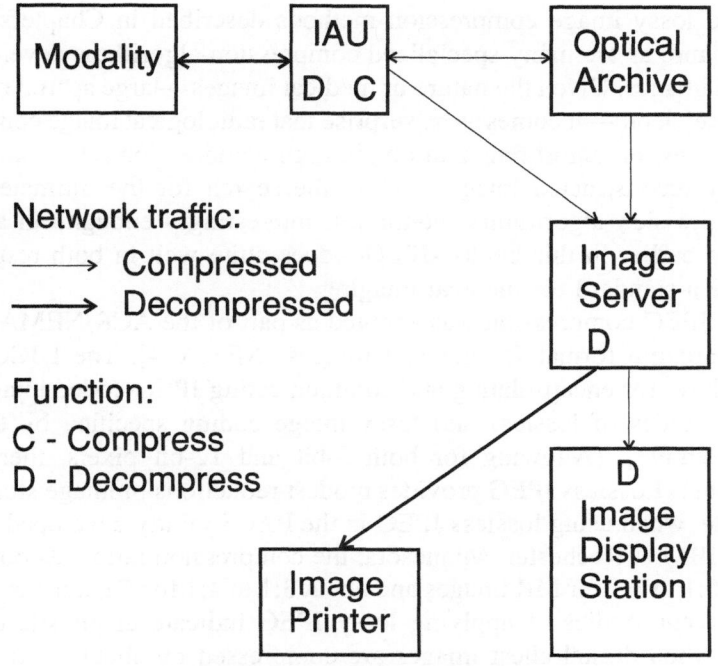

Figure 12.2 IMACS work flow.

12.5 IMACS Compression Issues

What type of data compression is appropriate for IMACS applications—lossless or lossy? The fundamental consideration is the physician's diagnostic capability; storing images in an IMACS must not degrade the radiologist's ability to read those images. In technology terms, it means that data compression cannot introduce image artifacts, or if it does, those artifacts must not contribute to an incorrect diagnosis. Consequently, only lossless compression is now used in clinical practice for images that are to be read by a radiologist. The reason that lossy compression is not being used is that it raises new legal and regulatory issues with which manufacturers, the healthcare industry, and the regulatory agencies are still struggling. We will say more about this in a moment. However, lossy compression is being used for medical image archives not intended for primary diagnosis—those images that have been read by a radiologist and are stored for reference purposes, or images used for teaching and medical research, for example.

Which compression algorithms are appropriate for medical images? Essentially, they *all* are, at least one might believe this is true judging from the wide variety of algorithms described in medical image literature references. A survey of medical imaging compression techniques appears in [Wong95]. All of the lossless and lossy image compression methods described in Chapters 4 and 5 are to be found, as are many specialized compression algorithms developed just for medical images. Given the nature of medical images—large spatial resolution and high pixel depth—it comes as no surprise that radiological image compression research focuses on algorithms that obtain high compression ratios and provide high-quality reconstructed images. While the search for the ultimate medical image compression algorithm(s) continues, interestingly enough, an algorithm encountered earlier in this book—JPEG—does quite well in both respects and has become a standard for medical imaging.

In 1993, JPEG compression was adopted as part of the ACR/NEMA DICOM V3.0 standard file format for medical images [NEMA94]. The DICOM V3.0 standard allows for encapsulating and communicating JPEG-coded images using any of the modes of lossless and lossy image coding specified by the JPEG standard [Penn93]. (Allowing for both 8-bit and 12-bit pixels, there are 29 combinations!) Lossless JPEG provides modest reductions in image storage size. For example, when using lossless JPEG in the PACS jointly developed by Mayo Clinic and IBM at Rochester, Minnesota, the compression ratio was observed to be about 2.5:1 to 3:1 for MR images and about 3:1 to 4:1 for CT images [Hang94, Pers94]. Recent studies of applying lossy JPEG indicate diagnostic quality is acceptable when digital chest images are compressed by about 10:1; for other types of medical images, compression ratios up to 20:1 cause no demonstrably statistically significant difference in diagnostic accuracy, whereas compression ratios up to 50:1 produce subtle loss in image quality [Wong95].

Another consideration gives JPEG the nod for medical imaging—it is robust and can deal with errors. Reliability is critical in medical systems; when digital image data is stored or transmitted, consideration must be given to the effect of errors and to means for error recovery. A bit of digital system design philosophy: Errors do occur in *all* digital data storage and transmission systems. Error-detection and error-correction techniques reduce the presence of errors in user data to *extremely* low levels. Granted, a well-designed digital system will allow only 1 in 10^x data bits to slip through uncorrected, but some do slip through, a fact that often is overlooked. The loss or alteration of a data bit might be lightly dismissed in some applications but not in medical imaging, particularly not when data compression is used.

The medical community has undertaken extensive studies to understand how data loss or alteration during storage or transmission affects the quality of compressed medical images [Pron91]. What they found is that all compression algorithms—both lossless and lossy—operating in the presence of errors affect image quality, some more than others. In these studies, the lossless algorithms described in Chapter 4 were especially hard-hit by the loss or corruption of a single bit, which sometimes corrupted an entire image. This is not surprising, because, as discussed earlier, these algorithms expect to operate in an error-free environment. JPEG stood up much better in that a single bit error within an 8×8 image block did not propagate outside the block, a situation much more acceptable for medical images. This is no accident, for JPEG designers included what they called restart markers in the JPEG data stream [Penn93]. These markers divide the compressed data stream into entropy-coded segments (the image data) and marker segments. The marker segments are uniquely decodable and allow a JPEG decoder to (optionally) implement error-recovery procedures that can localize the effects of an error to as little as a single 8×8 block.

There are unresolved problems with using data compression for medical images, problems that involve the stringent legal requirements and regulatory policies which govern the healthcare industry. Legal requirements relate to malpractice, and regulatory policies relate to the safety and quality of medical devices, including those that incorporate data compression. Lossless compression does not raise any legal issues. However, it provides only a modest reduction in image storage size, and it cannot solve the image transmission time problem for teleradiology. Lossy compression can do much better, but the question is, Can it be safely used for primary diagnosis? When medical images are subjected to lossy compression, radiologists, always aware of possible malpractice suits, must assure themselves that whatever loss of fine detail or subtle information may occur will not lead to incorrect diagnosis or interpretation. This is not a simple task, and, today, the lossy compression issue is far from being resolved. Not only are there different types of medical images, but there are a variety of diagnostic radiological tasks. Also, the acceptable degree of compression is task dependent, as learned from clinical validation tests in which radiologists subject compressed images to analysis by classical ROC (receiver operating characteristic) curves and other methods for evaluating image quality.[4] The acceptability of lossy compression poses problems for equipment manufacturers and regulators, too, but today the burden of proof falls on the medical community. The United States Food and Drug Administration (FDA) requires manufacturers of equipment that incorporates lossy data compression to explain its effects on image quality in their user manuals. Images obtained with this equipment must carry a statement that lossy compression was used and indicate the approximate compression ratio [Wong95]. Most of the IMACS products submitted to the FDA for marketing clearance contain compression [Zare93]. Although some contain lossy compression, one can expect the medical community to move slowly and carefully on incorporating lossy compression in IMACS intended for clinical practice.

In summary, to net out the impact of data compression in IMACS, lossless data compression today reduces the storage and transmission burden by 2–4 times. In the future, if legal and regulatory issues can be resolved, lossy compression will increase this to 10 times, or more. However, although it contributes to effective

---

[4] ROC is a method for evaluating the performance of a diagnostic imaging system [Cox92]. It allows the diagnostic accuracy radiologists achieve when using the system to be compared to a reference system. Neither this nor any other method presently available is able to fully characterize compression losses in radiological images [Wong95].

IMACS design, this amount of compression cannot wholly eliminate the time delay for moving large images across slow networks. Image management techniques such as prefetching and caching, and faster networks will continue to be needed.

12.6 Summary

This chapter examined medical imaging systems, a healthcare industry application where data compression is used for efficient data storage and for reducing transmission time. We learned the following:

- The healthcare industry increasingly relies on computers and communications and collecting electronic data for diagnosis and patient treatment.
- Efficient storage and communication of electronic medical images are crucial to cost-effective healthcare.
- Image management and communications system (IMACS) are being integrated into clinical practice. These distributed computing systems manage large collections of digitized medical images and related patient data.
- Digital medical images are large. They must be compressed to reduce storage costs and to shorten transmission time.
- For data compression to be most effective, images must be compressed immediately after they are captured and decompressed only when they are displayed or printed.
- The medical community has conducted extensive research on compression algorithms for medical images. High compression ratios, high-quality reconstructed images, and robust handling of image-corrupting errors during storage and transmission are important factors. JPEG deals with all these factors.
- JPEG compression has been adopted as part of the ACR/NEMA DICOM V3.0 standard file format for medical images. All lossless and lossy image coding modes specified by the JPEG standard are allowed.
- Lossless image compression is now widely used in clinical practice; the use of lossy compression is mostly restricted to medical image archives.
- The effects of using lossy compression for images that are to be read by a radiologist continue to be studied.

Part IV—Digital Systems

This part of the book is devoted to the integration of data compression in digital systems.

Chapter 13 discusses the decisions digital system designers face when integrating data compression. The chapter begins with design processes and guidelines for deciding whether to use data compression. Then key criteria are provided for selecting a compression algorithm and an implementation technique. The chapter concludes with a discussion of choosing locations for compression and decompression within the system dataflow.

Chapter 14 examines issues relating to managing compressed data. Techniques for handling compressed data in open systems and error-prone environments lead off the chapter. Then the interaction of compression with other system functions is examined. This is followed by an extensive investigation of both good and bad interactions between compression algorithms. Next, techniques for directly processing compressed data without first decompressing it are presented. The chapter concludes with a discussion of archiving compressed data.

Chapter 15 provides a look at data compression in future digital systems. It begins with a summary of trends and directions observed in earlier parts of the book. Then it examines future applications, technology, and marketplace conditions. The chapter and book are concluded with an examination of trends for future data compression algorithms and their implementation.

13

Digital System Design

In Part III of this book, we discovered that many applications and digital systems take advantage of data compression, be it for storage savings, bandwidth reduction, or transmission time savings. Incorporating data compression in a digital system requires careful design to assure it will provide the intended benefits and operate harmoniously with other system functions. In this chapter, we introduce decisions that designers face when choosing to integrate data compression in their digital systems.

Digital systems of varying complexity have been encountered throughout this book. From a physical perspective, there are simple self-contained systems, such as consumer products. There are more complex systems composed of several components, such as computer systems, and there are distributed systems, really a system of many interconnected systems. Table 13.1 provides some examples. Whatever the case, the design process starts (or should start) with the marketplace. Inputs from the marketplace define the need for data compression, if there is one. Marketplace requirements are the foundation for generating system requirements and specifications. They essentially establish the constraints and framework within which system designers must work, including the type of data compression that is acceptable and its impact on and visibility to end users.

Designing a digital system involves making trade-offs. System designers must wrestle with many factors. These include architectural considerations and compatibility with prior implementations for similar products. Also, software and hardware design, size, and packaging considerations. Then there are system performance requirements, application functional requirements, product cost considerations, and the list goes on. When data compression is part of the solution, system designers must first understand the problems it addresses, followed by a

Table 13.1 Digital systems.

Type	Structure	Examples
Simple	Self-containing product	Audio tape player Set-top box Digital camera Multifunction office machine
Complex	Multiple components	Desktop computer Multimedia server
Distributed	Interconnected systems	Radio or television broadcast chain Data communications network Telephone network

close inspection of the wake of interactions created by its introduction. These include additional hardware and software complexities, conflicts with other system functions, requirements for data interchange, and data quality compromises to name a few.

13.1 Data Compression—Do You Need It?

Essentially, the most important question that system designers can ask about data compression is whether it is needed. Are there alternatives that will address the storage, bandwidth, or transmission time reduction it provides—more simply, more economically, or with less disruption? That is, are there, in some sense, better alternatives? Surprisingly (at least in a book dedicated to promoting data compression), sometimes there are. Let us begin with some of the best reasons for using data compression:

- Standards call for data compression
- Competitive products use data compression
- The system cannot operate without data compression
- System specifications are improved
- System cost is reduced

Sometimes the marketplace dictates that data compression must be used; sometimes it does not. Interoperability with a standard that includes data compression leaves system designers no alternative. Going head-to-head in the marketplace with products that use data compression—and advertise it as an advantage—is almost as compelling a reason. Also, sometimes storage and transmission technology limits are unyielding, and data compression is the only practical solution. This is most evident among current applications where communications bandwidth is insufficient, or outrageously expensive. Then there are the gray areas—the cases where data compression is an option, one that may lead to competitive advantages. For instance, it may provide greater capacity, higher data rates, or more through-put; or it may simply reduce cost, providing yet another form of competitive advantage.

When data compression is an option, not a requirement, system designers must weigh its advantages, balancing them against the effect it has on other system functions and the complexity it adds to system design. In working through this process, a list of reasons for *not* using data compression may emerge. That list might include the following:

- More difficult-to-explain system operations and more complex user interfaces
- More complex hardware and software designs due to variable storage sizes, variable data rates, and the need for buffering
- More processing time and/or more VLSI circuitry
- Longer delay times for real-time data operations
- Increased sensitivity to storage and transmission errors
- More complex data recovery with or without errors

With lossy compression algorithms the list grows longer. Two important reasons not to use lossy compression are as follows:

- Loss of audio, image, and video quality
- Loss of VCR-like functions (random accessibility) for video data

Clearly, many very successful products have dealt with all these issues, but they paid a price, for data compression rarely is free. When data compression is optional, system designers sometimes may find it more cost-effective or satisfactory not to use compression, but to add the extra storage or buy the additional bandwidth it would save. Each situation must be carefully analyzed.

13.2   Selecting an Algorithm

Once a genuine need for data compression is established, system designers face the task of selecting a compression algorithm and adapting it to their application. Increasingly, the particular algorithm for an application is predetermined by prevailing official or de facto standards. In any event, system designers must still make implementation trade-offs, trade-offs that can affect the compression ratio and many other factors which determine how the algorithm will operate. Data compression algorithms frequently are compared just on compression ratio. Compression ratio is important, but a more thorough characterization includes the factors listed in Table 13.2, all of which are considered in this section.

Table 13.2 Compression algorithm characteristics.

Factor	Importance
Compression ratio	Determines storage and bandwidth required
Adherence to standards	Key to widespread adoption of an algorithm
Algorithm complexity, speed, and processing delay	Determines implementation, cost-performance, and application acceptability
Adaptive versus nonadaptive	Key to supporting applications characteristics and needs
Adaptivity and robustness	Defines allowable input data variations
Error tolerance	Key to success in error-prone environments
Encoder/decoder asymmetry	Key to supporting application communications style
Quality	Defines the acceptability of lossy compression
Multiple-coding limitations	Key to repeated usage of lossy compression
Scalability	Required for differing video display resolutions
Progressive resolution	Required for progressive image transmission at various resolutions
Operating bit rate	Defines acceptable range of data transmission speeds
Added function	Key to more application-friendly compression

Compression ratio

Since compressing data is what this is all about, one would think higher compression ratios are always better, but that is not so. As a rule, getting more compression means making bigger investments in algorithm complexity, processing power, and time. However, these trade-offs have limits: If the compression is lossless, the gains in compression and the added investment costs become marginal as the point is reached where all redundancy has been removed. When the compression is lossy, more compression means more information loss, which nearly always leads to lower-quality results. The most practical approach is to shoot for the minimum compression ratio needed, balancing system storage and bandwidth limits and making adjustments when it is not feasible or acceptable to do it all with compression.

Adherence to standards

Standards for data compression algorithms and their importance are focal points of this book. They exist and many applications demand they be used. Nevertheless, the existence of a standard does not rule out innovative implementations. Many standards for data compression algorithms really are nothing more than frameworks that describe the encoded bit stream and how it is to be transmitted between the encoder and decoder. Many examples throughout the book show that system designers are free to follow different paths in creating and sometimes in decoding those bit streams. They may choose to simplify the encoding process in the name of cost savings, to add complexity in the name of speed or transmission bandwidth reduction, and so on. The only real constraint is that the encoded bit stream conforms to the standard. Some may also choose to develop implementations that "enhance" the standard, but this user-beware strategy is fraught with danger because, in effect, it creates a new standard that defies interoperability.

If compressed information must be communicated between systems and between products from different manufacturers, then a standard for compression and decompression that everyone agrees to is the only choice. Many applications, as we have seen, have already settled on an official standard. But standard algorithms are not always the best choice for applications that have control over their environment, such as a self-contained application (described as a closed process in Section 3.4) that can, if it chooses to do so, implement built-in proprietary compression technology. In addition, there are many other reasons why selecting a proprietary algorithm makes good sense, including taking advantage of technology advances the standard algorithms do not offer to gain more compression, or higher-quality results, or finding a simpler implementation, or having a market advantage by being proprietary. There are also hazards in selecting a proprietary algorithm. What happens to your product if the algorithm vendor goes out of business and, therefore, can no longer provide regular updates and improvements or, equally important, fixes when problems arise? A solution gaining in popularity, at least for software, is to require that vendors place a copy of their code in escrow with an agreement that, if the unthinkable should arise, this information be made legally available to their customers [Seby96, WinW96].

Algorithm complexity, speed, and processing delay time

Algorithm complexity, speed, and processing delay relate to the computational workload and memory requirements that an algorithm imposes, to the need for parallel processing or other efficient processing techniques, and to how fast the algorithm will operate in whatever implementation chosen. These factors decide whether software, DSP, or VLSI hardware logic implementations are suitable for an algorithm and which one(s) will be needed to meet the performance requirements of an application. Two-way communications applications are most sensitive to processing delay time for encoding and decoding, because human interaction places limits on what is acceptable. One-way communications applications and storage applications, where processing delay times are largely irrelevant, are sensitive to processing speed, as throughput determines what level of performance is acceptable.

Adaptive versus nonadaptive

The questions about adaptive algorithms relate to how to design them and when to apply them. Adaptive algorithms continually adjust their parameters to match the data being encoded or decoded. If done properly, more compression will be obtained, as compared to nonadaptive algorithms that operate with static, fixed rules for encoding and decoding. There are some trade-offs to consider when selecting an adaptive algorithm: All adaptive algorithms depend on past history. They have a start-up time, requiring some number of bytes be processed before the algorithm can adjust to the data and the best compression is achieved. The start-up time is a fundamental limitation on the kinds of applications that can use adaptive compression algorithms. Some adaptive algorithms are designed to have shorter start-up times than others. When small, randomly accessed blocks of data are to be compressed, a short start-up time is an advantage, but nonadaptive or semiadaptive algorithms may be still better choices. Examples in Chapters 4 (see Table 4.2) and 6 (see Section 6.9) suggest that a few hundred bytes of data are needed to adapt lossless Lempel-Ziv compression algorithms. Lossy algorithms have start-up times too. For instance, MPEG (see Section 5.5) must encode at least one frame (an I-frame) before motion compensation and interframe prediction can work.

Adaptivity and robustness

Adaptivity and robustness refer to the ability of an algorithm to continually adjust to changes in the data and to produce quality results under adverse conditions. Adaptive algorithms have proven to be superior performers on symbolic data. Many of these algorithms, which were initially designed for text, are robust in the sense that they can handle (or can be extended to handle) graphics and other forms of information. For example, see the discussion of the IBM ADLC algorithm in Section 9.12. Most algorithms for diffuse data make limited use of this type of adaptivity. For example, the final stage of the JPEG algorithm allows adaptive Huffman and arithmetic entropy coding as options [Penn93]. However, the real opportunity for adaptivity is to deal with the variability of the input characteristics of audio, image, and video data. Diffuse data algorithms can be made more robust by applying adaptivity to varying characteristics such as data statistics, dynamic range, noise, frequency content, pixel-to-pixel correlation, and image resolution. Adaptivity can be applied at many steps of the algorithmic process, including transformation (to adjust the transform block size in transform coding, for example), coefficient selection, quantization step size, motion estimation and compensation, and so on.

Error tolerance

Error tolerance relates to the ability to encode and decode data successfully in the presence of errors that may occur during processing, storage, or transmission. Without question, data compression (coding) schemes are far more sensitive to transmission channel errors than all others. This stems from the fact that, totally apart from the needs of data compression, error control coding and recovery procedures are standard in the processing logic and storage devices used for most digital (computing) systems. These elements handle compressed data with the same aplomb as uncompressed data, with transparent error correction that assures near absolute accuracy, and with little or no increase in running time. Consequently, data compression algorithms intended for computing and storage applications include few if any special error control or recovery provisions.

This is not so for transmission channels. Here, the error rates often are much higher, meaning error recovery must be invoked with greater regularity. Another difference is the user (in this case the compression algorithm), not the transmission channel itself, may be responsible for system error control and recovery. Particularly for real-time transmissions, standard error control and recovery schemes are either far more intrusive or far less effective. For example, a packetized data network typically accomplishes transmission channel error recovery by resending corrupted packets. This form of system error recovery may not be practical for compressed data streams of audio and video data, where the latency of retransmission interferes with real-time playback. In this situation, a much more effective strategy is to limit the effects of a channel error to a small part of the data stream—a few seconds of audio, a small area of an image, or a few frames in a video stream. Section 14.2 will discuss techniques for doing this, but today, as a general rule, each compression algorithm for each application is forced to make additional specific provisions for error handling for each transmission channel. Numerous examples of what has been done are provided in Chapters 5 and 7. The price to be paid, unfortunately, is increased complexity and added bit rate (overhead) for error control and recovery.

Encoder/decoder asymmetry

Encoder/decoder asymmetry describes the expenditure of silicon and time for encoding in relation to the same factors for decoding. The basic idea of asymmetric coding is that a larger investment in encoding will result in fewer bits to be stored or transmitted. Asymmetric algorithms are frequently found in storage or broadcast applications, where encoding is done once and decoding is done many times. Most lossless algorithms are inherently symmetric and there is little than can or should be done to change them. Most lossy algorithms, by their very nature, are asymmetric because deciding what information to remove is frequently the most complex and time-consuming part of the encoding-decoding process. However, some of today's leading lossy algorithms allow trade-offs that will make them more or less asymmetric. Several applications illustrate that intelligently expending more encoding logic and time can result in both higher-quality audio, image, or video data and fewer bits to store or transmit. For example, see the discussion of DBS in Section 8.3 and CD-ROM publishing in Section 10.3.

Quality

Quality refers to the distortion that lossy coding introduces. Because lossy coding involves removing some data, compressed diffuse (speech, audio, image, and video) data may not retain all the quality of the original. As noted in some of the applications described earlier in this book, sometimes lossless compression of diffuse data is required when no loss of quality can be accepted, such as for nonhuman data processing or to meet legal requirements. But what is quality, particularly, what is quality when lossy psychoacoustical and psychovisual models are used for compression? For instance, image quality is a complex psychovisual combination of spatial resolution (detail, sharpness), temporal resolution (frame rate), and the effect of artifacts introduced by the compression process. Unfortunately, there are no good, easily applied quality measures for images or other data subjected to lossy compression.

Standard engineering measures of signal distortion, such as mean-squared error, frequency response, or anything that can be measured by linear instruments, frequently do not correlate well with how humans perceive quality, although, these measures are what engineers often resort to because little else is available. When humans are asked to examine a set of images and make decisions about their quality, they use subjective criteria. Subjective criteria such as whether an image is "visually lossless" are useful, but the downside is they have imprecise definitions. Subjective evaluations (for instance, see Section 12.5), despite their unreliability and time-consuming cost, are the best available tools for judging how objectionable the artifacts created by lossy coding systems are. The types of artifacts produced by these systems include the following:

- Audio distortion due to quantization error (bits/sample)
- Image softness due to low resolution

- Image fringing, blocking, or edge jaggedness
- Loss of image sharpness at edge transitions
- Random noise in images
- Video blurring due to limits in motion estimation

What is known today is that different algorithms create different artifacts, depending on their mode operation. Even a single given algorithm may exhibit different artifacts, depending on the bit rate at which it is operated. The presence of artifacts usually is more apparent at high compression ratios. Also, the objectionability of artifacts is highly dependent on the particular sound or image and the conditions under which it is presented to the listener or viewer.

Quality measures, perhaps, will be easier to develop for audio because we understand (or think we understand) quite well how the human ear perceives sound. But good quality measures for images and video are more difficult to develop. Although our understanding of the human visual system has increased significantly over the past century, it has also revealed many complexities of the visual system. This includes how shape, intensity, color, and motion are perceived. It also includes how we are affected by various media and different techniques to display images (for example, subtractive colors for printers and additive colors for displays), and so on. A simple and yet powerful model for visual processing, one that can be used for optimizing coding systems, remains a goal that still eludes the experts [Netr95].

Multiple-coding limitations

Multiple-coding limitations relate to the loss of quality that may result when data is repeatedly compressed and decompressed with lossy algorithms. Some applications may require that compression-decompression be repeatedly applied during transmission, or for storage on different media, or simply for processing such as when an image is rescaled, clipped, or cropped during document processing. Clearly, successive applications of lossless algorithms do not affect quality, but successive applications of most lossy algorithms cause additional degradation of audio, image, or video quality. Unfortunately, there are no general rules or guidelines that explain when multiple compression-decompression cycles can be safely used. Worse yet, as discussed in Chapter 14, when different algorithms are cascaded, the results can be unpredictable.

Scalability

Scalability, a term often restricted to video coding, may be broadly defined as the generation of bit streams that produce useful results even when only a subset has been decoded. Partial decoding of a video bit stream may be useful if the viewer wants an image of smaller size than the source, or the decoder lacks processing resources to decode the full bit stream, or insufficient channel capacity exists (perhaps momentarily) to carry the full signal. Existing television standards (NTSC, PAL, and SECAM), like early proposals for HDTV standards, make no provisions to decouple the parameters of encoding from decoding. This means that all receivers must support the same bandwidth, resolution, aspect ratio, and frame rate. With the coming of HDTV, scalability begins to make sense because not every viewer or receiver needs its full resolution and features. A small-screen receiver to be used for casual viewing would be more economical to build if it could decode a subset of the standard. Similar conditions exist for displaying video on computer workstations, where small screens and smaller-yet windows are the norms. Provisions for scalability are incorporated in the emerging U.S. HDTV standard [Chal95]. Essentially, what is required to achieve scalability within the context of the standard are spatial conversion, frame-rate change, and conversion between interlaced and noninterlaced formats [Basi95].

Progressive resolution

Progressive resolution, a form of scalability usually restricted to images, refers to coding and transmitting images at different resolutions or precisions. The idea is to code an image in several passes and sequentially provide these encodings to viewers. The coding may take the form of spectral selection, where image detail is grouped into bands of visual frequency coefficients. It may also be accomplished by successive approximation, where the precision of all image components is limited in early passes, and later passes extend the precision. Either way, transmission begins with an image that can be quickly sent at a low bit rate, allowing the viewer to recognize the image contents as soon as possible. The viewer, perhaps, may choose to halt the transmission of unnecessary detail or may choose to initiate actions for transmission of additional detail. Progressive presentation, besides providing an aesthetically pleasing sequence of images that holds the viewer's attention, allows more efficient browsing through a picture database. This is also known as hierarchical or pyramidal multiresolution coding as described in the Photo CD example that appears in Section 9.9; see also [Rabb91].

Progressive resolution techniques are being actively investigated; many different compression techniques are inherently progressive or can be adapted to operate progressively. However, today there are no strong solutions for managing image compression fidelity, either to satisfy end-user requirements for spatial or amplitude resolution or to meet end-user response time requirements, or to operate within available decompression time limits, or to match available transmission media bandwidth.

Operating bit rate

Operating bit rate refers to the number of bits per second transmitted from the encoder to the decoder. It is usually associated with real-time transmission of audio or video and, sometimes, with image transmission. An ideal compression algorithm would be able to operate over a wide channel-bandwidth range, providing the highest-quality audio, image, or video sustainable within available bandwidth. The algorithm would be tunable by adjusting a small set of compression parameters to trade off quality for bit rate. Some of today's algorithms, including JPEG, H.261, and MPEG, allow some amount of bit-rate tunability. Others, including nearly all speech coding algorithms, are designed to work only at a given bit rate.

Most compression algorithms are designed to work efficiently within a certain bit-rate range. They may become inefficient or inoperable for transmission rates that fall outside that range—inefficient in the sense that increasing the bit rate will not measurably improve quality, and inoperable in that there is a lower limit below which insufficient transmission bandwidth is available for sending the minimal required information. For example, the H.261 videoconferencing algorithm is designed to operate at not more than 1.92 Mbps and not less than 64 Kbps. At higher rates, there is simply little if any additional information that can be sent to improve picture quality, and at lower rates there is insufficient bandwidth for sending the minimum number of transformed video blocks and motion vectors.

Among those algorithms that can operate at varying bit rates, some require the bit rate be selected and remain fixed for the life of an application, whereas others support dynamically variable bit rates. Examples of the latter include MPEG-2 as implemented for DBS transmission (described in Section 8.3) and for DVD storage (described in Section 9.6). The JPEG hierarchical coding mode also essentially transmits data in this manner.

Added function

This catchall category includes functions that compression algorithms may include to make compression more tolerable for an application. Examples include the sort-order preserving and semiadaptive algorithms developed for database applications (described in Section 6.9).

13.3   Selecting an Implementation Technique

Implementations ranging from software to dedicated special-purpose hardware allow data compression to be adapted to diverse market segments and products, each having differing economics and differing compression needs. Historically, in the computer industry, early compression techniques were executed in software as programs of conventional instructions. In the 1970s, IBM researchers were among the first to define special microcoded CPU instructions and dedicated hardware to speed up data compression techniques such as Huffman coding [Momm74]. By the 1980s, the complexity of compression algorithms had grown, and with more applications demanding faster operation, several VLSI codec chips came to market [Arps88]. In the communications industry, dedicated codec hardware always has been the preferred implementation, essentially because real-time operations such as speech coding demand it and because computers and software that can operate in real time (or near real time) are relative newcomers in communications applications. In consumer-electronics products, where programmable computing technology is not always a given, hardware-implemented compression is often the method of choice.

The options

The optimal choice for implementation depends on the system requirements. Table 13.3 introduces four cost-performance options available to digital system designers for implementing data compression.

Table 13.3   Data compression implementations.

Option	Performance	Comments
CPU software	Low	Programmable
CPU accelerator	Medium - high	Programmable
DSP chip	Medium	May be programmable
ASIC codec chip	High	Fixed algorithm

CPU software compression is an easy way for computer-based products to introduce new function to the marketplace. For instance, when multiple data formats must be handled, a single hardware solution may be impractical. CPU software offers the cheapest and most flexible solution for many compression applications, as it can handle multiple formats and evolve most quickly to new formats. CPU software also is the right choice in situations calling for occasional usage. For example, when a data file is imported from another system in a heterogeneous computing environment, a software format translator is all that is needed. CPU software is not satisfactory in some situations because of computational complexity, resolution, or rate-of-delivery requirements; there one of the following solutions is often necessary.

Special-purpose CPU accelerators allow the flexibility of software programmability to be retained while providing vastly improved performance. These accelerators may take the form of specialized instructions added to the regular CPU chip, but specially designed coprocessor chips can be far more powerful. As learned in Section 9.11, both are available for multimedia computing applications where data compression and other audio, image, and video data operations require many times the performance of a regular CPU.

The DSP (digital signal processor) chip is a 1990s phenomenon finding its way into more and more applications. The primary advantage of a DSP chip is the specialized dataflow which allows high performance execution of real-time (signal) processing algorithms with far less expense and energy consumption than any CPU chip intended for general-purpose computing. Today's DSPs cost as little as $10, or less, and they are embedded in many portable products. They also offer the right cost-performance for high-volume, low-end home and small office environment applications such as audio products, modems, telephones, and FAX machines. They are used for implementing many diffuse data compression algorithms discussed in this book. (DSPs are not promoted as engines for implementing lossless symbolic data compression, although it is technically feasible.) The market for DSPs is about equally split between programmable chips that may be downloaded with various algorithms and fixed-function, algorithm-specific chips used for embedded applications where programmability is not required.

ASIC (application-specific integrated circuit) codec chips are appropriate when high-performance data compression solutions are required. In particular, ASIC codec chips may provide the only viable implementation of highly complex, computationally intense algorithms intended for real-time data compression applications. They also may be needed for simpler algorithms in applications where general-purpose computing logic is not available. When compared to the alternatives, ASIC codec chips can also be the lowest-cost solution for these applications. Data compression codec chips are available for almost all speech and audio algorithms, for JPEG and other image compression algorithms, and for video algorithms, including H.261 and MPEG. Chips also are available for many lossless data compression algorithms including Lempel-Ziv and binary arithmetic coding.

Choosing an option

Choosing an implementation for data compression is easy when the digital system design or the application itself dictates the correct choice. When a product does not include a general-purpose CPU, DSPs and ASIC codecs are the only choices. The same is true when software data compression performance is woefully inadequate. But there are gray areas, especially when a product does feature a CPU, one seemingly having enough performance to do software compression. In these situations, specialized data compression hardware could still be a wise choice. The issue is having a balanced design. One possible decision-making approach is to try to quantify the ratio between the operations-per-second devoted to compression versus those available for noncompression-related work. The larger this ratio, the more justified is hardware support for compression. Consider how this classification scheme might apply a hypothetical product built around a modern microprocessor: It would likely reveal that speech could be processed without special hardware. The same could be true for still-image processing if no hard real-time requirements are imposed. However, it would likely point to the need for compression hardware for high-quality video processing.

Future directions

To appreciate what future data compression implementations may be, consider what has happened in the past. Computer CPUs have become microprocessors—smaller, cheaper, and faster—and far more pervasive in products from all industries, even low-cost, mass-produced products. Microprocessors are now able to execute nearly all symbolic data compression algorithms at speeds that satisfy most applications and at costs that are affordable for scores of products. Simultaneously, compression algorithms have grown more complex—handling speech, audio, and video data types with real-time requirements. Where only a few short years ago it was inconceivable that *any* of these real-time algorithms could be executed in software, as a rule today's microprocessors have advanced to execute nearly *all* these algorithms with at least marginally acceptable performance.

Some type of compression hardware assist is necessary for many of today's algorithms, but time and technology march on. One can assert, with visionary clarity, that someday soon, all of *today's* data compression algorithms will operate quite adequately and cost-effectively in software on microprocessors of the future. Those microprocessors will somehow include the processing logic needed for executing the basic data manipulations on which today's algorithms are based. But it would be shortsighted to assume that all future implementations of data compression will be in software. They will not. Data compression algorithms, particularly those for video (and probably speech, audio, and maybe still images too) are going to grow still more complex. Continuing demand for higher-quality video images, transmitted at ever-lower bandwidth and stored evermore compactly, assure that algorithm development must continue. Thus, leading-edge algorithms will undoubtedly continue to require specialized hardware implementations.

13.4   Where To Do Data Compression

Location, location, location: With data compression, as in real estate, location is everything. As asserted throughout this book, from a technology perspective, the optimum location for data compression is close to the source or producer of data, and for decompression, close to the end user or consumer of data. As illustrated in Figure 13.1, this produces the maximum benefit by reducing bandwidth and minimizing storage (and processing time) for all hardware and software elements throughout the system. Clearly, some systems are so simple that no other choice is possible; the digital speech products described in Section 9.13 are a classic example. For almost all systems that handle video data, short of a hugely expensive investment in networks and storage, this is the only practical way to support the data rates needed for real-time display.

Deciding where to place compression and decompression can be far more complex for most digital systems, particularly, digital computer systems. Figure 13.2 shows the work flow for a database computer system. A human interacts

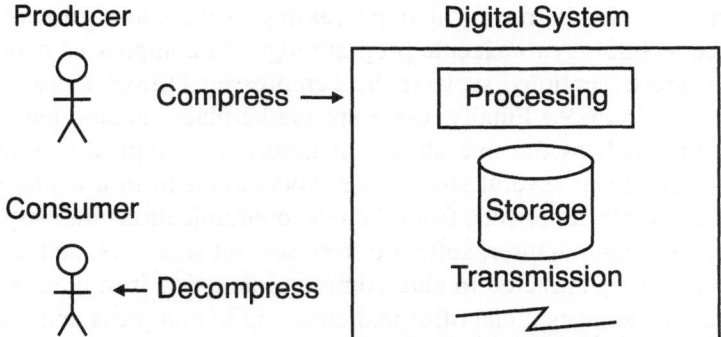

Figure 13.1 Optimal compression for a simple digital system.

with a workstation (WS) connected to a network, which, in turn, is connected to a server computer. Data enters the server through an I/O channel interface (IFAC). It passes through several software components, beginning with communications (COMM), through an application program (APPC), and then is passed to a database management system (DBMS), all of which run in the main storage (MSTG). Data is then routed through I/O channel interfaces to a disk subsystem where it enters a buffer (BUFF) and, subsequently, is passed through yet another interface to disk storage. Data is returned through these same elements in the reverse direction. Along this path there are many sites where it is possible to do compression/decompression functions (indicated by arrows), in hardware or in software.

This situation is quite different from earlier examples for several reasons. To begin with, the data rates and the amount of data for commercial database management applications are much lower; all components are quite able to operate without compression, but there are system cost and performance advantages when it is used. Another difference is that somewhere in this path, data must be processed—not simply passed along. At minimum, the application program, the DBMS code, and, usually, both must examine the data and make logical decisions based on its values. So, the strategy of compressing data when the producer generates it, and leaving it compressed until the consumer needs it, simply does

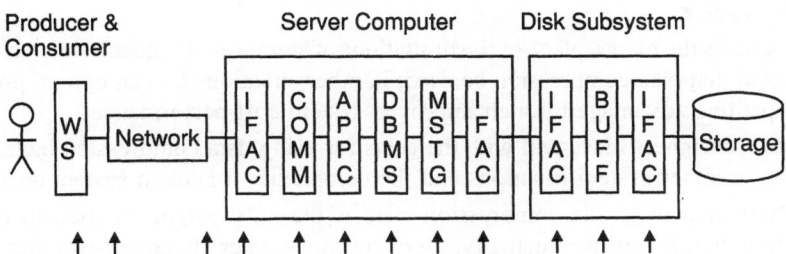

Figure 13.2 Work flow into and out of a database computer.

not work. At least this is true for data processing as we know it today because, generally, the technology to execute program logic on compressed data does not exist. (There are exceptions, such as the compressed DBMS index operations discussed in Section 6.9.) Finally, there are marketplace factors that come into play. A system such as the one shown in Figure 13.2 typically is assembled from components from several sources—a workstation from a manufacturer of computer peripherals, a network from the telecommunications industry, a server from a computer manufacturer, software from several suppliers, and so on. Each manufacturer may be attracted to data compression, using it in their product for the marketing advantages it can offer and choosing to compress and decompress at the product interfaces. Thus, data may be compressed and decompressed several times within this system, a situation that could be interpreted as wasted motion (or processing cycles), but there are valid reasons. It must be noted, from a technology viewpoint, that this is acceptable if the compression is lossless (which it is in business-oriented database computer systems).

In summary, the "rule" that data compression should be placed close to the source of data and decompression placed close to where data is used does not always apply. Sometimes marketplace decisions outweigh technical decisions, and in these situations data compression/decompression can be placed anywhere that adequate computing and storage resources are available and wherever the marketplace makes it profitable!

13.5 Summary

This chapter examined decisions that designers face when choosing to integrate data compression in their digital systems. We learned the following:

- Marketplace requirements define the need for data compression, the type of compression that is acceptable, and limits within which system designers must work.

- To assure data compression can be effectively integrated, system designers must understand not only the problems data compression addresses but also its interactions with other system functions.

- Essentially, the most important question that system designers can ask about data compression is whether it is needed or whether other alternatives may provide a better choice.

- Sometimes the marketplace or the limitations of storage and transmission technology demand that data compression be used; in other situations it is an option, providing competitive advantage through improved system cost-performance.

- System designers must deal with the costs for using data compression including its effect on other system functions and the complexity it adds to system design.

- All too frequently, the compression ratio is the only parameter used to evaluate compression algorithms; actually, there are many other characteristics that may be far more important in many system designs.

- Four cost-performance options are available for doing data compression, ranging from software to dedicated special-purpose hardware. The optimal choice for implementation depends on the system requirements.
- Software compression is becoming more powerful, but most leading-edge algorithms require some type of hardware assist and will continue to do so.
- The optimum location for data compression is close to the source or producer of data, and for decompression, close to the end user or consumer of data. But this cannot always be achieved for a variety of technical and marketing reasons.

14

Managing Compressed Data

In Part III—Applications we explored many digital systems and observed that the compression process and compressed data interact with the physical system and with other logical functions in the system. This chapter takes a closer look at some issues that digital systems designers face when managing compressed data.

14.1 Self-Identifying Compressed Data

Compressed data is essentially undecipherable unless the algorithm used for compression is known. The most efficient algorithms destroy all traces of regular data structure, producing data-dependent bit patterns that make it nearly impossible to do any data processing beyond storing or transmitting compressed data. Simple digital systems do not find this to be a problem because, usually, the system designers choose a single compression technique and they build knowledge about it into every part of the system. However, not all digital systems are so simple, nor are they created under such highly integrated conditions. When a system must handle data compressed by a variety of algorithms, or a single algorithm with different parameter settings, designers must assure that each element knows what compression has been applied to each piece of data. The same is true when the system is really a system of many systems.

Two choices are available: The first is to provide knowledge about compression, independent of the data. The second is to make data self-identifying, with attached standard header information that describes the algorithm and parameter settings used to compress the data. Both methods are used today. An example of the first approach can be found in the LAN-to-LAN internetworking bridges and routers described in Section 7.3, where a specific Lempel-Ziv dictionary is associated with each communications stream. Open systems, which demand interoperation between products from different manufacturers and even different industries, make self-identifying data increasingly important. The standards for these systems typically require that data begin with a header block recorded in uncompressed format. The compression algorithm and/or parameter settings identified in the header can be used to process the compressed data that follows. Some examples include the QIC standards for compressed tape cartridges discussed in Section 6.3, the JPEG standard for compressed images discussed in Section 5.4, and the H.261 and MPEG standards for compressed video discussed in Section 5.5.

In each of the above examples, the headers are intended to identify only one variety of compressed data: MPEG headers identify only MPEG-compressed video data, JPEG headers identify JPEG-compressed image data, and so on. Today, there is no universal standard header for compressed data that would allow unambiguous identification of any passing block on a data communications network or within a computer system. The need for this arises in open systems, both networks and the computers connected to them, where all varieties of compressed data may be present. Indeed, except for data communications networks running the IBM SNA/APPC protocol, little has been done to promote the exchange of compressed data between heterogeneous computer systems. Also, not much attention has been paid to having compressed data be self-identified within a computer system. Within computer systems, the common practice is for the application programs or the operating system to maintain knowledge about what compression applies. This is quite workable for traditional computers designed as self-containing systems. However, self-identifying data may provide a better solution for handling compressed data in more modular computers, where parts of the system such as communications or disk storage are independent subsystems.

14.2   Error-Proofing Compression Algorithms

Conventional wisdom says that compressed data is more sensitive to storage or transmission errors because its redundancy has been removed. Actually, the redundancy that compression removes was never intended for error control or recovery, but it does modestly contribute to limiting the effects of errors. For example, a single-bit error in the uncompressed message "This book is about compressing data" will garble only a single character. It will not corrupt the preceding characters and, unless a bit is lost during storage or transmission, not those that follow. When the data is compressed, depending on the algorithm, a single-bit error will likely do far more damage. In practice, all compression algorithms must be designed with some type of error control and recovery support. Although built-in error control certainly is useful for algorithms intended for storage applications, this is especially important for data transmission applications where errors are more frequent and recovery times are long.

The techniques used for error-proofing compression algorithms involve reinserting redundancy into the compressed data stream in a form that aids error control and recovery. Fortunately, long ago the computer and data communications industries developed general techniques that are now used to limit error propagation and to detect or correct errors in compressed data. Figure 14.1 shows the first of the two main techniques. It involves breaking the compressed data stream into blocks and, to each block, attaching header information recorded in an uncompressed format that describes the fixed or variable-length compressed data which follows. By periodically inserting headers, error propagation is limited, with each header providing a point in the data stream where resynchronization can occur and compression can be restarted. Some standards for transmitting compressed data use more than one layer of blocks. This makes sense when there is a natural correspondence with the data structure; for instance, each frame of video can be stored in a block, a group of frames can be stored as a higher-level block, and so on. Irrespective of the data structure, blocking data also makes sense when all we are looking for are tighter bounds on error control. For instance, as mentioned in Section 12.5, the JPEG standard allows inserting uncompressed synchronization points right down to the 8 × 8 pixel block level for applications where error control is a high-priority consideration.

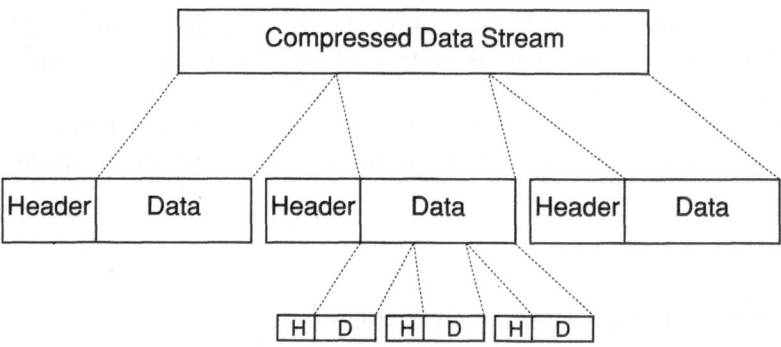

Figure 14.1 Block-structured compressed data stream.

The second main technique involves adding yet more redundancy to each block, to allow detection of errors occurring within the block or, more powerful yet, correction of any errors that may occur. This technique requires a field be added at the beginning, or end, or dispersed within each block in Figure 14.1. It will contain bits that provide a cyclic redundancy check (CRC) for error detection or an error-correcting code (ECC) for, as the name implies, correcting bits found to be in error within the block. For transmitting symbolic data, because it is more efficient, the preferred method is CRC combined with retransmission of corrupted blocks. ECC is usually reserved for those situations where retransmission is not feasible (and for storage applications). These codes are harder to generate, and to obtain acceptable levels of error correction, the length of the code may double the number of bits to be transmitted or stored [Stal94B]. For transmitting compressed audio, image, and video data, neither CRC nor ECC is used when it is deemed acceptable to tolerate the glitches that a corrupted block may introduce in the data stream. When that is not acceptable, CRC and ECC are used for transmitting and storing audio, image, and video data in the same way they are used for symbolic data. Examples of current applications include optional CRC for H.261 video [Tawb93], Dolby AC-3 audio [Davi93], and MPEG audio [Pan95], and standard ECC for DCC audio tape [Hoog94].

14.3   Interaction Between Compression and Other Functions

Data compression and many other functions do transformations on data in digital systems. Often these transformations are synergistic, but sometimes unexpected or undesirable interactions occur. The following are two examples drawn from the world of computer systems:

Compression and compaction

Compression and compaction are terms often used interchangeably. They are not exactly the same thing. Compression removes redundancy and/or information. Compaction removes unused bytes. Compaction allows more information to be stored on tape by combining records into larger blocks and eliminating interrecord gaps (Section 6.3). It is used to store more information on disk by reformatting records written in count-key-data format to eliminate gaps within records and, ignoring disk track boundaries, by packing records to eliminate unused space at the end of tracks (Section 6.4). Compaction allows databases to be stored more efficiently by using techniques such as removing end-of-record padding, packing two decimal numbers in a single byte, and many others (Section 6.9). In its purest form, compaction simply is a record-oriented data-reformatting operation.

Compression and compaction can be synergistic. As a practical matter, it is wise to remove irrelevant data with compaction before compressing the data. In this way, not only are there fewer bytes to compress, so compression will be faster, but also fewer bits are likely to be needed to represent the data.

Compression and encryption

The need for secure data storage and transmission channels continues to grow. In an age when financial transactions and all types of confidential personal and business information are routinely transmitted around the world, most applications require some degree of security to assure communications privacy. Usually, this is accomplished by encryption functions especially designed for the task, although data compression in itself can provide modest levels of privacy. By simply recoding messages, compression can make them appear as unintelligible gibberish to casual observers. But, assuredly, these encodings would be quickly cracked by all but the most inept computer hackers.

From time to time, researchers have considered how the transformations enacted by data compression and encryption can be combined to made compressed data more secure. Among all data compression algorithms, adaptive algorithms provide the greatest measure of privacy by constantly changing the rules of encoding throughout the message. One might think of an adaptive model as an encryption key, a key needed for decoding [Bell89]. With a little additional effort, one might find ways to systematically perturb adaptive compression processes in ways that can be equally systematically undone during decompression. Although these simple data scrambling techniques do not approach the level of security offered by formal encryption, they do offer inexpensive additional privacy for compressed data.

For truly secure data storage or transmission, a formal encryption technique is required, one that produces completely randomized data that can only be decoded with the encryption key. As indicated in Figure 14.2, when a system includes both encryption and data compression, there is one simple rule for system designers to follow:

- Compress first; then encrypt and
- Decrypt and then decompress

This order is absolutely necessary because true encryption completely randomizes data, and randomized data cannot be compressed by *any* compression algorithm, or at least by none of the algorithms presented in this book. In fact, data may expand. This restricts the locations where data compression can be done in a system that uses encryption. However, there is a synergy between compression and encryption in that compression reduces the number of bytes that must be encrypted. In systems that use software to encrypt data, this can be a real advantage because compression may greatly improve encryption performance. For systems that use hardware—if someone was to produce a chip that combines compression and encryption—there may be a performance advantage, too, in that a pipelined dataflow can execute these functions in tandem.

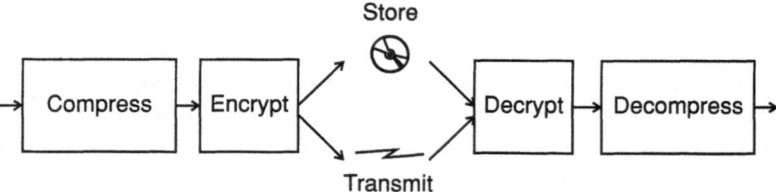

Figure 14.2 Compression and encryption.

14.4   Interaction Between Compression Algorithms

Data compression is used at many locations in complex digital systems. Just as with other functions that do data transformations, there may be interactions between data compression algorithms. Sometimes these interactions are synergistic, but, particularly for audio, image, and video data, all too often, unexpected or undesirable results occur. All is well when lossless algorithms are used; any type of data can be repeatedly compressed and decompressed losslessly without deterioration and, except for the time it takes, there are no adverse effects. It is even possible to losslessly compress already-compressed data a second or a third time; if the first compression was effective, subsequent compression may represent wasted motion, but it can be done without damaging the data in any way. However, when lossy algorithms are used, either to repeatedly compress and decompress data, or to compress already-compressed data, this definitely is not true. Following are two examples that illustrate the interactions between compression algorithms:

Losslessly compressing compressed data

The heading does not contain a typographical error. Indeed, this can happen in complex digital systems, as it definitely does within complex compression algorithms. For instance, a computer system is running DBMS (database management system) software that losslessly compresses its files. Those files are stored on a disk subsystem that also losslessly compresses data before storage. It is perfectly acceptable to cascade the two compression operations, applying compression to already-compressed data. The data will not be corrupted, but will the second compression shrink the files, leave their size unchanged, or expand them?

To answer this question, consider what is done to construct complex algorithms where multiple compression techniques are intentionally cascaded. Of the algorithms described in this book for processing audio, image, and video data, a large proportion consist of a front-end algorithm followed by a Huffman or arithmetic coding back-end. For some algorithms the front-end is lossless, but usually lossy compression is needed to reduce the number of bits fed to the back-end, whose job it is to encode those bits most efficiently. The same approach works for compressing symbolic data. In theory, it would be possible for a run-length coder to be applied to text, followed by a Lempel-Ziv dictionary algorithm that, in turn, is followed by a Huffman or arithmetic coder, and each would increasingly compress the data. (However, another arrangement might not.) In all these examples, the reason cascading compression techniques makes sense is each takes a different and complementary approach to removing redundancy.

Return now to our computer system example. If the cascade of lossless compression algorithms happens to match the one described above, all is well; compressing a second time will shrink the files or, at worst, leave their size unchanged. But if the DBMS and disk subsystem both use the same compression algorithm, say a lossless Lempel-Ziv algorithm, the data will likely expand. In this situation, and others where data may already be compressed by whatever type of algorithm, there are three known solutions for reapplying compression:

- Provide a priori knowledge to each stage of data compression (for example, by making data self-identifying). Apply compression only when data has not been previously compressed or has been compressed by a synergistic algorithm.
- Test compressibility, either through sampling or complete compression, and buffer the results until compressibility is determined. Then store or transmit whichever is smaller, the compressed results or the original data.
- Compress and accept the results, whatever happens.

The first solution requires a total system approach that is difficult to achieve unless standards for compression have been created which cover the entire system. The second solution, although highly effective, is expensive because of costs for buffering, multiple parallel-executing compression engines (or added running time), and decision-making logic. The third solution leads to unpredictable results and for that reason probably should be avoided.

Cascading lossy codecs in broadcasting

Nowhere are lossy compression algorithms, and the codecs (coder-decoders) that implement them, more valued than in broadcasting. Without compression for reducing the bandwidth and storage demands of audio and video data, the digital revolution in broadcasting could not have happened. Handling uncompressed digital signals certainly is not economical and, often, is impossible with the storage and transmission facilities available to broadcasters. From originating a broadcast, to delivering it to listeners and viewers, many signal processing steps are involved in what is termed the *broadcast chain*, steps where data compression is needed. To illustrate what makes up a broadcast chain and the role compression plays, the simplified example of network radio broadcasting shown in Figure 14.3 will be used. Locations for data compression and decompression are indicated by C and D, respectively, where in this chain there are four compress-decompress cycles. In practice, radio broadcast chains may be far more complex, necessitating even more compress-decompress cycles: Additional compressed transmission links may be needed for activities such as around-the-

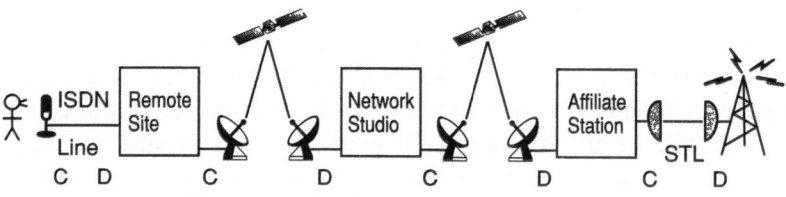

Figure 14.3   Radio broadcast chain.

world news gathering. Audio may need to be recorded and stored in compressed format at one or more sites in the chain for processing and for time-delayed broadcasting. The original interview or performance may be captured with a device such as a MiniDisc or DCC recorder that uses compression. Looking to the future, programs will be transmitted to listeners in compressed format via digital audio broadcasting (DAB). Each of these operations adds a compress-decompress cycle and, thus, four cycles can easily grow to six or more.

A natural question to ask is why is audio repeatedly compressed and decompressed; why not compress audio at the beginning and leave it compressed throughout the broadcast chain. The answer is that transmission links in the chain have differing bandwidth capabilities and requirements for compression. What is right for an ISDN line may not be what is needed for a satellite link or the microwave studio-to-transmitter link (labeled as STL in Figure 14.3). Also, broadcasters often do not own the transmission links, and the communications provider may be using compression for efficiency or to offer more attractive pricing. Then, too, broadcasters need decompressed audio at several steps along the way to allow mixing, editing, and processing to create the program delivered to listeners.

Sometime around 1990, manufacturers of professional broadcast radio equipment began offering lossy audio compression codecs that could be inserted wherever needed in the broadcast chain. Not incidentally, these products used several different lossy compression algorithms, most having adjustable parameters for sampling rates, bandwidths, and compression ratios as required for various applications. Anxious to reap the advantages of digital technology, broadcasters began using this gear throughout their broadcast chains.

Strange things began to happen. A broadcast chain might transmit radio broadcasts with perfect clarity and, suddenly, a particular musical selection or a speaker's voice would be badly distorted. Worse yet, sounds that were in no way part of the original signal would be heard and then disappear. Other more subtle or perhaps not so subtle lingering effects were observed, too, including degradation of the stereo image, swooshing background noises, and other unwanted, unnatural, and definitely unpleasing sound effects [Rana94]. Could the data compression codecs be the source of these problems? In 1993, Herb Squire, Director of Engineering at WQXR Radio in New York City, demonstrated to a meeting of the NAB (the National Association of Broadcasters) and to a joint meeting of the New York City chapters of AES and SMPTE (the Audio Engineering Society and the Society of Motion Picture and Television Engineers) that, indeed, they were. He devised an experiment that used a chain of codecs to produce tapes containing sonic effects which could only be attributed to the signal processing within the codecs. His demonstration made broadcasters, manufacturers, and engineers fully aware that lossy data compression was not the transparent technology they had thought it to be.

In the same time frame, acoustics engineers were busy at work in their laboratories developing more accurate tools and techniques for measuring and characterizing the sonic effects of cascading audio codecs [Cabo94]. Through their efforts, it now clear that the quantization noise generated by low-bit-rate coding, which each audio codec carefully places in regions of the frequency spectrum where louder sounds can mask it, grows louder with each reencoding and may become audible. At least one manufacturer, Audio Precision, Inc. of Beaverton, Oregon (there may be others) now provides test equipment and procedures that allow audio codec manufacturers and radio broadcasters to measure and quantify the effects of cascading. Laboratory tests of three circa-1994 audio codecs published by this manufacturer [Metz94] corroborated the in-the-field results cited above. These tests indicated that distortion may become audible in as few as three passes through even the best audio codecs. In tests where three different codecs were cascaded, the final result tended to be the worst-case summation of noise of all three codecs at every point in the audio frequency spectrum.

Although the radio broadcast industry's confidence in cascaded audio codes may have been temporarily shaken, since 1993 the codes and their application have been refined. Improved versions of older products have been introduced, as have new products that use more advanced audio compression algorithms. Broadcasters also are now better able to interpret manufacturers' specifications of both new and old products thanks to a classification scheme developed by the ITU-R [Fors94]. It characterizes audio codecs by the coding margin they provide between the true masking threshold and the actual level of coding noise under a given signal condition. This makes it easier to judge the suitability of a particular product for multigeneration coding applications. Broadcasters have also learned how better to use cascaded codecs. Experience has led to some practical guidelines for their application [Squi96]. These guidelines include the following:

- Be concerned when chaining three or more codecs that use differing algorithms, or three more codecs that use the same algorithm but with differing parameter settings (for example, different sampling rates or compressed bandwidths).

- At each step in cascaded applications, limit data reduction to not more than 4–6 times, using at least 256 Kbps of bandwidth. Place the lowest-bandwidth, highest-reduction codec early in the broadcast chain to make the task of those that follow less demanding.

- Use the lowest audio sampling rate allowed by the application to make the compression task less demanding. For example, use 24 KHz for AM and 32 KHz for FM broadcasts.

- Use lossy compression only as necessary, not for studio-to-transmitter links (because all broadcast signals, previously compressed or not, pass through this link) and not for archiving when audio quality is a concern.

Video broadcasters also use multiple codecs throughout their broadcast chains, essentially for the same reasons as radio broadcasters. A news report from the field may be recorded by a digital video camcorder that uses compression. The tape is then decompressed, allowing the news report to be recompressed and transmitted over compressed links to a studio. There, after decompression, the report is edited (which may require multiple compress-decompress cycles), and stored in compressed format for later broadcast. The video then may be decompressed and recompressed to be transmitted over yet another compressed link to broadcast stations, and so on.

A cascade of any of the lossy video algorithms discussed in this book can produce measurable and visible degradation beyond what a single codec produces. However, when compared to audio, most professional video products use data compression far less aggressively. The recording and transmission technology for video broadcasting, except the final link to home viewers, simply does not demand pushing compression technology so close to its limits. This reduces picture artifacts and makes the coding errors that do pile up less conspicuous. Then, too, visual coding errors may be less annoying in that our eyes are less sensitive to visual distortion than our ears are to audio irregularities. Incidentally, the same is true for cascaded lossy image compression algorithms whose effects can be treated as a subset of video.

There are two situations in which broadcasters may repeatedly compress and decompress video. The first includes storage applications where video is copied over and over, usually with the same algorithm; this happens frequently during professional (and consumer) video recording and editing. Video cameras, recorders, and editors use M-JPEG (motion-JPEG) or other frame-by-frame DCT-based intraframe compression. Modest compression ratios as low as 2:1 are used which, in practice, allows multigeneration copies to be made with essentially no loss of visual quality. The merits of this approach are easily demonstrated. One experimental study observed that during editing, a compression ratio of 4:1 or less maintains high-quality pictures throughout several compress-decompress cycles [Wilk94]. Under these conditions, most of the picture-quality degradation occurs during the first compress-decompress cycle. Even with the consumer camcorders described in Section 9.5 that conform to the DVC (digital video cassette) standard, where compression ratios are near 5:1, tests indicate no detectable loss of visual quality after 20 generations (compress-decompress cycles) [Roth96].

The second situation where cascaded codecs are used in video broadcasting is for transmission links, where various amounts of bandwidth reduction are important. Here, more aggressive compression is necessary, and a mixture of MPEG or other interframe coding algorithms may be repeatedly used. For these algorithms degradation can be reduced in several ways. The simplest is, obviously, to use the lowest possible compression ratio at each step throughout the chain. This means using the smallest possible GOP (group of pictures) size, resulting in more I-pictures and higher quality (and higher data rates). (See Figure 5.16 and related discussion that explains GOP and the role of I-, P-, and B-pictures.) Maintaining the same GOP size and synchronizing the algorithms throughout the chain also contributes to better quality. In this way, at each encoding cycle I-, P-, and B-pictures will be recoded as, respectively, I-, P-, and B-pictures. Experimental studies confirming the merits of these techniques also provide some additional insights [Wilk94]; for example, it was observed that the best results were obtained when each MPEG codec used identical adaptive schemes and buffer control techniques. Furthermore, when different algorithms (in this instance MPEG and wavelets) were used in mixed combinations, the final picture degradation was a difficult-to-characterize mix of artifacts from all the algorithms.

14.5   Operating on Compressed Data

The normal paradigm for processing compressed data is to first decompress it, then process it, and, when required, recompress it. Generally, processing means examining the data and making logical decisions based on its values, manipulating the data in ways other than simply storing and transmitting it. What if data could be processed without decompressing it? Not spending CPU cycles or hardware time decompressing and compressing data would provide a performance advantage, especially for more sophisticated algorithms. Having fewer data bytes to manipulate would require less storage, which not only could make processing faster but also greatly reduce the cost for manipulating high-volume data such as images and video.

Generally, compressed data is not amenable to processing because computer programming standards and conventions assume known, unchanging, value-insensitive data formats. But in special cases it is possible to work directly on compressed data—well, almost directly—as evident by the compressed DBMS index operations described in Section 6.9 and the applications in this section. The secret to operating on compressed data is to recognize that data compression algorithms, however complex they may be, lay down data in orderly, well-structured bit patterns. Given the motivation, and processing speeds that are 10–100 times faster are good motivators, sometimes these bit patterns can be operated on by undoing just a few of the compression steps. Thus, the wasted motion of complete decompression and recompression can be avoided.

Transcoding

Transcoding is the process of converting compressed data from one compressed format to another. There are many examples: Transcoding is often required when compressed data files are exchanged in heterogeneous computing environments. Transcoding is required when speech is transmitted through various communications links; for instance, a conversation between a cellular telephone and a standard telephone must be transcoded between differing wireless and wireline standards. Videoconferences between sites using codecs that conform to different standards, or even the same standard but different transmission rates, must be transcoded. The same is true for HDTV transmission, where pictures may be transmitted in one standard format and displayed in another. Yet another example is video edited in M-JPEG format that must be transcoded to MPEG for storage or transmission. Within multimedia computer systems, video data must be trans-coded between different prevailing standards.

Sometimes, transcoding can be accomplished without completely decompress-ing and recompressing data. Not only is this faster, but for speech, audio, image, and video data there may be less chance of quality loss. The cascading of codecs in broadcast chains, described in Section 14.4, is an example that illustrates the hazards of compression-decompression in transcoding. In that application, for a variety of reasons, including the unpredictable combination of equipment and the differences between compression algorithms, the only feasible solution was complete decompression followed by recompression. However, in many situa-tions, transcoding is a preplanned, orderly process where, often, the compression formats are not very different. They may share the same technology elements, making them at least somewhat compatible, and this makes complete decompres-sion-recompression unnecessary. Some examples include the variable-rate speech coding standards discussed in Section 5.2, where transcoding is accomplished by simply stripping or adding back low-order bits from each sample [Noll95]. For image and video compression techniques that begin with DCT transformation, including JPEG, H.261, and MPEG, transcoding can be done without completely decompressing the bit stream. Hardware codec manufacturers use this to advan-tage to produce chips that can efficiently transcode between any of the three standards [Cata95]. For example, to transcode a bit stream produced by an editor that uses M-JPEG compression, if no rescaling is required all that must be done is unwind the back-end encoding steps of JPEG (see Figure 5.9) and then perform the back-end encoding steps of H.261 or MPEG (see Figures 5.15 and 5.16). Because the DCT step is computation intensive, this method of transcoding is much faster.

Video editing

The job of video editing is to turn raw inputs into finished products. Editing in the digital domain requires that, frame by frame, and scene by scene, transforma-tions be applied to manipulate pixels. The transformation may be something simple like changing image brightness. It may involve segmenting a continuous video stream into individual scenes, or it may mean dissolving one video scene into the next to create a continuous video stream. It can also involve combining multiple video streams to create composite images and a single video stream. Using workstation-based tools, stored video may be edited in non-real time to produce the final product, but for live broadcasts editing must be done in real time. Either way, operating on fully decompressed digital video inhibits rapid processing because of the data size and the time for decompression and recom-pression.

As a result, researchers are beginning to find ways to operate directly on compressed digital video [Chan95]. Efforts focused on M-JPEG and other DCT-based compression algorithms have met with success, in that direct manipulation of DCT-transformed images cuts the operational overhead by up to two orders of magnitude. Most commonly, the back-end Huffman or arithmetic entropy coding step of JPEG must be undone. See Figure 14.4 (and also Figures 5.8 and 5.9). Then standard algebraic operations—adding a scalar value to each pixel, multiplying each pixel by a scalar value, adding pixels, or multiplying pixels—can be performed on the run-length-encoded DCT-transformed pixels [Smit93]. This shortcut bypasses most of the image encoding and decoding time, resulting in faster algorithms for many image-transformation editing operations including those mentioned above. Some operations merely need to examine images; examples include detecting where scene transitions occur in a video stream or where edge transitions occur within an image. These operations, too, can be directly executed on the DCT-transformed pixels [Yeo95].

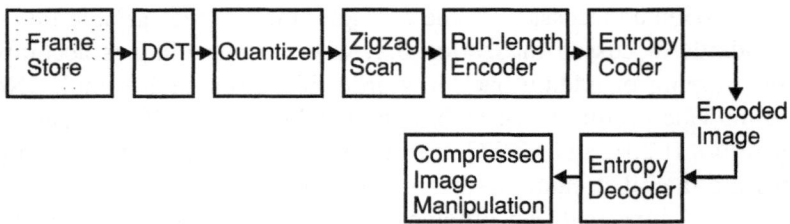

Figure 14.4 Operating on compressed images.

The value of direct operation on compressed video for real-time applications was made clear by a prototype videoconferencing system developed at IBM Research [Edge92, Sant92]. A PC desktop multimedia collaborative system was demonstrated that allowed several users to share and edit online information and to see each other in video windows displayed at every user workstation. By operating on the compressed video streams arriving at each workstation, the number of operations to create a composite display image was reduced by two orders of magnitude (cut from about 100 million computer operations per second to about 1 million operations per second). Composing the display image involved working directly on the DCT-transformed 8 × 8 pixel blocks to resize, move, hide, or overlap video windows and combine them with windows containing text. Waiting to decode the video streams until after composing the picture that each user viewed allowed a single decoder to be used at each workstation, no matter how many incoming video streams were present.

14.6 Archiving Compressed Data

Maintaining an accurate historical record of past activities is essential in almost all endeavors; the place where those records are kept is called an archive. Any organization that commits information to a digital system needs a digital archive. With digital systems, where long-term information is stored on magnetic and optical media, data compression cuts the amount of storage required and reduces the cost for maintaining the archive. Table 14.1 describes the archiving applications encountered earlier in this book.

Table 14.1   Archiving applications.

Application	Reference	Information Stored	Compression	
			Lossless	Lossy
Computer systems	Chapter 6	Text	✓	—
Telemetry systems	Section 7.9	Binary data Images	✓	Images
Publishing	Section 10.2	Text Images	✓	Images
Entertainment	Section 11.3	Speech Audio Images Video	✓	[1]
Healthcare	Section 12.5	Medical images	✓	[1]

Notes:
[1] Depends on quality requirements.

The ideal data compression for archiving (or any other use) would transform information into a format that requires very little storage, easily compresses and decompresses—instantly, and reproduces the same quality as the original. Unfortunately, the algorithms discussed in this book may do only one or two of these things well, at the expense of the others. For many applications, small size, simplicity, and high speed are most important. But for archiving, quality outweighs all other factors. The crucial question about using data compression for archiving is what kind is safe and appropriate. Only lossless compression can be used for symbolic data. Losing or altering even a single bit in character text, numeric data, or a computer program spells disaster for business, computer programming, database, electronic mail, and scientific applications that deal with exact representations of information. Speech, audio, image, and video data applications do not share this requirement and, most often, depend on lossy compression to make them practical. But does that dependency extend to archiving—is it safe to use lossy compression for archiving speech, audio, image and video data?

In many of the speech, audio, image, and video archives cited above, there is essentially no other practical choice. Lossy compression is needed because storage costs or access times for uncompressed or lossless-compressed versions of the original information are too great. But there are other situations where, as part of the archiving process, one might consider applying lossy compression but should not:

- Applying lossy compression is unacceptable if legal requirements for storage of the original information or complete reconstruction of the original information (from a lossless-compressed version) is mandatory.
- Applying lossy compression is undesirable if future needs for the archived data are unknown.
- Applying lossy compression may be undesirable if the archived data must be postprocessed.
- Applying lossy compression may be undesirable when data is known to have been previously compressed and decompressed by some (perhaps unknown) lossy algorithm. The only safe way to avoid the unwanted interactions or degradations that lossy recompression may cause is to store the data in its as-received, uncompressed format (or to use lossless compression).
- When lossy-compressed data is received, there is no other choice but to archive it in its as-received format.

From a technologist's viewpoint, it is important to think carefully about what is being thrown away by lossy compression. The current standards for speech, audio, image, and video compression are totally focused on what the human ear can hear and what the eye can see. An unspoken design maxim for compression standards is that it is acceptable to throw away anything humans cannot hear or see, given the listening or viewing conditions for which the standards are designed. However, humans in other situations and other kinds of sensors may respond differently. If all the information thought to be unheard by the human ear or invisible to the human eye is thrown away, then information may have been discarded that might be usable to humans placed in another situation. This information also may be vital to some machine automata in making significant decisions based on the sound or image.

A simple illustration of when lossy compression is not appropriate involves an imaging system (see Section 6.13) where, currently, the archived images are viewed at workstations. One approach is to create the archive using a lossy algorithm such as JPEG. For maximum storage and transmission efficiency, the images should be compressed to the resolution and quality needed for existing displays. But requirements often do change; for instance, users may decide they want to print copies of the images on high-resolution image printers. Unfortunately, the archive does not contain print-quality images. A wiser choice when setting up this image archive, one that anticipates future needs, is to initially capture images at the highest possible quality and archive them with lossless compression. By creating a working copy of the archive, processed with lossy compression to the resolution and quality needed for current equipment, the imaging system can operate efficiently (although at the expense of added storage capacity). When needs change, it will be relatively easy to rebuild the working copy, at least far easier than rescanning the original images, if that is still possible.

Other examples of when lossy compression is not appropriate for archiving involve computer-aided postprocessing techniques: Digital images of fingerprints may be subjected to automated feature extraction of minutia, followed by OCR (optical character recognition). Computer-assisted interpretation of scanned medical images, involving automated techniques such as heightening the effect of small differences in brightness, may prove to be valuable diagnostic tools. In these and other situations, features that are invisible to the human eye can be highly important for extracting more information from the image. Furthermore, as the volume of online speech, audio, image, and video material increases, the need for computer-aided searching of sound and picture libraries will increase. The way computers best do character, pattern, and scene recognition and do content searches on speech, audio, image and video libraries may use information that escapes the human senses. For instance, edge detection in images can use information outside the human sense range to increase the confidence in prediction of unbroken curves. In essence, postprocessing requirements and methods must be known and evaluated before any lossy compression algorithm can be declared acceptable for archiving.

Another aspect of addressing the use of lossy compression for archiving deals with the rapid progress made in lossy algorithms, progress that can be expected to continue. Advances in speech, audio, image, and video compression have not only greatly reduced the transmission data rate (and storage sizes) but also have brought improvements in higher-quality data with fewer discernible artifacts. So long as lossy algorithms continue to improve, using even the best of today's algorithms to archive data may seen an unwise decision a few short years down the road.

From the viewpoint of the organization that owns it, a digital archive represents a big investment. Recouping that investment means letting people use and share all kinds of archived information in whatever way that is most effective. This may require providing speech, audio, image, and video at various presentation resolutions. In some circumstances, it may be essential to recover or completely reconstruct the original information, or to construct a new lossy-encoded version of the original information at a greater or lesser level of detail. To fulfill these needs, speech, audio, image, and video data must be stored at a quality level that will never cause regrets.[1]

---

[1] Another important aspect of building a durable archive is to select media that will survive for the expected life of the archive. Two examples of media whose life span proved too short, due to unstable chemical composition, are nitrate-based movie film and early magnetic tapes. Having working machines to read the archived media is equally important too. Included on the lengthy list of nearly extinct devices are 7-track computer tape drives, 8-track audio players, Betamax VCRs, and more.

14.7 Summary

This chapter examined issues that digital systems designers face when managing compressed data. We learned the following:

- Making compressed data self-identifying is important in all digital systems but most valued in open systems such as networks and servers where data may come from various sources.
- Each of today's major compression standards makes its data self-identifying; however, there is no universal standard format allowing the exchange of all types of compressed data.
- All compression algorithms need some type of error control and recovery support, especially those intended for transmission applications where, compared to storage applications, the error rate is higher and the recovery time is longer.
- Error-proofing compression algorithms involves reinserting redundancy into the compressed data stream. Breaking the data stream into self-identifying blocks and adding error-detecting or error-correcting bits within blocks are two widely used techniques.
- Data compression may interact with other system functions that do data transformations. Where data compression is placed in the dataflow determines if it will act synergistically with other functions.
- Data compression algorithms may interact with each other. When data is repeatedly compressed and decompressed, as it may be in complex digital systems, unexpected or undesirable results may occur.
- Repeated application of lossless compression may be beneficial or be simply a waste of time.
- Repeated application of lossy compression may reduce data quality or, even worse, corrupt data beyond repair.
- Experience with using lossy codecs in broadcasting, where data must be repeatedly compressed and decompressed, has contributed to a better understanding of the effects of lossy audio compression on data quality and how to deal with them.
- Generally, compressed data must be decompressed before it can be processed, but this is not always necessary. Direct operations on compressed data are often much faster and result in substantial savings in storage.
- Examples of directly processing compressed data include transcoding from one compressed format to another and video editing with speedups ranging from 10 to 100 times.
- The crucial question about using data compression for archiving is what kind is safe and appropriate. Lossless compression is always safe. Sometimes lossy compression is more appropriate, but in the light of future needs for the archived data, it may not be safe. Regrettably, the effects of lossy compression cannot be undone.

15

A Window On The Future

In this chapter, we will look at data compression for future digital systems. Surely, few, if any, of the pioneers working with data compression in the 1950s could have envisioned the diversity of today's applications or that it would be so vital to their existence and viability. In the intervening years, increasingly more powerful data compression has developed at a pace equal to and sometimes ahead of the VLSI technology needed for its implementation. With continuing progress in both algorithms and electronics, future digital systems can be expected to be wrapped evermore tightly around what has become a core technology, data compression.

15.1 Trends and Directions

Throughout this book we have explored events and developments relating to data compression during the last half of the 20th century. With very little foresight, it can be anticipated that the following will be true heading into the 21st century:

- Multimedia will be a part of every client and server computer.
- A wide range of consumer products will have digital multimedia capability.
- Advances in storage technology will be evolutionary, with optical storage continuing to be the key low-cost storage for multimedia data.
- Computer networks will be enabled for text, speech, audio, image, and video data.
- All communications networks and channels, even those that today are devoted to moving analog data, will be well advanced toward digital delivery of all forms of data.

- Data compression will continue to be a vital technology because applications will continue to demand more storage and bandwidth than digital systems can deliver without it.
- Standards will continue to evolve to match advances in compression technology and to meet application needs.
- Almost all of today's compression algorithms will be done in software, and very low-cost compression hardware will be available if software is not sufficient.
- Today's leading-edge speech, audio, image, and video compression technology will be widely used but will be recognized as trailing-edge technology because of new advances.
- Breakthroughs will have occurred, increasing compression by at least an order of magnitude but only in some niche applications.

Let us now explore the implications.

15.2 Future Applications

It is not unrealistic to expect the digital revolution to continue for many years to come. Some projections suggest that it may take up to 30 years for existing products such as television and telephones to fully transition to digital technology. Along the way, there will appear new applications and new computer-based products from all industries that deal with all forms of digitized data. These products will make more creative, more effective uses of human senses, increasing our capacity to discover, absorb, and respond to information. Improved forms of speech recognition and more effective uses of audio, still images, and video will capitalize on our senses of sound and sight. Along with improved forms of handwriting recognition, our tactile sense will perhaps be more fully utilized through touch devices such as transducers and sketchpads. Expanding the capabilities for interaction between people and machines, hopefully, will result in more effective communications between people.

It is hard to predict what the new applications will be or which ones will be big winners in the marketplace, but assuredly they will be driven by how people live, do business, and choose to be entertained. Witness the growth in FAX and other applications generated by the revolution in the workplace. As people move into the home office, set up the electronic office, or become mobile workers, new kinds of tools of handling digital information are required. For instance, some believe personal digital assistants (PDAs) will become essential business tools for the 21st century. For many years, both computer and communications prophets have served up tantalizing visions of a take-it-anywhere, communicate-with-anyone PDA, having Solomon-like knowledge to assist with or manage everyday business activities. At the very least, they say, PDAs will speed up time-consuming tasks such as reading mail, scheduling meetings, arranging travel, and filling out expense reports. In more advanced incarnations, foreseen by the most visionary of visionaries, PDAs will act as intelligent advisors assisting humans in making decisions. To accomplish this, PDAs will need to be part computer, part communications, part entertainment devices employing all multimedia data types. The first PDAs put on the market in the 1990s fell far short of these lofty goals, being little more than electronic notepads with a wireless communications link. Handwriting recognition, the most advanced function they offered, proved disappointing in that it did not work all that well for everyone. It can be argued that to close the gap between the PDAs of the 1990s and high-function visionary products, what is needed is better technology, not better visions. Clearly, the PDAs of the 1990s pushed the limits of packaging, processing, storage and communications technology. To deal with these limitations and allow PDAs to reach their full potential, more effective data compression is needed. Perhaps it must go beyond today's data compression, doing more than entropy coding and data reduction to tame the demands of multimedia data.

Television provides yet another example where opportunity exists for innovation. Television has become an indispensable part of our lives, whether for entertainment, business videoconferencing, or educational training. Compared to standard television, HDTV is a better way to convey real-time video information in that it provides the audience with a heightened sensation of reality and "being there." But it, like all existing television systems, offers a two-dimensional view of the world. People see and experience a three-dimensional (3-D) real world, so it is natural to ask if television should not also produce pictures in three dimensions. Today, at best, 3-D television is little more than a concept confined to experimental systems found in research laboratories. However, visionaries believe it will soon be ready for applications including videoconferencing, virtual reality, and robotics. Although various methods exist for capturing and displaying 3-D television images, much remains to be done before any can be put into practical use. Display technology is a key hurdle. So are improved compression methods for storage and transmission because 3-D television, as shown in Table 15.1, requires two to N times or more bandwidth than conventional television [Moto95]. Research on bandwidth reduction for 3-D television has just started. As a hint for what is to come, consider that like multichannel audio compression, which exploits the correlation between audio channels, 3-D television compression will exploit the correlation that exists between the channels needed to produce pictures for both the left and right eyes.

PDAs and 3-D television are but two examples for possible future digital systems. At the heart of the innovations promised by these systems is improved interaction between people and machines. This will be accomplished by increasing the intelligence of machines and by delivering information in forms that humans can more readily absorb. For digital system designers, this means applying ever-larger doses of processing power—and storing and transmitting more digital bits. Just as with multimedia computers and many other products that have improved the coupling between humans and machines, these products will not be practical without data compression.

Table 15.1   Three-dimensional television display methods.

Display Method	Television Screen Display	Viewpoint Movement[1]	Information Required[2]
Conventional TV; user wears glasses	Yes	No	2
Striped lenticular screen with parallax barrier	Yes[3]	One dimensional	N
Fly-eye lens	Not yet	Two dimensional	N^2
Holography	Not yet	Three dimensional[4]	N^3

Notes:
[1] The televised scene is observable from different viewpoints depending on viewer position with respect to the display.
[2] Times conventional television (approximate). N = number of viewpoints.
[3] Moving picture quality is poor for current technology.
[4] Provides depth perception.

15.3   Future Digital System Technology

Because of the ongoing revolution in the price and computing capability of digital technology, the factors that now make data compression an economical alternative to storage capacity and communications bandwidth will continue to prevail. Several forces are at work: Historically, the cost for computing power has declined at the same rate or, perhaps, somewhat faster than the cost for either storage capacity or communications bandwidth. The introduction of small form-factor magnetic disks, high-density optical discs, and optical-fiber communications links may have temporarily upset the balance, but system costs have been largely unaffected in that storage and transmission capacity enhancements (and processing speed enhancements too) have been eaten up by new applications and programming techniques. It still is possible to squeeze more circuits onto VLSI chips, conceivably an easier task (or cheaper) than stuffing more bits onto storage media or pushing more bits through communications links; therefore, the trends of the past are projected to continue well into the 21st century.

The cost improvement in computing power, resulting from higher levels of VLSI integration, will allow more powerful compression algorithms to be included in every system almost for free. How? By integrating data compression macros on-chip with other microprocessor functions, logic circuits that might have otherwise gone unused will provide the primitive operations needed for compression.

This will make data compression of no more special significance than floating-point addition or multiplication are today. With higher levels of integration comes more speed, making it feasible to do all but the most complex compression in software.

Then, too, there are situations where no more storage capacity is affordable or no more communications bandwidth is available at any price. Portable products where power consumption is critical will continue to make data compression an economical alternative to increased storage capacity. Communications applications where optical fiber cannot be applied will continue to most dramatically illustrate the value of data compression. For applications that must communicate via radio waves, including radio and television broadcasting, PDAs, and other mobile computing products, there simply is no more room in the already over-crowded radio-frequency spectrum. This in itself seems sufficient to assure the boom in data compression for more efficient transmission will continue.

15.4 Living in a Changing World

As there will be new applications, and those applications will demand better data compression, so too will new standards for storing and transmitting compressed data be needed. This poses some interesting problems for all who depend on data compression standards, not only existing standards but new standards too. With continually changing technology and applications, will today's standards be historical relics in a few short years? They could be. Probably the most endearing benefit of the recent explosion in data compression standards activity is the stability it brings. When a standard exists, it is not easily displaced unless it cannot support a new application, or unless new compression methods exhibit far superior performance. Among today's standards, those that have avoided overspecification and have planned for evolution are likely to survive the longest. The H.261 videoconferencing standard, which allows users to pick a nonstandard compression algorithm if they so choose, and the MPEG video standard, which really is a family of standards, are good examples. However, even these standards will fall by the wayside unless they can adapt to more advanced coding methods sure to appear sometime in the future.

For manufacturers building products where standards are transitory, how do you survive? And where competing standards exist, which should you back? Software compression seems to provide answers to both questions. True, building software programmability into a product *may* cost more and software *may* not be a solution for the most complex compression algorithms, but it offers some assurance that the product can survive changes in standards and user preferences.

15.5 Future Compression Algorithms

There is a great need for better compression algorithms for all types of diffuse data, particularly for video. When compared to symbolic data, diffuse data requires orders-of-magnitude more storage or transmission capacity, even with state-of-the-art compression. This difference is painfully obvious where there is a choice of using symbolic or diffuse data, such as the multimedia application described in Section 2.2. (See Figure 2.5.) Also, as we have learned, the quality of decompressed diffuse data sometimes falls short of expectations. Thus, it is not surprising that the research community has, for all practical purposes, declared symbolic data compression algorithms to be "good enough" and moved on. We will explore one important part of their efforts.

With video data having the greatest need for improved compression, appropriately, video is receiving much attention. To appreciate where the next generations of video compression algorithms are headed, let us consider two data processing techniques that usually are not thought of as data compression per se. The first is optical character recognition (OCR), a technology refined by over 30 years of practical applications. OCR is an image processing technique that reduces images containing characters, represented as two-dimensional arrays of bits, to strings of ASCII or EBCDIC characters. The second is speech recognition, a technology with an equally long history but only recently becoming sufficiently mature for practical applications. Speech recognition is a processing technique that reduces spoken words and phrases to strings of ASCII or EBCDIC characters. Speech synthesis is a complementary processing technique that converts text (represented as ASCII or EBCDIC characters) into machine-generated speech. Few practical applications have been found for a technique to complement OCR.[1]

Both OCR and speech recognition can represent diffuse data far more compactly than any conventional data compression technique. They do this by extracting the information contained in diffuse data, converting it to symbolic data. To accomplish this, both OCR and speech recognition are driven by models for what should be recognized. These models are vastly different, but there are some common elements. OCR systems contain templates that specify what characters should look like and rules specifying how they are used within a language or application environment. Speech recognition systems contain models for spoken utterances and rules for grammar and semantics.

Underlying these models are so-called cognitive processes, techniques that mimic the human brain in how it ascribes meaning to visual, auditory, and other sensory inputs. One can think of cognitive processing as information compression, a step (or several steps) beyond conventional data compression [Wolf93C]. According to artificial intelligence research, three concepts are involved in cognitive processing: pattern matching, unification, and metrics-guided searching [John95B]. Patterns are found within a block of data and matched or unified

---

[1] Until recently, there was no worldwide standard for ASCII text data. This created a problem when exchanging ASCII-encoded data between countries observing differing standards. One solution was to FAX the data, scan the received documents, and use OCR to convert the data into the ASCII format observed in the receiving country.

with similar patterns learned from previous experience. Among these patterns, the best match(es) is located by search procedures that use some type of distance measure, a metric. When a match is found, the original pattern can be dispensed with, allowing a greatly compressed representation of its information to be stored or transmitted as a tag identifying the pattern. Cognitive processing is a far more powerful compression tool than are conventional data compression techniques. As you probably have guessed, the cost for this is significantly more computing power.

Figure 15.1 provides another perspective of cognitive processing as data compression. Recognition can be viewed as a compression operation that transcends what has been termed the cognition barrier [Arps79], transforming diffuse data to an equivalent symbolic data representation. Generation, the complementary operation, can be viewed as a decompression operation. Another parallel can be drawn between cognitive processing and data compression: Just as lossy compression does not always faithfully represent information, the recognition process is imperfect too. When data is transformed from diffuse to symbolic formats, both information loss and recognition errors may occur. Although lossy compression may slightly corrupt the information contained in diffuse data, recognition may substitute wholly incorrect and inappropriate symbolic data. For many applications the consequences of recognition errors are far more serious; incorrectly recognized characters and speech have been and continue to be inhibitors to OCR and speech recognition. Recognition technology is getting better, but many applications still require human assistance to get acceptable accuracy.

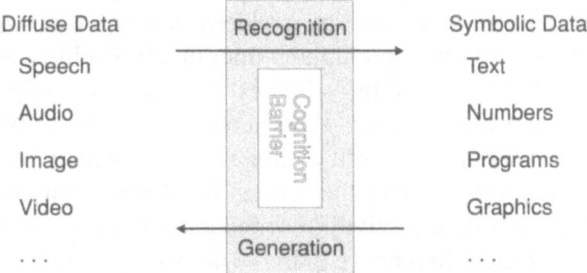

Figure 15.1   Cognitive processing.

With this background, let us turn to the next generation or generations of video compression algorithms now being explored. ITU-T and ISO video compression standards for the late 1990s (MPEG-4 for instance) are likely to move beyond perceptual coding, DCTs, and quantization. They are expected to employ coding methods that rely on or are closely related to cognitive processing techniques and make greater use of knowledge about the human visual system. There are several approaches, but the general idea for all is the same—analyze the scene, its structure, and content, then encode and transmit parameters that describe the scene. The simplest of these techniques analyzes a scene to discover humanly recognizable objects, describes them and their behavior in time, and then encodes and transmits information about object behavior. These are called object-based coding techniques [Ebra95]. More complex schemes involve both analysis and synthesis where objects in the scene are described by models, and it is the model parameters that are encoded and transmitted. As shown in Figure 15.2, the decoder maintains a copy of the model, and it uses the passed parameters to synthesize a representation of the objects in the scene. These are called model-based coding techniques where, for example, the model may be that of a human face or something more complex. Still more advanced video coding techniques, using even greater injections of recognition and human intelligence, have been proposed [Pear95].

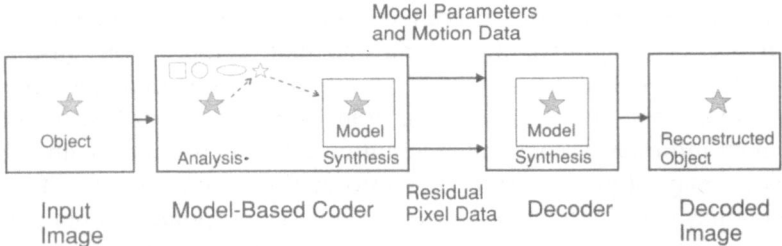

Figure 15.2   Model-based coding.

However, there are many unresolved issues to be addressed before any of these advanced video coding techniques are ready to leave the laboratory and be nominated as standards: Implementability, as always with new and surely more complex algorithms, is an obvious concern, but one that assuredly will be solved with the passage of time and higher-function VLSI chips. A more difficult issue for all advanced video coding schemes that make assumptions about the scene content, and especially model-based coding, is generality. In particular, most of the experimental model-based coding techniques have been designed for "talking head" applications, where the human head and shoulders are modeled and coded. Although highly effective for videoconferencing and videotelephone applications, these coding schemes are likely to do poorly when the scene contains other types of objects. The parallel between these model-based video coding techniques and vocoders, which work well on human voices and not on general audio signals, is apparent. Thus, MPEG-4, the next video coding standard that professes to apply to any video source material, whether based on model-based coding or something else, will require algorithms that generalize to a range of objects, including but not limited to human faces.

15.6   Conclusion

The purpose of this book has been to show that data compression is an invaluable technology for efficiently representing information in digital systems. Lossless compression for text and other symbolic data has developed over nearly four decades and, barring developments unforeseen by information theory today, lossless compression algorithms have reached maturity. So, too, have its implementations been perfected, making lossless compression feasible for nearly all applications. On the other hand, the most spectacular progress in lossy compression for diffuse data—speech, audio, image, and video—has occurred roughly within the last 10 years. Being far less mature, and in no way having yet reached limitations predicted by any theory, the discovery of better algorithms for diffuse data is all but inevitable. Clearly, with better algorithms, with more effective and economical implementations, there is great potential for even more widespread deployment of diffuse data compression. The future prospects for data compression are exciting!

Acronyms and Abbreviations

ACATS Advisory Committee on Advanced Television Service

ACR/NEMA American College of Radiology/National Electrical Manufacturers Association

ADPCM Adaptive Differential Pulse Code Modulation

ADSL Asymmetric Digital Subscriber Line

AES Audio Engineering Society

ALDC Adaptive Lossless Data Compression

AM Amplitude Modulation

ANSI American National Standards Institute

APPN Advanced Peer-to-Peer Networking

ASCII American national Standard Code of Information Interchange (a byte-oriented character encoding scheme)

ASIC Application-Specific Integrated Circuit

ATM Asynchronous Transfer Mode

ATRAC Adaptive TRansform Acoustic Coding

ATV Advanced (digital) Television

BLDC Bit-mapped Lossless Data Compression

BMCP Bidirectional Motion-Compensated Prediction

BTC Block Truncation Coding

BTI British Telecom International

B-tree Balanced-tree

CCD Charge-Coupled Device

CCIR Consultative Committee for International Radio

CCITT Consultative Committee for International Telephony & Telegraphy

CD Compact Disc

CDMA Code-Division Multiple Access communications

CDPD Cellular Digital Packet Data

CD-E Compact Disc—Erasable

CD-I Compact Disc—Interactive

CD-R Compact Disc—Recordable

CD-ROM Compact Disc—Read Only Memory

CD-ROM XA Compact Disc—Read-Only Memory eXtended Architecture

CELP Code-Excited Linear Predictive coding

CIF Common Intermediate Format for H.261 video

CISC Complex Instruction-Set Computer

CLI Compression Laboratories Inc.

CPU Central Processing Unit

CR Computed Radiography.

CRC Cyclic Redundancy Check error-detecting code

DAB Digital Audio Broadcast

DAR Digital Audio Radio

DARS Digital Audio Radio Services

DAT Digital Audio Tape

DAVIC Digital Audio-Video Council

dB Decibel

DBCS Double Byte Character Set (a double-byte-oriented character encoding scheme)

DBMS DataBase Management System

DBS Direct Broadcast Satellite

DCC Digital Compact Cassette tape

DCT Discrete Cosine Transform

DECnet Digital Equipment Corporation networking

DF Digital Fluorography

DFT Discrete Fourier Transform

DICOM Digital Imaging and Communications in Medicine

DOS Disk Operating System

DPCM Differential Pulse Code Modulation

DSA Digital Subtractive Angiography

DSP Digital Signal Processor

DSS Digital Satellite System

DVB Digital Video Broadcast

DVC Digital Video Cassette (a VCR format)

DVCR Digital VCR

DVD Digital Video Disc

DVI Digital Video Interactive

D-VHS Data-Video Home System (a VCR format)

DWT Discrete Wavelet Transform

EBCDIC Extended Binary-Coded Decimal Interchange Code (a byte-oriented character encoding scheme)

ECC Error-Correcting Code

FAX Facsimile

FBI U.S. Federal Bureau of Investigation

FCC Federal Communications Commission

FM Frequency Modulation

fps frames per second

FS Federal Standards (U.S. Federal Government)

GB GigaBytes

GBS GigaBytes per Second

GHz GigaHertz

GIF Graphics Interchange Format

GII Global Information Infrastructure

GOP Group of Pictures (for MPEG compression)

GSM Groupe Spéciale Mobile

GUI Graphic User Interface

HDC Hardware Data Compression (a data compression algorithm for IBM 3430 tape)

HDTV High-Definition Television

Hz Hertz

IAU Image Acquisition Unit

IEC International Electrotechnical Commission

IDRC Improved Data Recording Capability (an IBM-developed data compression algorithm for tape)

IMACS Image Management And Communications System

ISDN Integrated Services Digital Network

ISO International Organization for Standardization

IIT Integrated Information Technology

ITU-R International Telecommunication Union—Radio

ITU-T International Telecommunication Union—Transmission

ITU-T G.711 ITU-T standard for general telephony speech coding

ITU-T G.721 ITU-T standard for general telephony speech coding

ITU-T G.722 ITU-T standard for wide-band speech coding

ITU-T G.723 ITU-T standard for general telephony speech coding

ITU-T G.726 ITU-T standard for general telephony speech coding

ITU-T G.727 ITU-T standard for speech coding on packet-oriented networks

ITU-T G.728 ITU-T standard for general telephony speech coding

ITU-T G.729 ITU-T standard for cellular telephony speech coding

ITU-T H.261 ITU-T standard for motion video compression for videotelephony and videoconferencing on ISDN

ITU-T H.262 ITU-T standard for motion video compression for high-resolution videoconferencing over ATM

ITU-T H.263 ITU-T standard for motion video compression for videotelephony over PSTN analog telephone lines

ITU-T H.320 ITU-T standards series for videotelephony and videoconferencing on ISDN

ITU-T H.323 ITU-T standards series for data, audio, and videoconferencing over packet-switched networks

ITU-T H.324 ITU-T standards series for videotelephony over PSTN analog telephone lines

ITU-T T.120 ITU-T standards for data and graphics conferencing

ITU-T T.4 ITU-T Group 3 compression algorithm for FAX

ITU-T T.6 ITU-T Group 4 compression algorithm for FAX

ITU-T T.81 ITU-T standard for JPEG image compression

ITU-T T.82 ITU-T standard for JBIG image compression

ITU-T V.42bis ITU-T standard for modem data compression

I/O Input/Output

JBIG Joint Bi-level Image experts Group (a compression algorithm for image data)

JDC Japanese Digital Cellular

JPEG Joint Photographic Experts Group (a compression algorithm for still, continuous-tone image data)

KB KiloBytes

KHz KiloHertz

Kbps Kilobits per second

LAN Local-Area Network

LCD Liquid-Crystal Display

LD-CELP Low Delay—Code-Excited Linear Predictive coding

LEC Local Exchange Carrier (telephone company)

LMDS Local Multipoint Distribution System

LPAS Linear-Prediction-based Analysis-by-Synthesis coding

LPC Linear Predictive Coding

LRU Least-Recently Used

LZS Lempel-Ziv-Stacker (a compression algorithm for symbolic data)

LZW Lempel-Ziv-Welch (a compression algorithm for symbolic data)

M Million

MAN Metropolitan-Area Network

Mbps Megabits per second

MB MegaBytes

Mb Megabits

MBONE Multicast Backbone

MBS MegaBytes per Second

MCP Motion-Compensated Prediction

MD MiniDisc

MDCT Modified Discrete Cosine Transform

MDDS Multipoint Multichannel Distribution System

MH Modified Huffman coding

MHz MegaHertz

MIPS Millions of Instructions Per Second

mm Millimeter

MMR Modified Modified Read coding

MO Magneto-Optical

MPLP MultiPulse-excited Linear Prediction coding

MP-MLQ MultiPulse Maximum Likelihood Quantization coding

MR Modified Read coding

MS-DOS Microsoft Disk Operating System

MPEG Motion Picture Experts Group (an algorithm for motion video compression)

M-JPEG Motion-JPEG (a video compression technique)

NAB National Association of Broadcasters

NASA National Aeronautics and Space Administration

NII National Information Infrastructure

NM Nuclear Medicine

NTSC National Television Signal Committee (U.S. analog television transmission standard)

OCR Optical Character Recognition

OLTP Online Transaction Processing

OSI Open-Systems Interconnection

OSTA Optical Storage Technology Association

PACS Picture Archive and Communications System

PAL Phase Alternation Line (a European analog television transmission standard)

PASC Precision Audio Subband Coding

PC Personal Computer

PCI Peripheral Component Interface (a PC local bus)

PCM Pulse Code Modulation

PCMCIA Personal Computer Memory Card International Association

PD Phase-change Dual

PDA Personal Digital Assistant

PEL Picture Element

PET Positron Emission Tomography

Pixel Picture Element

POTS Plain Old Telephone Service

PSI-CELP Pitch Synchronous Innovative—Code-Excited Linear Predictive coding

PSTN Public Switched Telephone Network

QCELP Quantized Code-Excited Linear Predictive coding

QCIF Quarter-Common Intermediate Format for H.261 video

RAID Redundant Arrays of Independent Disks

RAM Random Access Memory

RAU Report Acquisition Unit

RBOC Regional Bell Operating Companies

READ Relative Element Address Designate coding

RGB Red-Green-Blue color components

RISC Reduced Instruction-Set Computer

ROC Receiver Operating Characteristic

ROM Read-Only Memory

RPE-LTP Regular Pulse Excitation— Long-Term Prediction coding

RPM Revolutions Per Minute

SDTV Standard-Definition Television

SECAM Sequential Couleur Avec Memoire (a European analog television transmission standard)

SG3 A PictureTel Corporation data compression algorithm for videoconferencing

SMDS Switched Multimegabit Data Service

SMPTE Society of Motion Picture and Television Engineers

SMR Signal-to-Mask Ratio

SNA IBM System Network Architecture

SPECT Single Photon Emission Computerized Tomography

STDM Statistical Time-Division Multiplexing

S-VHS Super Video Home System (a VCR format)

TCP/IP Transmission Control Protocol / Internet Protocol

TDM Time-Division Multiplexing

TDMA Time-Division Multiple Access communications

Telco Telephone company

TIA Telephone Industry Association (North American)

TV Television

T-1 A digital data transmission system operating at 1.544 Mbps

UHF Ultra-High-Frequency television channel assignment

U.S. United States

VCELP Vector-sum Excited Linear Predictive coding

VCR Video Cassette Recorder

VHF Very-High-Frequency television channel assignment

VHS Video Home System (a VCR format)

VLSI Very Large-Scale Integration

VRAM Video Random Access Memory

WAN Wide-Area Network

WORM Write-Once Read Many

X.25 A packet-switching network protocol

YUV Luminance-chrominance-chrominance color components

3M Minnesota Mining and Manufacturing Company

References

[AHA95] AHA3410 StarLite™ 25 Mbytes/Sec Simultaneous Lossless Data Compression/ Decompression Coprocessor IC, Advanced Hardware Architectures AHA3410 Product Brief, 1995.

[AMNE94] Sinatra Dials Up Duets, *America's Network*, February 15, 1994, p. 16.

[ANAS94] Dimitris Anastassiou, Digital Television, *Proceedings of the IEEE*, 82(4):510–519 (April 1994).

[ANDE94] Don Anderson, *PCMCIA System Architecture*, Richardson, TX, MindShare Inc. (1994).

[ANDL96] Prabhat K. Andleigh and Kiran Thakrar, *Multimedia Systems Design*, Upper Saddle River, NJ, Prentice-Hall, Inc. (1996).

[ANTO92] Marc Antonini, Michel Barlaud, Pierre Mathieu, and Ingrid Daubechies, Image Coding Using Wavelet Transform, *IEEE Transactions on Image Processing*, 1(2):205–220 (April 1992).

[ANTO95] Michael Antonoff, Digital Snapshots from My Vacation, *Popular Science*, 246(6):72–76 (June 1995).

[ANTO96] Michael Antonoff, More Wireless, *Video*, October 1996, pp. 14–15.

[APIK91] Steve Apiki, Lossless Data Compression, *Byte*, 16(3):309–312, 314, 386–387 (March 1991).

[ARAV93] Rangarajan Avavind, Glenn L. Cash, Donald L. Duttweller, Haush-Ming Hang, Barry G. Haskell, and Atui Puri, Image and Video Coding Standards, *AT&T Technical Journal*, 72(1):67–89 (January/February 1993).

[ARMS94] Larry Armstrong, Ira Sager, Kathy Rebello, and Peter Burrows, Home Computers, *Business Week*, November 28, 1994, pp. 89–94.

[ARNS96] Catherine Arnst and Michael Mandel, The Coming Telescramble, *Business Week*, April 8, 1996, pp. 64–66.

[ARPS79] Ronald B. Arps, Binary Image Compression, In William K. Pratt (editor), *Image Compression Techniques*, pp. 219–276, San Francisco, Academic Press Inc. (1979).

[ARPS88] R. B. Arps, T. K. Truong, D. J. Lu, R. C. Pasco, and T. D. Friedman, A Multi-Purpose VLSI Chip for Adaptive Data Compression of Bilevel Images, *IBM Journal of Research and Development*, 32(6):775–795 (November 1988).

[ARPS94] Ronald B. Arps and Thomas K. Truong, Comparison of International Standards for Lossless Still Image Compression, *Proceedings of the IEEE*, 82(6):889–899 (June 1994).

[BAIN95] Rupert Baines, Getting Information to Everyone's Home, *Electronic Engineering Times*, October 2, 1995, pp. 48, 65.

[BANE95] Bernard Banet, Encyclopedias on CD-ROM: The Market Advances, *The Seybold Report on Desktop Publishing*, 9(6):3–16 (February 6, 1995).

[BARR93] Jim Barry, Small Dish, Big Picture, *Video*, August 1993, pp. 30–33, 46.

[BASI95] Carlo Basile, Alan P. Cavallerano, Michael S. Deiss, Robert Keeler, Jae S. Lim, Wayne C. Luplow, Woo H. Paik, Eric Petajan, Robert Rast, Glenn Reitmeier, Terrence R. Smith, and Craig Todd (The Grand Alliance authors), The U.S. HDTV Standard: The Grand Alliance, *IEEE Spectrum*, 32(4):36–45 (April 1995).

[BEAC94] Frank Beacham, Hype, Hope & Reality: Why the Video Superhighway Will Take Longer & Cost More Than Anyone Believed, *Video*, August 1994, pp. 36–39.

[BEER93] Jeffrey Beer, Video For Windows, Microsoft's Latest Multimedia Winner, *CD-ROM Professional*, 6(5):44–46 (September 1993).

[BELL89] Timothy C. Bell, John G. Cleary, and Ian H. Witten, Modeling for Text Compression, *ACM Computing Surveys*, 21(4):557–592 (December 1989).

[BELL90] Timothy C. Bell, John G. Cleary, and Ian H. Witten, *Text Compression*, Englewood Cliffs, NJ, Prentice-Hall, Inc. (1990).

[BELL95] Trudy E. Bell, Remote Sensing, *IEEE Spectrum*, 32(3):24–31 (March 1995).

[BELL96] Trudy E. Bell, John A Adam, and Sue J. Lowe, Communications, *IEEE Spectrum*, 33(1):30–41 (January 1996).

[BENS94] Jim Benson, Searching for Stock Photos Online, *Macworld*, 11(8):124 (August 1994).

[BLAH95] Donald E. Blahut, Texas E. Nichols, William M. Schell, Guy A. Story, and Edward S. Szurkowski, Interactive Television, *Proceedings of the IEEE*, 83(7):1071–1085 (July 1995).

[BOUR95] Cynthia Bournellis, Internet '95: The Internet's Phenomenal Growth is Mirrored in Startling Statistics, *Internet World*, 6(11):47–52 (November 1995).

[BOYD95] Rick Boyd-Merritt, Iterated Claims Advances in Fractal Compression, *Electronic Engineering Times*, April 24, 1995, p. 105.

[BRAH95] Robert Braham, The Digital Backlot, *IEEE Spectrum*, 32(7):51–63 (July 1995).

[BRCA93] Fox Movietone Counts on Digital, Archives in 0S and 1S, *Broadcasting & Cable*, 123(44):D4 (November 1, 1993).

[BROW95] Chappell Brown, Video Processing Goes Parallel, *Electronic Engineering Times*, July 24, 1995, p. 37.

[BRYA94] Marvin Bryan, *DiskDoubler & AutoDoubler*, New York, Windcrest Books/ McGraw-Hill, Inc. (1994).

[BRYA95] John Bryan, Compression Scorecard, *Byte*, 20(5):107–108, 110, 112 (May 1995).

[BURR92] Michael Burrows, Charles Jerian, Butler Lampson, and Thimothy Mann, On-line Data Compression in a Log-structured File System, *ASPLOS-V Proceedings, Fifth International Conference on Architectural Support for Programming Languages and Operating Systems*, ACM/IEEE, Boston, MA, October 12–15, 1992, pp. 2–9.

[BUSC95] David D. Busch, Point and Shoot (Eight Digital Cameras), Getting the Picture, *Windows Sources*, 3(11):139–143 (November 1995).

[CABO94] Richard C. Cabot, Performance Assessment of Reduced Bit Rate Codecs, Presentation at the Audio Engineering Society Conference "Managing the Bit Budget," London, England, May 1994, available from Audio Precision, Inc., Beaverton, OR.

[CAHN91] Robert. S. Cahn, P.C. Chang, P. Kermani, and Arron Kershenbaum, INTREPID: An Integrated Network Tool for Routing, Evaluation of Performance, and Interactive Design, *IEEE Communications Magazine*, 29(7) 40–47 (July 1991).

[CAHN92] Robert S. Cahn and Arron Kershenbaum, Architectural Studies of Data Compression Using the INTREPID Network Design Tool, IBM Research Report RC18348, September 1992.

[CAPP85] Vito Cappellini (editor), *Data Compression and Error Control Techniques with Applications*, London, Academic Press, Inc. (1985).

[CATA95] Anthony Cataldo, AT&T boosts APV Programmability to Support Multiple Video Codecs, *Electronic News*, May 8, 1995, p. 48.

[CHAL95] Kiran Challapall, Xavier Lebegue, Jae S. Lim, Woo H. Paik, Regis Saint Girons, Eric Petajan, Vinay Sathe, Paul A. Snopko, and Joel Zdepski, The Grand Alliance System for US HDTV, *Proceedings of the IEEE*, 83(2):158–174 (February 1995).

[CHAN95] Shih-Fu Chang and David G. Messerschmitt, Manipulation and Compositing of MC-DCT Compressed Video, *IEEE Transactions on Selected Areas in Communications*, 13(1):1–11 (January 1995).

[CHEN93] Cheng-Tie Chen, Video Compression: Standards and Applications, *Journal of Visual Communication and Image Representation*, 4(2):103–111 (June 1993).

[CHEN94] Walter Y. Chen and David L. Waring, Applicability of ADSL to Support Video Dial Tone in the Copper Loop, *IEEE Communications Magazine*, 32(5) 102–109 (May 1994).

[CHEN95] J. M. Cheng and L. M. Duyanovich, Fast and Highly Reliable IBMLZ1 Compression Chip and Algorithm for Storage, *Proceeding of Hot Chips VII*, Stanford University, CA, August 13–15, 1995.

[CHIA94] Tihao Chiang and Dimitris Anastassiou, Hierarchical Coding of Digital Television, *IEEE Communications Magazine*, 32(5):38–52 (May 1994).

[CHIA95] Leonardo Chiariglione, The Development of an Integrated Audiovisual Coding Standard: MPEG, *Proceedings of the IEEE*, 83(2):151–157 (February 1995).

[CHIL95] Jeff Child, Data-Compression Chips Get Specific, *Computer Design*, 34(8):46–48 (August 1995).

[CHIM92] William J Chimiak, The Digital Radiology Environment, *IEEE Transactions on Selected Areas in Communications*, 10(7):1133–1144 (September 1992).

[CICI93] Walter S. Ciciora, Scenarios for Compression on Cable, *1993 International Television Symposium*, Vol. 242, pp. 435–443, 1993. [Also in Theodore S. Rzeszewski (editor), *Digital Video Concepts and Applications Across Industries*, pp. 295–303, Piscataway, NJ, IEEE Press (1995).]

[CICI95] Walter S. Ciciora, Inside The Set-Top Box, *IEEE Spectrum*, 32(4):70–75 (April 1995).

[CLAR95] Don Clark, Chip Makers Make Gains Regarding Images, Sound, *Minneapolis Star Tribune*, October 15, 1995, p. D3 (an article reprinted from the *Wall Street Journal*).

[COCO95] Donna Coco, Compositing and Special Effects: Graphics Software Offers Film and Video Makers Powerful Features, *Computer Graphics World*, 18(5):46–50 (May 1995).

[CODY93] W. F. Cody, H. M. Gladney, M. B. Heritage, D. B. Hildebrand, and J. D. Reinke, Can Hospitals Afford Digital Storage for Imagery? IBM Research Report RJ9413, June 1993.

[COHN91] D. L. Cohn, P. M. Greenwalt, M. R. Casey, and M.P. Stevenson, Using Kernel Level Support for Distributed Shared Data, *Proceedings of the Symposium on Experiences with Distributed and Multiprocessor Systems, UNENIX*, Atlanta, GA, June 24–25, 1992.

[COLE94] Bernard C. Cole, Motion-Video ICs Boost Multimedia PCs, *Electronic Engineering Times*, January 30, 1995, pp. 52, 54.

[COLE95] Bernard C. Cole, Set-top Is Pandora's Box, *Electronic Engineering Times*, January 30, 1995, pp. 52, 54.

[COLL93] Andrew Collier, Group to Advocate Multimedia, *CommunicationsWeek*, June 28, 1993, p. 8.

[COME96] Richard Comerford, Interactive Media: An Internet Reality, *IEEE Spectrum*, 33(4):29–32 (April 1996).

[CONN95] RAM Doubler For Windows, Connectix Corporation, San Mateo, CA, 1995.

[COOP82] David Cooper and Michael F. Lynch, Text Compression Using Variable-to-Fixed-Length Encodings, *Journal of the American Society for Information Science*, January 1982, pp. 18–31.

[COOP93] Johnathan Coopersmith, Facsimile's False Starts, *IEEE Spectrum*, 30(2):46–49 (February 1993).

[CORT95] Amy Cortese, Once Again, Software Is Seething, *Business Week*, January 9, 1995, p. 76.

[COSM93] Pamela C. Cosman, Karen L. Oehler, Eve A. Riskin, and Robert M. Gray, Using Vector Quantization for Image Processing, *Proceedings of the IEEE*, 81(9):1326–1341 (September 1993).

[COST92] Terry Costlow, Compressed Data Makes Iceberg Hot, *Electronic Engineering Times*, February 3, 1992, p. 14.

[COST96] Terry Costlow, Kodak-Led Group Sets Digital-Image Format, *Electronic Engineering Times*, June 10, 1996, pp. 4, 142.

[COVE78] Thomas M. Cover and Roger C. King, A Convergent Gambling Estimate of the Entropy of English, *IEEE Transactions on Information Theory*, 24(4):413–421 (July 1978).

[COY95] Peter Coy and Neil Gross, Cowboys Vs. Committees, *Business Week*, April 10, 1995, pp. 104–106.

[COX92] Jerome R. Cox, Jr., Edward Muka, G. James Blaine, Stephen M. Moore, and R. Gilbert Jost, Considerations in Moving Electronic Radiography into Routine Use, *IEEE Transactions on Selected Areas in Communications*, 10(7):1108–1120 (September 1992).

[CRAF95] David J. Craft, ADLC and a Pre-Processor Extension, BDLC, Provides Ultra Fast Compression for General-Purpose and Bit-Mapped Image Data, In James A. Storer and Martin Cohn (editors), *Data Compression Conference 1995*, p. 440, Los Alamitos, CA., IEEE Computer Society Press (1995).

[CROU93] Paul E. Crouch, J. Al Hicks, and John J. Jetzt, ISDN Personal Video, *AT&T Technical Journal*, 72(1):33–40 (January/February 1993).

[CROT95] Cameron Crotty, CompuServe GIF Uproar:On the Menu: Royalty Surprise, *Macworld*, 12(5):38 (May 1995).

[CRUT94] Laurence Crutcher and John Grinham, The Networked Video Jukebox, *IEEE Transactions on Circuits and Systems for Video Technology*, 4(2):105–120 (April 1994).

[CUMM96] Joanne Cummings, Drumming Up Support, *Network World*, 13(3):C27-C28 (January 15, 1996).

[CUTA90] Al Cutaia, *Technology Modeling of Future Computer Systems*, Englewood Cliffs, NJ, Prentice-Hall, Inc. (1990).

[DALL90] William J. Dallas, A Digital Prescription for X-ray Overload, *IEEE Spectrum*, 27(4):33–36 (April 1990).

[DARL95] Charles B. Darling, Routers Can Save Your WAN Dollars, *Datamation*, 41(13):64–67 (July 1, 1995).

[DAVI93] Mark F. Davis, The AC–3 Multichannel Coder, *Proceedings of the 95th Convention of the Audio Engineering Society, Inc.,* October 7–10, 1993, Reprint Publication No. S93/9951.

[DAVI94] Robert P. Davidson, *Broadband Networking ABCs for Managers: ATM, BISDN, Cell/Frame Relay to Sonet*, New York, John Wiley & Sons, Inc. (1994).

[DAVI95] Mark F. Davis (Dolby Laboratories, Inc.), AC–3 Bit Lengths, private communication, June 23, 1995.

[DEIT83] Harvey M. Deitel, *An Introduction to Operating Systems*, Reading, MA, Addison-Wesley Publishing Company, Inc. (1983)

[DICK95A] Glen Dickson, Digital Goes to Work for Adlink, *Broadcasting & Cable*, 125(45):108 (November 6, 1995).

[DICK95B] Glen Dickson, Garth Goes Digital, *Broadcasting & Cable*, 125(46):88 (November 13, 1995).

[DOYL94] T. C. Doyle, Stac Wins Patent Suit, Microsoft to Pay $120M, *Computer Reseller News*, February 28, 1994, p. 3.

[DSPG95] Truespeech™ 6.3, 5.3, 4.8 Kbps Algorithm ITU G.723, DSP Group, Inc. Publication TS 6.3–4/11/95, 1995.

[DURR94] Michael Durr, Fast Imaging on Slow Networks, *Datamation*, 40(24):61–62 (December 15, 1994).

[EARL93] Scott H. Early, Andrew Kuzma, and Eric Dorsey, The VideoPhone 2500— Video Telephony on the Public Switched Telephone Network, *AT&T Technical Journal*, 72(1):22–32 (January/February 1993).

[EBRA95] Touradj Ebrahimi, Emmanuel Reusens, and Wei Li, New Trends in Very Low Bitrate Video Coding, *Proceedings of the IEEE*, 83(6):877–891, (June 1995).

[EDGE92] Computer Conferencing: IBM Scientists Demo Prototype of Affordable Computer Conferencing Systems, *EDGE Work-Group Computing Report*, 3(128):2 (November 2, 1992).

[EDGE95A] Storage: HARC Unveils Cutting-Edge Compression Technology, *EDGE Work-Group Computing Report*, 6(250):35 (March 6, 1995).

[EDGE95B] DBS: Primestar, Tempo & Advanced Communications Seek Reversal of FCC Staff Order Limiting Competition in High-Power DBS, *EDGE, on & about AT&T*, 10(357):10 (May 29, 1995).

[EDGE95C] Chips: DSP Group Introduces Digital TAD Processors for Flash Memory, *EDGE, on & about AT&T*, 10(364):24 (July 17, 1995).

[EDGE95D] Satellite Launch: AlphaStar Digital Television Launched on AT&T Satellite; Communications Satellite Carries 14 Transponders for AlphaStar Digital DTH System, *EDGE, on & about AT&T*, 10(375):22 (October 2, 1995).

[EDGE96] New Satellite: EchoStar-I Lift-Off Successful, *EDGE, on & about AT&T*, 11(389):5 (January 1, 1996).

[EDWA94] Stephen E. Edwards, David Neeff, Rosanne Rossello, and Andrew Tribute, Nexpo, II: Electronic Delivery, Output, Digital Photography, Image Databases, *The Seybold Report on Publishing Systems*, 23(22):3–57 (August 15, 1994).

[EET95A] Video Dialtone Gets Bell Boost, *Electronics Engineering Times*, February 20, 1995, p.2.

[EET95B] MPEG Licensing Unit Planned, *Electronics Engineering Times*, April 3, 1995, p. 2.

[EET96] MPEG License Group Nearly Set, *Electronics Engineering Times*, May 6, 1996, p. 2.

[ELNE95] DBS Systems Drive Set-Top Demand, *Electronic News*, 41(2082):28 (September 11, 1995).

[ELTI92] Pictures of the World in A Spin, *Electronics Times*, September 10, 1992, p. 23.

[ELTI93] Microsoft Facing Suit over Data Compression, *Electronics Times*, February 4, 1993, p. 6.

[FORS94] Steven E. Forshay, Audio Compression 101, *Broadcast Engineering*, September 1994, pp. 78–90.

[FOST94] Bill Foster, Sonopress: Part 2 Archiving, *One to One*, May 1994, p. 63.

[FOX95] Barry Fox, The Digital Dawn in Europe, *IEEE Spectrum*, 32(4):50–53 (April 1995).

[FRAN92] Bob Francis, Double Your Drives with Data Compression, *Datamation*, 38(24):49–51 (December 1, 1992).

[FREN95] Jeff Frentzen, Standards Emerge for Internet-Based Audio Technology, *PC Week*, 12(32):10 (August 14, 1995).

[FRIT95] Mark Fritz, Multimedia Motherboard-Bound: Digital Signal Processing Chips and the Quest for Integrated Multimedia, *CD-ROM Professional*, 8(12):32–52 (December 1995).

[FTL94] International Company News: Microsoft Ordered to Pay Patents Damages, To Pay $120 mil to Stac Electronics for Patent Infringement of Data Compression, *Financial Times Ltd. (London)*, February 24, 1994, p. 34.

[GAFF95] Adam Gaffin, Confusion Reigns on the Web Over GIF Patent Claims; New Graphics Formats Under Development, *Network World*, 12(2):4 (January 9, 1995).

[GEMM95] D. James Gemmell, Harrick M. Vin, Dilip D. Kandlur, P. Venkat Rangan, and Lawrence A. Rowe, Multimedia Storage Servers: A Tutorial, *IEEE Computer*, 28(5):40–49 (May 1995).

[GERS93] Nahum D. Gershon and C. Grant Miller, Dealing with the Data Deluge, *IEEE Spectrum*, 30(7):28–32 (July 1993).

[GERS94] Allen Gersho, Advances in Speech and Audio Compression, *Proceedings of the IEEE*, 82(6):900–918 (June 1994).

[GIBB95] Mark Gibbs, Web Sites: The Good, the Bad and the Complete Waste of Bandwidth, *Network World*, 12(51):36–38, 41 (December 18, 1995).

[GOUL95] Michael A. Goulde, World Wide Web Servers, *Open Information Systems*, 10(9):3–34 (September 1995).

[GREE95A] Tim Greene, SDSL Promises T–1 Bandwidth over Standard Telephone Lines, *Network World*, 12(40):17, 22 (October 2, 1995).

[GREE95B] Tim Greene, Modem Can Deliver Video on Demand in Blink of an Eye, *Network World*, 12(44):19–20 (October 30, 1995).

[GREE96] Tim Greene, Beam Your ATM Traffic over to Foreign LANs, *Network World*, 13(15):25 (April 8, 1996).

[GREH93] Rick Grehan and Stan Wszola, Shrink to Fit, *Byte*, 18(4):150–156,158, 160, 162 (April 1993).

[GROS95] Neil Gross, Peter Burrows, and Robert D. Hof, Internet Lite: Who Needs a PC? *Business Week*, November 13, 1995, pp. 102–103.

[GUEN96] David R. Guenette, Document Imaging, CD-ROM, and CD-R: A Starting Point, *CD-ROM Professional*, 9(4):32–44 (April 1996).

[GURU84] Anura Gurugé, *SNA Theory and Practice*, Maidenhead, Berkshire, England, Pergamon Infotech Limited (1984).

[HABI92] Ali Habibi, Future Trends in Image Coding, *SPIE Applications of Digital Image Processing XV*, 1771:406- 412 (1992).

[HALH91] Basil R. Halhed and D. Lynn Scott, Videoconferencing Market Trends, *Business Communications Review*, 21(10):51–56 (October 1991).

[HAMA95] Jukka Hamalainen, Video Recording Goes Digital, *IEEE Spectrum*, 32(4):76–80 (April 1995).

[HANG94] N. J. Hangiandreou, B. Williamson, D. Gehring, K. R. Persons, F. J. Reardon, J. R. Salutz, J. P. Felmlee, M. D. Loewen, and G. S. Forbes, Current Status of the Joint

Mayo Clinic-IBM PACS Project, *Medical Imaging VIII: PACS Design and Evaluation, SPIE Proceedings*, Edited by R. G. Jost, et al., 2165:519–526 (1994).

[HARA95A] Yoshiko Hara and Terry Costlow, Digital Compression to Seek Spotlight at NAB, *Electronic Engineering Times*, April 3, 1995, p. 24.

[HARA95B] Yoshiko Hara, Digital Camcorders Due from Two, *Electronic Engineering Times*, August 14, 1995, p. 16.

[HARK82] John Harker, Byte Oriented Data Compression Techniques, *Computer Design*, 22(10):95, 95, 98, 100 (October 1982).

[HARR93] Matthew Harris, *The Disk Compression Book*, Indianapolis, IN, Que Corporation (1993).

[HECK94] Christine Heckart, Myriad of Factors Blur Desktop Video Picture, *Network World*, 10(5):50, 53, 54, 57, 58 (October 31, 1994).

[HELD91] Gilbert Held and Thomas R. Marshall, *Data Compression: Techniques and Applications, Hardware and Software Considerations*, New York, John Wiley & Sons, Inc. (1991).

[HEYW95] Peter Heywood, Compression and Routers, Together at Last, *Data Communications*, 24(5):55–56, 61–63 (April 1995).

[HINE95] John R. Hines, Program Notes: Look the GIF Horse in the Mouth, *IEEE Spectrum*, 32(3):20 (March 1995).

[HOF95] Robert D. Hof and Peter Burrows, Intel: Far Beyond the Pentium, *Business Week*, February 20, 1995, pp. 88–90.

[HOFF70] R. L. Hoffman and K. Fukunaga, Pattern Recognition Signal Analysis For Mechanical Diagnostics Signature Analysis, *IEEE Conference Record of the Symposium on Feature Extraction and Selection in Pattern Recognition*, Chicago, IL, October 5–7, 1970, pp. 226–235.

[HOFF92] Eric Hoffert, Mark Krueger, Lee Mighdoll, Micheal Mills, Johnathan Cohen, Doug Camplejohn, Bruce Leak, Jim Batson, David Van Brink, Dean Blackketter, Michael Arent, Rich Williams, Chris Thorman, Mitch Yawitz, Ken Doyle, and Sean Callahan, Quicktime™: An Extensible Standard for Digital Multimedia, *IEEE COMPCOM Proceedings*, Vol. 37, pp. 15–20, Spring 1992. [Also in Theodore S. Rzeszewski (editor), *Digital Video Concepts and Applications Across Industries*, pp. 552–557, Piscataway, NJ, IEEE Press (1995).]

[HOOG94] Abraham Hoogendoorn, Digital Compact Cassette, *Proceedings of the IEEE*, 82(10):1477–1489 (October 1994).

[HOPK94] Robert Hopkins, Choosing an American Digital HDTV Terrestrial Broadcasting System, *Proceedings of the IEEE*, 82(4):554–563 (April 1994).

[HOWA95] Bill Howard, Multimedia Marvels, *PC Magazine*, 14(8):189–191, 196, 199–202, 206–208, 210, 215–218 (April 25, 1995).

[HUFF52] D.A. Huffman, A Method for the Construction of Minimal Redundancy Codes, *Proceedings of IRE*, 40(9):1098–1101 (September 1952).

[HUNE89] Bryan L Huneycutt, Spaceborne Imaging Radar—C Instrument, *IEEE Transactions on Geoscience and Remote Sensing*, 27(2):164–169 (March 1989).

[HUNT93] M. A. Hunt, Wavelets Accelerate Fingerprinting Methods, *Electronic Engineering Times*, September 27 1993, p. 74.

[IBD95] Double Your PC Pleasure by Doubling Your RAM, *Investor's Business Daily*, June 1, 1995.

[IBM1] AS/400 Basic Backup and Recover Guide, IBM Publication SC41–0036–02, 1993.

[IBM2] IBM AIX Version 4.1, IBM Product Announcement, July 26, 1994.

[IBM3] AS/400 Central Site Distribution Guide, IBM Publication SC41–9993, 1995.

[IBM4] AS/400 CL Programming Guide, IBM Publication SC41–8077, 1995.

[IBM5] Enterprise Systems Architecture/390 Data Compression, IBM Publication SA22–7208, 1993.

[IBM6] AS/400 Machine Interface Function Reference, IBM Publication SC41–8226, 1994.

[INTE94] DiskMizer, Data Compression Software and Utilities for VMS User's Guide, Intersecting Concepts Inc., Agoura Hills, CA, 1994.

[IYER94] Balakrishna Iyer and David Wilhite, Data Compression Support in Databases, IBM Technical Report TR03.547, April 1994.

[JACO90] Van Jacobson, Compressing TCP/IP Headers for Low-Speed Serial Links, Network Working Group Request for Comments RFC 1144, Lawrence Berkeley Laboratory, Berkeley, CA, February 1990.

[JACQ93] Arnaud E. Jacquin, Fractal Image Coding: A Review, *Proceedings of the IEEE*, 81(10):1451–1465 (October 1993).

[JOHN94] Stuart J Johnston, Microsoft Settles for Piece of the Stac, *Computerworld*, 28(26):30 (June 27, 1994).

[JOHN95A] R. Colin Johnson, Impressive Compression, *Electronic Engineering Times*, January 30, 1995, p. 56.

[JOHN95B] R. Colin Johnson, Is Cognition Really Compression? *Electronic Engineering Times*, October 30, 1995, pp. 47, 52.

[JULI95] Egil Juliussen, Small Computers, *IEEE Spectrum*, 32(1):44–47 (January 1995).

[JURG92] Ronald K. Jurgen, Consumer Electronics, *IEEE Spectrum*, 29(1):52–54 (January 1992).

[JURG93] Ronald K. Jurgen, Consumer Electronics, *IEEE Spectrum*, 30(1):65–67 (January 1993).

[JURG96] Ronald K. Jurgen, Broadcasting with Digital Audio, *IEEE Spectrum*, 33(3):52–59 (March 1996).

[KALS95] David Kalstrom, Optical, CD Recordable: Some WORMS Run Faster, *Computer Technology Review*, 15(2):36–37 (February 1995).

[KARN95] James Karney, CapaCD Boosts CDs Beyond 650 MB, *PC Magazine*, 14(8):42 (April 25, 1995).

[KARV95] Anita Karve, Hooray for Hollywood, *LAN Magazine*, 10(2):125–130 (February 1995).

[KEIZ92] Andreas Keizers, Dietrich Meyer-Ebrecht, and Ferdinand Vossebürger, A Fiber-Optic Line-Switching Network with a 140 Mb/s User Data Rate, *IEEE Journal in Selected Areas of Communication*, 10(7):1197- 1202 (September 1992).

[KHER95] Gerry Khermouch, Large Computers, *IEEE Spectrum*, 32(1):48–51 (January 1995).

[KLEI95] Kenneth R. Klein, Jr., Mahendra Pratap, and Jerry A. Prestinario, Combining Voice and Data on a POTS Line, *AT&T Technology*, 10(1):24–27 (Spring 1995).

[KOBB95] Bennett Z. Kobb, Telecommunications, *IEEE Spectrum*, 32(1):30–34 (January 1995).

[KOBI95A] James Kobielus, Drawing a Bead on Desktop Conferencing, *Network World Collaboration*, May/June, 1995, pp. 11, 12, 14, 18, 23.

[KOBI95B] James Kobielus, Standards, Floodwalls Will be Key to Making Internet Packet Video Viable, *Network World*, 12(26):36 (June 26, 1995).

[KODA94] PHOTO CD INFORMATION BULLETIN: Fully Utilizing Photo CD Images, Article No. 4, Photo YCC Color Encoding and Compression Schemes, 1994, available via ftp from the Eastman Kodak Company WWW site as: *ftp://ftp.kodak.com/pub/photo-cd/general/pcd045.txt*.

[KODA96] FlashPix Architecture Combines New, Existing Technologies to Make Digital Imaging Popular, June 3, 1996, available from the Eastman Kodak Company WWW site.

[KRAU95A] Reinhardt Krause, JVC Format, Sans MPEG, Attracts Thompson, Hitachi, *Electronic News*, April 10, 1995, p. 1.

[KRAU95B] Reinhardt Krause, 3DO May Diverge into PCs, DVDs (Digital Video Disk Players), *Electronic News*, September 18, 1995, p. 22.

[KROE88] David M. Kroen and Kathleen A. Dolan, *Database Processing:Fundamentals, Design, Implementation*, Chicago, Science Research Associates, Inc. (1988).

[LABR95] Don Labriola, Desktop Videoconferencing Candid Camera, *PC Magazine*, 14(8):221–226, 230, 231, 236, 238, 240–242, 244–246, 251–254 (April 25, 1995).

[LANG81A] Glen G. Langdon, Jr., Tutorial on Arithmetic Coding, IBM Research Report RJ3128, IBM Research Laboratory, San Jose, 1981.

[LANG81B] Glen G. Langdon, Jr. and Jorma Rissanen, Compression of Black-White Images with Arithmetic Coding, *IEEE Transactions on Communications*, 29(6):858–867 (June 1981).

[LANG95A] Mark Langner and Tom Brennan, Up in the Air, *Network World*, 12(38):49–50, 52 (September 18, 1995).

[LANG95B] Larry Lange, Real-Time Video Set for the Net, *Electronic Engineering Times*, December 11, 1995, p. 22.

[LARG95] David Large, Creating A Network For Interactivity, *IEEE Spectrum*, 32(4):58–63 (April 1995).

[LARO94] Judy Larocque, Client-Server Trends, *IEEE Spectrum*, 31(4):48–50 (April 1994).

[LEAC96] Norvin Leach, Stac Pulls Plug on Future Stacker Developments, *PC Week*, 13(17):8 (April 29, 1996).

[LEAV95] Neal Leavitt, Trends in Desktop Videoconferencing, *Enterprise Communications*, April 1995, pp. 24–31.

[LEE95] Ruby B. Lee, John P. Beck, Joel Lamb, and Kenneth E. Severson, Real-Time Software MPEG Video Decoder on Multimedia-Enhanced PA 7100LC Processors, *Hewlett-Packard Journal*, 46(2):60–68 (April 1995).

[LELL92] D. Lellouch and L. Levinson, Offline Data Compression in a Large Experiment,

References 385

Proceedings of the International Conference on Computing in High Energy Physics '92, Anney, France, September 21–25, 1992, pp. 884–887.

[LEOP95A] George Leopold, Bell Atlantic Granted Long-Distance-TV OK, *Electronic Engineering Times*, March 27, 1995, p. 18.

[LEOP95B] George Leopold, Battle to Be First on Air with Digital Radio Erupts (USA Digital Radio Group Plans FCC Petition), *Electronic Engineering Times*, April 24, 1995, p. 16.

[LEOP95C] George Leopold, Davic Group Close to Adopting Set-Top Standard, *Electronic Engineering Times*, May 15, 1995, p. 10.

[LEOP95D] George Leopold and Junko Yoshida, SDTV Seen as Way for Broadcasters to Compete, *Electronic Engineering Times*, June 19, 1995, pp. 14, 20.

[LEOP96] George Leopold and Loring Wirbel, Deregulation: Dial D for Danger, *Electronic Engineering Times*, February 12, 1996, pp. 1, 118.

[LEVI95] Harry Levinson, Compression Technology and Channel Extension, *Enterprise Systems Journal*, 10(4):60–64 (March 1995).

[LEWI94] Ted G. Lewis, Where is Computing Heading? *IEEE Computer*, 27(8):59–63 (August 1994).

[LIDD96] Dave Liddell, (IBM Corporation), Document Imaging Systems, private communication, October 1, 1996.

[LIEB95] Jörg Liebeherr, Multimedia Networks: Issues and Challenges, *IEEE Computer*, 28(4):68–69 (April 1995).

[LIEB96] Carl Liebold, Telcos Look to Enter Homes Via DSL, *Electronic Engineering Times*, March 4, 1996, pp. 52, 106.

[LIN95] David W. Lin, Cheng-Tie Chen, and T. Russell Hsing, Video on Phone Lines: Technology and Applications, *Proceedings of the IEEE*, 83(2):175–193 (February 1995).

[LINH93] Gordon Linhoff and Craig Stanfill, Compression of Indexes with Full Positional Information in Very Large Text Databases, *Proceedings of the Sixteenth Annual International ACM SIGIR Conference on Research and Development in Information Retrieval*, Pittsburgh, PA, June 1993, pp. 88—95.

[LITZ88] Michael J. Litzkov, Miron Livny, and Matt W. Watka, CONDOR—A Hunter of Idle Workstations, *Proceedings of the 8th International Conference on Distributed Computing Systems*, San Jose, CA, June 1988, pp. 104–111.

[LUTH91] Arch C. Luther, *Digital Video in the PC Environment, Second Edition*, New York, McGraw-Hill Book Company (1991).

[LYNC85] Thomas J. Lynch, *Data Compression Techniques and Applications*, Belmont, CA, Wadsworth Inc. (1985).

[MALL93] Jim Mallory, Microsoft Countersues Stac Electronics, *Newsbytes News Network*, February 25, 1993.

[MALL94A] Jim Mallory, Stac Awarded $120 Million in Microsoft Suit, *Newsbytes News Network*, February 24, 1994.

[MALL94B] Jim Mallory, Stac Electronics President Reacts to Court Awards, *Newsbytes News Network*, February 28, 1994.

[MALL94C] Jim Mallory, Microsoft Ships DOS 6.22 with New Data Compression, *Newsbytes News Network*, June 6, 1994.

[MANN95] George Mannes, The Need for Speed: A New Breed of Modems Makes Data Transfer Less Costly, *Popular Mechanics*, 172(9):77–79, 119 (September 1995).

[MARR95] Michel Marriott, Regina Elam, Ellise Pierce, and Steve Rhodes, Flight of the Digital Dish, *Business Week*, January 9, 1995, p. 61.

[MART77] James Martin, *Computer Data-Base Organization, 2nd edition*, Englewood Cliffs, NJ, Prentice-Hall, Inc. (1977).

[MBR95] MPC Level III Standard Under Development, *Multimedia Business Report*, 4(12):1–2 (March 31, 1995).

[MCCO92] Kenneth R. McConnell, Dennis Bodson, and Richard Schaphorst, *FAX: Digital Facsimile Technology and Applications, Second Edition*, Norwood, MA, Artech House, Inc. (1992)

[MCCO94A] John A. McCormick, *The New Optical Storage Technology—Including Multimedia, CD-ROM, and Optical Drives*, Burr Ridge, IL, Irwin Professional Publishing (1994).

[MCCO94B] Chris McConnell, Otari's MiniDisc Tackles Cart Market, *Broadcasting & Cable*, 124(34):36–37 (August 22, 1994).

[MCCO94C] Chris McConnell, FoNet Reach Growing, *Broadcasting & Cable*, 124(40):47–48 (October 3, 1994).

[MCWI95] Gary McWilliams, Peter Burrows, and Kathy Rebello, PCs: The Battle For The Home Front, *Business Week*, September 25, 1995, pp. 110–112, 114.

[MEER92] Jan van der Meer, The Full Motion System for CD-I, *IEEE Transactions on Consumer Electronics*, 38(4):910–920 (November 1992). [Also in Theodore S. Rzeszewski (editor), *Digital Video Concepts and Applications Across Industries*, pp. 541–551, Piscataway, NJ, IEEE Press (1995).]

[MESS95A] Ellen Messmer, PictureTel to Unveil Group Share Data Collaboration Software, T120 Causes IMTC, PC WG Battle, *Network World*, 12(4):4 (January 25, 1995).

[MESS95B] Ellen Messmer, Spec Near Completion for Video Over Analog Phone Lines, *Network World*, 12(10):17 (March 6, 1995).

[MESS96] Ellen Messmer, Microsoft Plays Conferencing Matchmaker, *Network World*, 13(33):29 (August 12, 1996).

[METZ94] Bob Metzler, Cascaded CODECS, *AUDIO.TST*, 9(3):1–5 (September 1994) (a publication of Audio Precision, Inc., Beaverton, OR).

[MILL94] Matthew D. Miller, A Scenario for the Deployment of Interactive Multimedia Cable Television Systems in the United States in the 1990's, *Proceedings of the IEEE*, 82(4):585–589 (April 1994).

[MITC95] Peter W. Mitchell, The High End: The Sound of Dolby AC–3, *Stereo Review*, July 1995, p. 100.

[MITC96] Joan L. Mitchell (IBM Corporation), JPEG Committee Activities, private communication, April 28, 1996.

[MOHA95] Suruchi, Mohan, Ease into Multimedia, *Computerworld*, 29(2):52 (January 9, 1995).

[MOKH95] Nicolas Mokhoff, IBM Shows Multipoint Video via the Net, *Electronic Engineering Times*, December 11, 1995, p. 16.

[MOMM74] Jacques H. Mommens and Josef Raviv, Coding for Data Compaction, IBM Research Report RC5150, November 26, 1974.

[MONS91] Robert A. Monsour and Douglas L. Whiting, Data Compression Breaks Through to Disk Memory Technology, *Computer Technology Review*, Spring 1991, pp. 39, 40, 42, 44.

[MOTO95] Toshio Motoki, Haruo Isono, and Ichiro Yuyama, Present Status of Three-Dimensional Television Research, *Proceedings of the IEEE*, 83(7):1009–1021 (July 1995).

[MUKH91] Amar Mukherjee, N. Ranganathan, and M. Bassiouni, Efficient VLSI Designs for Data Transformation of Tree-Based Codes, *IEEE Transactions on Circuits and Systems*, 38(3):306–314 (March 1991).

[MUST94] Linda Musthaler, Modularity Eases the Imaging Purchase, *Network World*, 11(50):55–64 (December 12, 1995).

[NASR88] Nasser M. Nasrabadi and Robert A. King, Image Coding Using Vector Quantization: A Review, *IEEE Transactions on Communications*, 36(8):957–97 (August 1988).

[NELS92] Mark Nelson, *The Data Compression Book*, Redwood City, CA, M&T Books, A Division of M&T Publishing, Inc. (1992)

[NEMA94] Digital Imaging and Communications in Medicine (DICOM V3.0), NEMA Standards Publications PS3.1- 3.9, NEMA, Washington, DC, 1994.

[NESD95] Paul Nesdore, A Perspective on the Perspective on GII, *Digital News & Review*, 13(4):6 (April 10, 1995).

[NETR95] Arun N. Netravali and Barry G. Haskell, *Digital Pictures Representation and Compression, Second Edition*, New York, Plenum Press (1995)

[NEWS93] Don't Videophone Us, We'll Videophone You: American Tel & Tel Videophones Are Incompatible with British Telecom Videophones, *New Scientist*, April 17, 1993, p. 19.

[NICE96] Bob St. Nice, Friendly Skies, *Video*, May, 1996, p. 10.

[NISH94] Shuzoh Nishida, Yukihiko Haikawa, Ichiroh Nakata, Hirotoshi Yamamoto, Hidenori Minoda, and Takeshi Tanaka, New Developments for the Mini Disc System, *IEEE Transactions on Consumer Electronics*, 40(3):774–780 (August 1994).

[NOLL95] Peter Noll, Digital Audio Coding for Visual Communications, *Proceedings of the IEEE*, 83(6):925–943 (June 1995).

[NORM95] Dennis Normile, Music on a Card, *Popular Science*, 246(4):48 (April 1995).

[NSci93] Will Patent Challenge Stymie Software Giant? *New Scientist*, March 6, 1993, p. 20.

[OCON95] Mike O'Connor, Extending Instructions for Multimedia, *Electronic Engineering Times*, November 13, 1995, pp. 82, 94.

[OKA92] Kenichiro Oka and Masaru Onishi, Implementation of Image Compression for Printers, *SPIE Color Hard Copy and Graphics Arts Processing*, 1670:450–454 (1992).

[OSTA95] Optical Storage Technology Association, Data Interchange and Optical Standards, *Computer Technology Review*, 15(4):36, 44 (April 1995).

[OZER94] Jan Ozer, Video Codecs for Multimedia Applications Are Not Created Equal, *Computer Technology Review*, Spring/Summer 1994, pp. 88–93.

[OZER95A] Jan Ozer, *Video Compression for Multimedia*, Cambridge, MA, Academic Press, Inc. (1995).

[OZER95B] Jan Ozer, Indeo and MPEG Gird for the Next Big Battle, *CD-ROM Professional*, 8(2):56–64 (February 1995).

[OZER95C] Jan Ozer, Decoding MPEG Encoders: How People Will Buy MPEG and What That Means for Publishers, *CD-ROM Professional*, 8(11):78–92 (November 1995).

[PAN94] Davis Pan, An Overview of the MPEG/Audio Compression Algorithm, *SPIE Digital Video Compression on Personal Computers: Algorithms and Technologies Proceeding*, Volume 2187, pp. 260–272 (1994).

[PAN95] Davis Pan, A Tutorial on MPEG/Audio Compression, *IEEE Multimedia*, 2(2):60–74 (Summer 1995).

[PARK94] Lorne Parker, Audiographics Technology, In Patrick S. Portway and Carla Lane (editors), *2nd Edition Guide to Teleconferencing & Distance Learning*, pp. 35–39, Livermore, CA, Applied Business teleCommunications (1994)

[PATT90] David A. Patterson and John L. Hennessy, *Computer Architecture: A Quantitative Approach*, San Mateo, CA, Morgan Kaufmann Publishers, Inc. (1990).

[PEAR95] Donald E. Pearson, Developments in Model-Based Video Coding, *Proceedings of the IEEE*, 83(6):892–906 (June 1995).

[PENN88] W. B. Pennebaker, J. L. Mitchell, G. G. Langdon, Jr., and R. B. Arps, An Overview of the Basic Principles of the Qcoder Adaptive Binary Arithmetic Coder, *IBM Journal of Research and Development*, 32(6):717–726 (November 1988).

[PENN93] William B. Pennebaker and Joan L. Mitchell, *JPEG Still Image Data Compression Standard*, New York, Van Nostrand Reinhold (1993).

[PERE95] Christine Perey, Desktop Video Conferencing is Here Today! *Digital Video Magazine*, 3(9):51, 52, 54, 56–61 (September 1995).

[PERS94] K. R. Persons, F. J. Reardon, D. G. Gehring, and N. J. Hangiandreou, Performance of the Mayo-IBM PAC system, *Medical Imaging VIII: PACS Design and Evaluation, SPIE Proceedings*, edited by R. G. Jost, et al., 2165:811–819 (1994).

[PETE85] James L Peterson and Abraham Silberschatz, *Operating System Concepts, Second Edition*, Reading, MA, Addison-Wesley Publishing Company, Inc. (1985).

[PIET96] Bill Pietrucha, CAI Demos Digital Network's Capabilities, *Newsbytes*, July 22, 1996.

[POHL95A] Ken C. Pohlmann, The Battle of the Balcony, *Stereo Review*, April 1995, p. 24.

[POHL95B] Ken C. Pohlmann, Bit Streams: MPEG Coding in Theory and Practice, from 22,300 Miles in Space, *Video*, September 1995, pp. 18–20, 22.

[POHL95C] Ken C. Pohlmann, The Big One: Toshiba's Family of SD SVDs Pushes the Technology Envelope, *Video*, November 1995, pp. 19–21, 24.

[POHL95D] Ken C. Pohlmann, DirecTV's Castle Rock Facility Races Along Digital's Cutting Edge: Like A Rock, *Video*, December 1995, pp. 20, 21, 24.

[Pohl96] Ken C. Pohlmann, Signals: Phone Home, *Stereo Review*, September 1996, pp. 38–39.

[PORT94] Patrick S. Portway and Carla Lane (editors), *2nd Edition Guide to Teleconferencing & Distance Learning*, Livermore, CA, Applied Business teleCommunications (1994)

[PORT96] Otis Port, Digital Finds Its Photo Op, *Business Week*, April 15, 1996 pp. 71–72.

[PRES93] Larry Press, The Internet and Interactive Television, *Communications of the ACM*, 36(12):19–23, 140 (December 1993).

[PRNE93] IBM and Laser-Pacific Media Corp. Announce Joint Development Agreement, *PR Newswire*, January 6, 1993, p. 1.

[PRON91] Nikos B. Pronios and Gregory S. Yovanof, Effects of Transmission Errors on Medical Images, *Medical Imaging V: PACS Design and Evaluation, SPIE Proceedings*, edited by R. G. Jost, et al., 1446:108–128 (1991).

[PROS94] Theodor A. Prosch and Suddeutscher Rundfunk, The Digital Audio Broadcast Single Frequency Network Project in Southwest Germany, *IEEE Transactions on Broadcasting*, 40(4):238–246 (December 1994).

[PRSO94] APT Wins Export Award, *Pro Sound News Europe*, May 1994, p. 21.

[QIC89] QIC Development Standard: Data Compression Format for ¼-Inch Data Cartridge Tape Drives, *Quarter- Inch Cartridge Drive Standards, Inc. Publication QIC–122, Revision A*, October 18, 1989.

[QUIA94] Barry Quiat, Is WAN Compression Right for You? *Network Computing*, May 1, 1994, p. 172.

[RABB91] Majid Rabbani and Paul W. Jones, *Digital Image Compression Techniques*, Bellingham, WA, SPIE Optical Engineering Press (1991)

[RAIT87] T. Raita, An Automatic System for File Compression, *The Computer Journal*, 30(1):80–86 (1987).

[RANA92] David Ranada, Inside DCC, *Stereo Review*, November 1992, pp. 98–102.

[RANA93] David Ranada, Inside Mini Disc, *Stereo Review*, March 1993, pp. 47–51.

[RANA94] David Ranada, Digital Chaos, *Stereo Review*, May 1994, pp. 70–73.

[RAPP94] Theodore S. Rappaport (editor), *Cellular Radio & Personal Communications*, Piscataway, NJ, IEEE Press (1994).

[REGH81] H. K. Reghbati, An Overview of Data Compression Techniques, *IEEE Computer*, 14(5):71–75 (April 1981).

[RENS95] Barbara Renshaw, It's Time for Multifunctional Devices, *Electronic Engineering Times*, September 11, 1995, pp. 56, 80.

[RICH91] N. D. Richards, Showing Photo CD Pictures on CD-I, *Philips Research Labs-Redhill Review 1990*, pp. 11- 14, 1991. [also in Theodore S. Rzeszewski (editor), *Digital Video Concepts and Applications Across Industries*, pp.561–565, Piscataway, NJ, IEEE Press (1995).]

[RIGG95] Michael Riggs, Digital Surround Comes Home, *Stereo Review*, May 1995, pp. 62–68.

[RISS79] J. J. Rissanen and G. G. Langdon, Jr., Arithmetic Coding, *IBM Journal of Research and Development*, 23(2):149–162 (1979).

[RODR94] Ardor A. Rodriguez and Ken Morse, Evaluating Video Codecs, *IEEE Multimedia*, 1(3):25–33 (Fall 1994).

[ROHR93] Linda Rohrbough, Stac Cuts 20% of Staff, *Newsbytes News Network*, May 26, 1993.

[ROSE95] Steve Roselaren, Publishing Beyond Paper, *Macworld*, 12(12):96–102 (December 1995).

[ROTH95] Cliff Roth and DV Nation: The Digital Video Format Debuts with Camcorders from Panasonic and Sony, *Video*, November 1995, pp. 78–80.

[ROTH96] Cliff Roth, Generation Excellence: Even After 20 Generations, DV Format Tapes Still Look Pristine, *Video*, January 1996, pp. 82–83.

[SANT92] Brian Santo, IBM Videoconferencing for Less, *Electronic Engineering Times*, November 9, 1992, p. 18.

[SANT93] Brian Santo, "Video Dialtone" Calls for ADSL, *Electronic Engineering Times*, July 12, 1993, pp. 1, 80, 82.

[SAYO92] Khalid Sayood, Data Compression in Remote Sensing Applications, *IEEE Geoscience and Remote Sensing Society Newsletter*, September 1992, pp. 7–15.

[SAYO95] Khalid Sayood, *Introduction to Data Compression*, San Francisco, Morgan Kaufmann Publishers (1995).

[SCAN94] Ed Scannell and Stuart J Johnston, Ruling Means DOS to Lose Compression, *Computerworld*, 28(9):4 (February 28, 1994).

[SCHA94] Richard Schaphorst, Status of ITU and ISO/MPEG4 Video Coding Standards at Very Low Bit Rates, *Digital Video Compression on Personal Computers: Algorithms and Technologies, SPIE Proceedings*, edited by Ardor A. Rodriguez, 2187:280–287 (1994).

[SCHA95] George Schaub, Pictures Bit-by-Bit, *Popular Mechanics*, 172(8):60–64, 107 (August 1995).

[SCHÄ95] Ralf Schäfer and Thomas Sikora, Digital Video Coding Standards and Their Role in Video Communications, *Proceedings of the IEEE*, 83(06):907–924 (June 1995).

[SCHM94] Julie Schmit, High-Tech Tool Changing Way Firms Work, *USA Today*, July 20, 1994, pp. 1B–2B.

[SEYB93] HP LaserJet 4L and ML Set Low Price Point: New Features, "Green" Products, *The Seybold Report on Desktop Publishing*, 7(10):8–9 (June 1, 1993).

[SEYB95A] Kodak Digital Imaging Strategy, Part 2: Alliances, Standards, Open Licensing, *The Seybold Report on Desktop Publishing*, 9(9):7–9 (May 8, 1995).

[SEYB95B] Methods for Image Management, *The Seybold Report on Publishing Systems*, 24(18):S44-S49 (May 15, 1995).

[SEYB95C] Servers, Workflow, and Managing Images, Files and Data, *The Seybold Report on Publishing Systems*, 24(21):20–36 (July 21, 1995).

[SEYB95D] Publishing on the World Wide Web, *The Seybold Report on Publishing Systems*, 25(1):8–18 (September 1, 1995).

[SEYB96] P.Ink Bankrupt; Scitex Declines Rescue Effort, *The Seybold Report on Publishing Systems*, 28(2):1–2 (February 21, 1996).

[SHER92] Mostafa Hashem Sherif and Duncan K. Sparrell, Standards and Innovation in Telecommunications, *IEEE Communications Magazine*, 30(7):22–28 (July 1992).

[SHIV96] Jube Shiver, Jr., MCI Wins License for Satellite TV Service, *Los Angeles Times*, January 26, 1996, p. D1.

[SIMO95] Keneth A. Simons, A High Standard (a letter to the editor appearing in Forum), *IEEE Spectrum*, 32(4):8 (April 1995).

[SLAT95] Michael Slater, MICRO SCENE: Nefarious Scheme for Pentium? *Electronic Engineering Times*, February 20, 1995, p. 72.

[SMIT93] Brian C. Smith and Lawrence A. Rowe, Algorithms for Manipulating Compressed Images, *IEEE Computer Graphics & Applications*, 13(5):34–42 (September 1993).

[SNYD70] Martin Snyderman and Bernard Hunt, The Myriad Virtues of Text Compaction, *Datamation*, 16(23):36–40 (December 1, 1970).

[SOMO95] Stephan Somogyi, MPEG–2 Primer: Video Compression Scheme, *Digital Media*, 5(3):12–15 (August 7, 1995).

[SPAN94] Andreas S. Spanias, Speech Coding: A Tutorial Review, *Proceedings of the IEEE*, 82(10):1539–1582 (October 1994).

[SQUI96] Herb Squire (WQXR radio, New York City), The Application of Lossy Data Compression Codecs to Radio Broadcasting, private communication, January 23, 1996.

[STAL94A] William Stallings and Richard Van Slyke, *Business Data Communications, 2nd edition*, New York, Macmillian Publishing Company (1993)

[STAL94B] William Stallings, *Data and Computer Communications, 4th edition*, New York, Macmillian Publishing Company (1994)

[STEE91] George H. Steele, Optical Disk Data Compression Foments Storage Revolution, *Computer Technology Review*, Spring 1991, pp. 53–54, 56–57.

[STOR93] James A. Storer and Martin Cohn (editors), *Data Compression Conference 1993*, Los Alamitos, CA, IEEE Computer Society Press (1993)

[STOTEK1] StorageTek Iceberg 9200 Storage System Introduction, Storage Technology Corporation Publication 3074061, second edition, January 1995.

[STOTEK2] StorageTek Iceberg 9200 Storage System Reference, Storage Technology Corporation Publication 3074062, first edition, January 1995.

[STRY94] David J. Strybel, *SuperStore: An Illustrated Tutorial*, New York, Windcrest Books/McGraw-Hill, Inc. (1994)

[SUGI95] Akihiko Sugiyama, Masahiro Iwadare, Nobuhiro Ohdate, Takashi Manabe, Hideto Takano, Osamu Kitabatake, and Eiji Hirao, The Silicon Audio: An Audio-Data Compression and Storage System with a Semiconductor Memory Card, *IEEE Transactions on Consumer Electronics*, 41(1):186–194 (February 1995).

[SULL95] Joe Sullivan, T.120 Conferencing Standards Ease Data Sharing, *Network World*, 12(25):49 (June 19, 1995).

[TAKI95A] Jonathan Takiff, Small Dish Mania: How DSS is Bringing Digital Sizzle to Satellite Television, *Video*, April 1995, pp. 46–48, 70, 78.

[TAKI95B] Jonathan Takiff, Digital Surround, The Next Big Sound? *Video*, May 1995, pp. 36–39, 74, 76, 78, 80.

[TAKI96] Jonathan Takiff, Deep Dish: Belly Up for the Hot News on DBS Satellite Systems, *Video*, June 1996, pp. 29–38.

[TANE92] Andrew S. Tanenbaum, *Modern Operating Systems*, Englewood Cliffs, NJ, Prentice-Hall, Inc. (1992).

[TAYL95A] Kieran Taylor, Subrate Voice/Data Muxes Keep WAN Costs in Check, *Data Communications*, 24(9):91–96, 98 (July 1995).

[TAYL95B] Kieran Taylor and Kevin Tolly, Desktop Videoconferencing: Not Ready for Prime Time, *Data Communications*, 24(5):64–68, 70, 72–74, 76, 80 (April 1995).

[TAWB93] W. Tawbi, F. Horn, E Horlait, and J. B. Stefani, Video Compression Standards and Quality of Service, *The Computer Journal*, 36(1):43–54 (1993).

[THOM92] Clark Thomborson, The V.42bis Standard for Data-Compressing Modems, *IEEE Micro*, 12(5):41–53 (October 1992).

[TODD94] Craig C. Todd, Grant A. Davidson, Mark F. Davis, Louis D. Fiedler, Brian D. Link, and Steve Vernon, AC–3: Flexible Perceptual Coding for Audio Transmission and Storage, *Proceedings of the 96th Convention of the Audio-Engineering Society,* March 1994, preprint 3845.

[TOLL94A] Kevin Tolly, Testing Remote Token Ring Bridges, *Data Communications*, 24(5):93–96, 98,100, 102,104 (April 1994).

[TOLL94B] Kevin Tolly, Testing Remote Ethernet Bridges, *Data Communications*, 24(5):81–85, 88–89 (April 1994).

[TREV92] S. T. Treves, Eman S. Hashem, Bhairav A. Majmudar, Karl Mitchell, and Dennis J. Michaud, Multimedia Communications in Medical Imaging, *IEEE Transactions on Selected Areas in Communications*, 10(7):1121–1134 (September 1992).

[TROW94] Toby Trowt-Bayard, *Videoconferencing: The Whole Picture*, Chelsea, MI, Flatiron Publishing, Inc. (1994)

[TROW91] Dave Trowbridge, "Compressionware" Offers Soft and Hard Choices, *Computer Technology Review*, 11(7):1, 18, 26, 30 (July 1991).

[TURL95] James L. Turley, MPEG Choices for PCs Abound, *Microprocessor Report*, 9(10):9–12 (July 31, 1995).

[UPI92] Federal Communications Commission Approves TV-On-Phone-Line Rule, UPI news release, Washington DC, July 16, 1992.

[VALK92] J. P. J. de Valk (editor), *Integrated Diagnostic Imaging—PACS in Medicine 1980–2000*, New York, Elsevier Science Publishers (1992).

[VARB93] TenX Technology Inc. OptiXchange 940 Subsystem, *Varbusiness*, April 1993, p. 77.

[VENB92] Jack Venbrux, Pen-Shu Yeh, and Muye N. Liu, A VLSI Chip Set for High-Speed Lossless Data Compression, *IEEE Transactions on Circuits and Systems for Video Technology*, 2(4):381–391 (December 1992).

[VIZA93] Frank Vizard, Electronics: Dial a Picture, *Popular Mechanics*, 170(6):106, 110 (June 1993).

[WALD94] Michael Wald, DOS 6, 6.2 Recall May Go Through, *Computer Retail Week*, June 20, 1994, p.5.

[WALL91] Gregory K. Wallace, The JPEG Still Picture Compression Standard, *Communications of ACM*, 34(4):30–44 (April, 1991).

[WALL96] Bob Wallace, 56K Modems on Deck, *Computerworld*, 30(38):1,135 (September 16, 1996).

[WARN96] R. M. Warner Jr.and Earl Masterson: A Fresh Slant on Videorecording, *IEEE Spectrum*, 33(2):51–57 (February 1996).

[WARR95] Rich Warren, DSS at Home, *Stereo Review*, January 1995, pp. 105, 106, 108, 110.

[WEBB93] Dave Webb, AMD/C-Cube Deal, *Electronic Buyers News*, January 4, 1993, p. 12.

[WEBC96] WebCrawler's Web Size, April 1996, available from the Global Network Navigator, Inc. WWW site as *http://webcrawler.com/WebCrawler/Facts/Sizes.html*.

[WEBE93] David Weber, Trimming Numerical Fat, *Embedded Systems Programming*, 6(8):60–62, 64, 66–69 (August 1993).

[WEBE96] Sam Weber, Consumer Formats Flocking to Flash, *Electronic Engineering Times*, July 22, 1996, pp. 53, 54, 58, 60.

[WEIN94] Fred W. Weingartem, Public Interest and the NII, *Communications of the ACM*, 37(3):17–19 (March 1994).

[WELC84] Terry A. Welch, A Technique for High-Performance Data Compression, *IEEE Computer*, 17(6):8–19 (June 1984).

[WHIT67] H. E. White, Printed English Compression by Dictionary Encoding, *Proceedings of the IEEE*, 55(3):390- 396 (March 1967).

[WILK94] J. H. Wilkinson and J. J. Stone, Cascading Different Types of Video Compression Systems, *IEE Colloquium on Cascading Audio and Video Data Compression Systems* (Digest No. 1994/055), 1994, pp. 2/1–2/4.

[WILL91] Shawn Willett, Data Compression: Buyers Beware of Expansive Claims, *Digital News*, March 18, 1991, pp. 29, 31.

[WILS94A] Ron Wilson and Loring Wirbel, HP to Launch Multimedia Workstations, *Electronic Engineering Times*, January 17, 1994, p. 4.

[WILS94B] Ron Wilson, IBM Cites 40-Mbyte/s Lossless Compression, *Electronic Engineering Times*, June 27, 1994, p. 93

[WILS95A] Ron Wilson, Triton Chip Set Aims for Signal-Processing Speed, *Electronic Engineering Times*, January 30, 1995, pp. 1, 96.

[WILS95B] Ron Wilson, NSP Challenges DSP in PC Architecture, *Electronic Engineering Times*, February 20, 1995, p. 22.

[WILS95C] Ron Wilson and Junko Yoshida, "Hot Chips" This Year Are Multimedia Processors, *Electronic Engineering Times*, August 7, 1995, pp. 1, 88.

[WILS95D] Ron Wilson, Intel to Relaunch NSP Multimedia, *Electronic Engineering Times*, November 13, 1995, pp. 1, 234.

[WILS95E] Ron Wilson, Audio Chips Pile It On, *Electronic Engineering Times*, November 20, 1995, p. 78.

[WILS95F] Ron Wilson, Speaking of Silicon: Data Compression Advances, *Electronic Engineering Times*, November 27, 1995, p. 118.

[WILS95G] Ron Wilson, DEC Primes Video for Pentium, *Electronic Engineering Times*, December 4, 1995, pp. 18, 110.

[WILS96] Ron Wilson, Graphics Controllers Take Multimedia Turn, *Electronic Engineering Times*, September 30, 1996, p. 4.

[WINW96] OLE Controls on a Roll, But Market Hurdles Remain, *Windows Watcher*, 6(2):1 (February 1996).

[WIRB94] Loring Wirbel, The 64-Gbit Question: Exactly What Is NII? *Electronic Engineering Times*, January 17, 1994, pp. 28, 63.

[WIRB95] Loring Wirbel and Junko Yoshida, MCI, Partners Define Video-Phone Set-Top Box, *Electronic Engineering Times*, October 30, 1995, p. 10.

[WITH92] Peter H. N. de With, Marcel Breeuer, and Peter A. M. van Grinsven, Data Compression Systems for Home-Use Digital Video Recording, *IEEE Transactions on Selected Areas in Communications*, 10(1):97–121 (January 1992).

[WITT94] Ian H. Witten, Alistair Moffat, and Timothy C. Bell, *Managing Gigabytes— Compressing and Indexing Documents and Images*, New York, Van Nostrand Reinhold (1993)

[WOLF92] Andrew Wolfe and Alex Chanin, Executing Compressed Programs on an Embedded RISC Architecture, *IEEE SIGMICRO Newsletter*, 23(1–2):81–91 (December 1992).

[WOLF93A] Alexander Wolfe, New Standard Sought for Video Compression, *Electronic Engineering Times*, July 5, 1993, pp. 1, 66.

[WOLF93B] Richard M. Wolfe, The Electronic Cinema: A Market Analysis, In *HDTV Issues: Where We Are And Where We Are Going*, NTU Advanced Technology and Management Programs, Live Satellite Broadcast MC930729B1, July 29, 1993.

[WOLF93C] J. Gerard Wolff, Computing, Cognition and Information Compression, *AI Communications*, 6(2):107–127 (June 1993).

[WOLF95A] Alexander Wolfe, Embedded Insights: Patent Nonsense? *Electronic Engineering Times*, March 20, 1995, p.70.

[WOLF95B] Alexander Wolfe, Intel Takes P6 on a Multimedia Ride, *Electronic Engineering Times*, July 31, 1995, pp. 1, 162.

[WOLF95C] Alexander Wolfe, Sun, IBM, Microsoft Take on SGI: Three Look to Star in Hollywood Role, *Electronic Engineering Times*, August 14, 1995, pp. 1, 114.

[WONG95] Stephen Wong, Loren Zaremba, David Gooden, and H. K. Huang, Radiologic Image Compression—A Review, *Proceedings of the IEEE*, 83(2):194–219 (February 1995).

[WUEB95] Michael Wuebker (CompuServe Incorporated), GIF Development, private communication, February 28, 1995.

[WYLI95] Margie Wylie, An Oxymoron to Watch: Why Wireless Cable is Hot After 20 Years of Obscurity, *Digital Media*, 5(6):15–19 (November 6, 1995).

[YEO95] Boon-Lock Yeo and Bede Liu, Rapid Scene Analysis on Compressed Video, *IEEE Transactions on Circuits and Systems for Video Technology*, 5(6):533–544 (December 1995).

[YOSH93A] Junko Yoshida, HDTV Fires up Imagination But Flattens Vision, *Electronic Engineering Times*, March 29, 1993, p. 43.

[YOSH93B] Junko Yoshida, Group Backs "Karaoke-CD" Video Format, *Electronic Engineering Times*, May 31, 1993, p. 4.

[YOSH94A] Junko Yoshida, MPEG Sees Unexpected Patent Woes, *Electronic Engineering Times*, January 3, 1993, pp. 1, 64.

[YOSH94B] Junko Yoshida, MPEG "Patent Pool" to Entice New Users? *Electronic Engineering Times*, April 4, 1994, pp. 1, 82.

[YOSH94C] Tadao Yoshida, The Rewritable MiniDisc System, *Proceedings of the IEEE*, 82(10):1490–1500 (October 1994).

[YOSH95A] Junko Yoshida, Developers Like the Sound of 3-D Audio, *Electronic Engineering Times*, May 1, 1995, p. 14.

[YOSH95B] Junko Yoshida, Computer Quintet Urges Single DVD, *Electronic Engineering Times*, May 8, 1995, pp. 1, 8.

[YOSH95C] Junko Yoshida, TV Rushing into Multichannel Future, *Electronic Engineering Times*, June 19, 1995, pp. 18, 26.

[YOSH95D] Junko Yoshida, Finally, Digital TV for Japan, *Electronic Engineering Times*, July 31, 1995, pp. 2, 164.

[YOSH95E] Junko Yoshida, Feuds Fulminate as Feds Finish up HDTV, *Electronic Engineering Times*, August 7, 1995, pp. 1, 88.

[YOSH95F] Junko Yoshida, Videodisk's Hollywood Connection, *Electronic Engineering Times*, August 28, 1995, p. 8.

[YOSH95G] Junko Yoshida and Brian Fuller, Novel Technologies to Drive Multimedia Processors, *Electronic Engineering Times*, October 9, 1995, pp. 1, 152.

[YOSH96] Junko Yoshida, Intel, Microsoft Get Behind Internet Phone, *Electronic Engineering Times*, July 22, 1996, p. 14.

[ZARE93] L. A. Zaremba and R. A. Phillips, Image Compression—Regulatory Issues and Policies, *Presentation at American Association of Physicists in Medicine (AAPM) 1993 Annual Meeting*, Washington, DC, August 1993.

[ZAND93] Ahmad Zandi, Bala Iyer, and Glen Langdon, Sort Order Preserving Data Compression for Extended Alphabets, *DCC93: Proceedings of the Third Data Compression Conference*, pp.330–339, Los Alamitos, CA, IEEE Computer Society Press (1993).

[ZIEG93] Bart Ziegler, American Telephone & Multimedia? *Business Week*, September 6, 1993, pp. 78–79.

[ZIV77] Jacob Ziv and Abraham Lempel, A Universal Algorithm for Sequential Data Compression, *IEEE Transactions on Information Theory*, 23(3):337–343 (May 1977).

[ZIV78] Jacob Ziv and Abraham Lempel, Compression of Individual Sequences via Variable-Rate Coding, *IEEE Transactions on Information Theory*, 24(5):530–536 (September 1978).

[ZOLL95] Robert A Zollo, New Media Interchange Standards For Rewritable Optical Systems, *Computer Technology Review*, 15(1):44 (January 1995).

[ZOU92] William Y. Zou, Digital HDTV Compression Techniques for Terrestrial Broadcasting, *HD World Review*, 3(3):4–10 (1992).

Index